Clinical Nephrology

3rd Edition

Clinical Nephrology

3rd Edition

WOO KENG THYE

Emeritus Consultant Physician
Department of Renal Medicine, Singapore General Hospital
Clinical Professor, National University of Singapore

World Scientific

NEW JERSEY · LONDON · SINGAPORE · BEIJING · SHANGHAI · HONG KONG · TAIPEI · CHENNAI

Published by

World Scientific Publishing Co. Pte. Ltd.

5 Toh Tuck Link, Singapore 596224

USA office: 27 Warren Street, Suite 401-402, Hackensack, NJ 07601

UK office: 57 Shelton Street, Covent Garden, London WC2H 9HE

British Library Cataloguing-in-Publication Data
A catalogue record for this book is available from the British Library.

ISBN-13 978-981-4340-80-9 (pbk)
ISBN-10 981-4340-80-4 (pbk)

Typeset by Stallion Press
Email: enquiries@stallionpress.com

Printed in Singapore.

For
May, Bernardine, Geraldine
Bernard, Adeline and Anne.

My Teachers and Students,
past, present and future.

Yesterday this time, we sat at length
Analysed, dissected, polished ink stones
Bared the sinews of our thoughts
Between the bristles of the brush
And grains of rice-paper.

Preface

Over the past 30 years, Dr Woo has been teaching Renal Medicine to medical students and doctors. This book is written in response to their request to put together a series of tutorials and lectures in Renal Medicine to serve their needs for a textbook of Clinical Nephrology.

He has given a comprehensive review of Renal Medicine pertaining to Clinical Nephrology. The topics range from glomerulonephritis, urinary tract infection, hypertension and renal stones to renal failure, dialysis and transplantation, thus providing the student with a broad perspective of Renal Medicine. In addition, tables on local incidence and statistics are provided. This is important as all the available books on Renal Diseases have been written by overseas authors in the West, quoting data and statistics which are quite different from our local scene. Local data on disease incidence and patterns are important as there exist widely differing patterns of geographical distribution among various types of renal diseases in different parts of the world.

This book is also written for the practising doctor or clinician who is looking for a basic handbook to serve as a reference for current concepts and practice in clinical nephrology. It is written in simple language with discussions on clinical problems occurring in daily practice.

The knowledge in this book is graded. Many chapters will be relevant to medical students. However, depending on the requirements of the reader, whether he is a medical student or postgraduate doctor preparing for his M Med (Internal Medicine) Examination, he will be able to find within this book chapters relevant to his needs.

In this 3rd Edition the book has undergone extensive revision not only to bring it up to date with current practice of Nephrology but also provide more details and greater breadth and depth in order to meet the requirements of the Specialist Accreditation Board of Renal Medicine in Singapore so that the Advanced Trainee in Nephrology can use it as a text to supplement his knowledge of Nephrology. Therefore all the previous chapters have been revised and additional chapters on Clinical Trials and Renal Therapeutics, Cardiorenal Syndrome, Geography and Evolution of Glomerulonephritis, Aging Kidney, Poisoning and Renal Research incorporated. In keeping with present trends Acute Kidney Injury is used in place of Acute Renal Failure. Classification of Chronic Kidney Disease (CKD) with eGFR and new nomenclature for Lupus Nephritis and IgA Nephritis have also been introduced.

1st October 2010

About the Author

Dr Woo Keng Thye is Emeritus Consultant Physician and Advisor to the Department of Renal Medicine, Singapore General Hospital and Clinical Professor at the National University of Singapore.

For the past 35 years, he has been teaching Renal Medicine to medical students. He has also been a lecturer in Renal Medicine for the Master of Medicine Course in Internal Medicine. He is a past President of the Singapore Society of Nephrology as well as a former Head of the Dept of Renal Medicine. He obtained his training in Nephrology at the Royal Melbourne Hospital in Australia.

The book on Clinical Nephrology is Dr Woo's first comprehensive textbook on kidney diseases. Besides this, he has written several other books on kidney diseases: Know Your Kidneys, All You Need to Know about Your Kidneys, 101 Questions & Answers about your Kidneys and Handbook on Clinical Nephrology. In addition, he has written several literary books: *Risen Ash* (a collection of poems), *Web of Tradition, Winds of Change* (novels), *Encounter and Other Stories* (a collection of short stories), *Reincarnation* and Other Stories and *Obsession* and Other Stories.

Acknowledgements

It gives me great pleasure to acknowledge the contributions of the following:

Medical students and doctors whose needs have led me to write this book.

Ms Irene Ow for her secretarial assistance.

Mr Steven Patt, Editor, World Scientific Publishing, for his editorial assistance.

Ms Lim Hui Chee, Graphic Designer, World Scientific Publishing, for her assistance in the cover design.

Clinical Professor Dr Gilbert Chiang, Emeritus Consultant Pathologist, Singapore General Hospital, for his contribution in renal histopathology.

Contents

CHAPTER 1

Structure and Function

ANATOMY OF THE KIDNEYS

The kidneys are a pair of bean-shaped organs located at the back of the body about the level of the waist. They receive their blood supply from the main artery of the body called the aorta. Each kidney measures 10–15 cm in length and weighs about 160 gm. Urine is conducted from the kidneys along two tubes known as the ureters which join the urinary bladder in the pelvis. The capacity of the bladder varies from 500 to 750 ml. Each kidney is made up of 1 million units called nephrons. Each nephron consists of two parts, the glomerulus which is a bunch of capillaries with thin walls serving as a filter, and the tubule which drains the glomerulus (Figs. 1.1 & 1.2).

The glomerular tuft is made up of a coil of capillaries which is fed by an afferent arteriole and drained by an efferent arteriole. The tuft lies in a space known as Bowman's capsule which is spherical and opens directly into the proximal tubule. The glomerular tuft and capsule is lined by epithelial cells. Ultrafiltration occurs across the capillary tuft and the fluid passes into the proximal tubule. Between the afferent and the efferent arterioles of the glomerulus lies the juxta-glomerular apparatus which lies in the area bounded by the two arterioles, the distal tubule of the same nephron and the lacis cells lying between the two arterioles.

Within the glomerular tuft are the mesangial cells and mesangial matrix. The mesangial cells have a supportive and phagocytic function and have been referred to as the third reticulo-endothelial

1

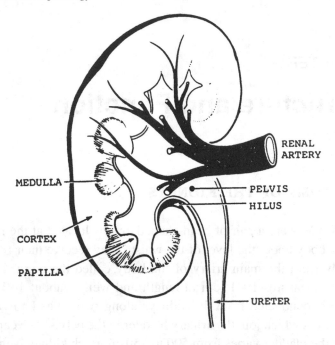

MEDULLA

RENAL
ARTERY

PELVIS

HILUS

CORTEX

PAPILLA

URETER

Fig. 1.1   The gross structure of the cut surface of the kidney

system. They are capable of contraction and are involved in the pathogenesis of IgA nephritis and diabetic nephropathy. Factors or agents that cause increased mesangial cell contractility predispose to mesangial sclerosis and therefore glomerulosclerosis. The capillary loops abound around the core of mesangial cells and matrix. The wall of these capillary loops consists of three layers, the epithelial cells, the glomerular basement membrance and the endothelial cells (Fig. 1.3).

The term "proliferative glomerulonephritis" refers to a proliferation of one of the three types of cells within the glomerulus: mesangial cells, endothelial cells or epithelial cells; and hence the different types of proliferative glomerulonephritis (GN): Mesangial Proliferative GN, Endocapillary Proliferative GN and Crescenteric GN. In Crescenteric GN, there is now evidence to show that macrophages from the circulation as well as those in situ within the glomeruli gain entry into the glomerular tuft and

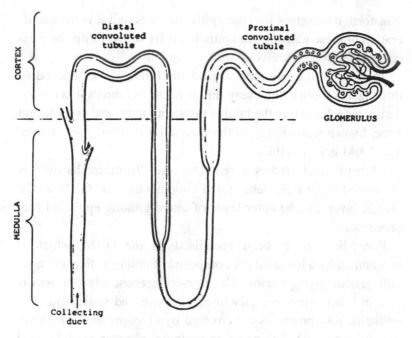

Fig. 1.2 Diagram of a nephron

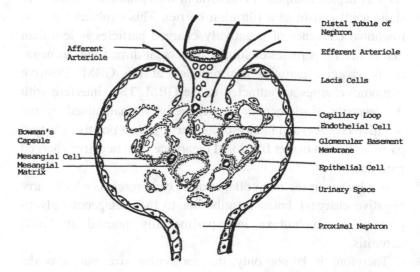

Fig. 1.3 Diagram of a glomerus

transform themselves into the epithelial cells and it is the proliferation of these transformed epithelial cells which forms the crescents in Crescenteric GN.

The glomerular basement membrane (GBM) is composed of three layers (notice that many things occur in "threes"): a central dense zone, known as the lamina densa, an inner and outer lucent zone, known respectively as the lamina rara interna and externa. The GBM is 80 nm thick.

Ultrastructural studies reveal that the "filtration barrier" is composed of an inner fenestrated endothelium, the GBM as the middle layer and the outer layer of interdigitating epithelial foot processes.

Pores have never been visualised on the GBM, which is biochemically a hydrated gel composed of collagen-like and non-collagenous glycoproteins. The non-collagenase glycoprotein is rich in hydroxyproline, galactose, mannose and sialic acid. The epithelial foot processes are covered by glycoproteins which are rich in sialic acid. The negative (anionic) charges of sialic acid help to keep the foot processes apart. The negative charges on the basement membrane (due to the presence of glycosaminoglycans, such as heparan sulphate) and around the epithelial slits (due to sialic acid) constitute a filtration barrier. This explains why the fractional clearance of negatively charged particles is less than that of neutral particles of similar molecular dimensions as negatively charged particles are repelled at the GBM. Positive (cationic) charges are attracted to the GBM. They interfere with the integrity of glomerular permselectivity (maintained by the negative charges) and induce proteinuria. Hence positive charged particles have a higher fractional clearance than negative charged particles.

Antibodies to the non-collagenous glycoproteins (which carry negative charges), but not antibodies to the collagenous glycoproteins, are nephrotoxic in experimentally induced anti-GBM nephritis.

Therefore it is not only the molecular size but also the electrostatic charge which determines a particle's exclusion from glomerular filtration. Loss of the charge barrier results in the loss of glomerular permselectivity and causes proteinuria.

Intrathoraxic Kidney with Right Bochdalek's Hernia

1. A 55 year old Taiwanese presented to A & E Unit with epigastric discomfort and a plain film of the abdomen showed an elevated right hemidiaphragm. Computed tomography revealed a right sided intrathoraxic kidney without hydronephrosis and right hemidiaphragm with herniation, consistent with congenital right Bochdalek's hernia.
2. The patient was treated conservatively and pain resolved.
3. Bochdalek's hernia is the most common form of diaphragmatic hernia occurring in 1 in 2500 births. Intrathoraxic kidney is even rarer, presenting in 1 in 10,000 births, more common on the left and among males.
4. No specific intervention is required.
5. Reference: Chung SD *et al.* Intrathoraxic kidney with right Bochdalek's hernia. Kidney Int 2009, **77**:166.

FUNCTIONS OF THE KIDNEYS

Each day the two kidneys excrete about 1.5 to 2.5 litres of urine. One of the most important functions of the kidney is to regulate the amount of water and salt excreted. About 99% of the filtered salt is reabsorbed by the tubules. The output of salt is regulated to maintain a normal and constant salt level in the body. The renal tubules also reabsorb dissolved substances like glucose and amino acids, the building blocks of proteins. The kidney has the important task of ridding the body of excess acid and potassium.

There is a minimum amount of soluble waste we must excrete through our kidneys each day. They are mainly nitrogenous waste products, principally urea. These products are poisonous and they are the substances retained in the body when the kidney fails.

The kidney is also a producer of certain hormones. Renin is one of them. Renin by itself is inactive but it acts on angiotensin I to produce angiotensin II which causes blood vessels to constrict thereby raising the blood pressure. Another hormone produced by the kidney is the active form of vitamin D which is necessary for strong and healthy bones as it promotes the absorption of calcium from the bowels. Without it we suffer from rickets. Erythropoietin, the third hormone produced by the kidney is necessary for the formation of red blood cells in the bone marrow. Patients with diseased kidneys are anaemic because they lack erythropoietin. Prostaglandins, another hormone, regulates the blood flow and blood pressure.

The main function of the kidneys is to make urine which contains the waste products of our metabolic processes. By regulating the rate at which these substances are excreted the kidneys are able to maintain the internal environment or the "milieu interieur". The production of urine depends on the renal plasma flow and the glomerular filtration. Hence the measurement of the glomerular filtration rate (GFR) is an index of renal function.

In addition to various substances **which are cleared by the kidneys,** there are others which are filtered **and reabsorbed like glucose** and sodium, and some which are secreted **or excreted by the renal tubules**.

Renal Handling of Sodium

Sodium is filtered at the glomeruli and actively reabsorbed by the tubules. About 80% of filtered sodium chloride and water are reabsorbed by the proximal tubules. The sodium which reaches the distal tubule is reabsorbed by an ion exchange mechanism. Potassium and hydrogen ions are passed into the tubular lumen and sodium ions are removed actively from the lumen. This exchange mechanism is enhanced by aldosterone. Therefore altogether about 99% of filtered sodium is reabsorbed. The volume of the extracellular fluid is determined by the sodium content of the body which is regulated by the kidneys.

Renal Handling of Potassium

1. The majority of potassium is reabsorbed in the proximal tubules and that which is found in the urine is derived from potassium exchanged for sodium reabsorbed in the distal tubules and the collecting ducts.
2. Potassium is simultaneously reabsorbed and secreted along the nephron. Variations in secretion in the distal nephron segments play a major role in regulating potassium secretion. Such secretion is modulated by sodium, acid base factors, hormones and diuretics [Giebisch G *et al.* Renal and extra renal regulation of potassium. Kidney Int 2007, **72**:397–410].

Kidney Regulation of Acid-Base Balance

The extracellular fluid is maintained at a pH between 7.35 to 7.45. Two forms of acid which are continuously produced by the body require buffering and subsequent excretion.

i. Carbon dioxide which is formed as a result of cellular metabolism combines with water to form carbonic acid. In the lungs, carbonic acid dissociates and CO_2 is eliminated in the expired air.
ii. Fixed acids are acids which cannot be excreted via the lungs. They are also produced by the body's metabolic processes. The hydrogen ions produced by these fixed acids are buffered by bicarbonate ions in the body. The role of kidneys is to "regenerate" the bicarbonate which has been used up in the buffering of fixed acids.

Acidification of the Urine and Excretion of H⁺

In normal persons, renal acidification maintains the plasma bicarbonate at physiologic concentrations by reclaiming all the filtered bicarbonate and excreting endogenously produced non-volatile or fixed acids.

This mechanism takes place at 3 sites.

i.   *At the Proximal Tubules*:
     85% to 90% of filtered bicarbonate is reclaimed. For each mole of Na^+ reabsorbed, one mole of H^+ is excreted and one mole of bicarbonate is generated and returned to the blood.

     Secreted H^+ titrates HCO^{3-} to H_2CO_3 in the tubular lumen.

     $$H_2CO_3 \xrightarrow{\text{carbonic anhydrase}} H_2O + CO_2$$

ii. *At the Distal Tubule*:
     10% to 15% of filtered bicarbonate is titrated with secreted H^+. The urine pH is now about 6.2. Also titrated are the urinary buffers:

     $$Na_2HPO_4 \rightarrow NaH_2PO_4$$
     $$NH_3 \rightarrow NH_4$$

     Titratable Acid = Measure of H^+ excreted as NaH_2PO_4

iii. *At the Collecting Duct*:
     5% of bicarbonate is reabsorbed. The secretory capacity for H^+ is small but the large gradient generated for H^+ secretion enables the kidney to reduce the urinary pH to values of 5 or less and excrete NH_4 and titratable acid at a rate equal to the endogenous production of the fixed acids.

     Therefore,

     $$\text{Net Acid Excretion} = \text{Titratable Acid} + NH_4$$
     $$- \text{Bicarbonate excreted}$$

In Metabolic Acidosis

Bicarbonate is titrated to extinction in the proximal tubule. The secretion of H^+ at the distal tubule is not buffered by delivered bicarbonate as the gradient of H^+ at the lumen-peritubule is decreased. Urine pH is less than 5, net H^+ excretion is increased, but total H^+ secretion is decreased.

In Metabolic Alkalosis

The amount of bicarbonate delivered to the distal tubule exceeds the H^+ secretory capacity. Urine pH is 8. Bicarbonaturia swamps H^+ excretion, though the total H^+ secretion is increased.

Adequacy of Gradient-Generating and Acid-Excreting Ability

The adequacy of gradient-generating and acid-excreting ability is evaluated by measurement of urinary pH, titratable acid and ammonium during metabolic acidosis, either spontaneous or induced by means of the ammonium chloride loading test (short or long test).

With small reduction in plasma bicarbonate concentration, e.g. 3 to 4 mEq/l, normal subjects decrease urinary pH to less than 5.3, titratable acid increased to more than 25 and ammonium to more than 39 mEq per minute. Urine pH of 5.3 and below denotes ability to acidify the urine and urine pH above 5.3 denotes inability to acidify the urine.

In non-azotemic renal acidification defect, the urinary pH is high during acidosis and excretion rates of titratable acid and ammonium is reduced. The serum chloride increases as bicarbonate decreases. This defect is termed "Renal Tubular Acidosis" by Pines and Mudge.

Concentration of Urine

There is a progressive increase in tissue osmolarity from cortex to papillary tip. In the kidney the loops of Henle function as countercurrent multipliers. Fluid in the descending limb becomes progressively more concentrated during its passage from the cortico-medullary junction to the tip of the loop. In the ascending limb, sodium is reabsorbed more rapidly than water and the fluid passing to the distal convoluted tubule is more dilute than that which enters the descending limb. A gradient between the limbs is created by the transport of sodium unaccompanied by equivalent amounts of water out of the ascending limb into the interstitial fluid. Water then diffuses out of the descending limb so concentrating the contents of the limb until an equilibrium is reached in which the concentration of the fluid at any point in the descending limb is the same as that of the interstitial fluid at the same level and slightly higher than that at the corresponding point of the ascending limb.

The collecting ducts pass through the medulla. In the presence of antidiuretic hormone (ADH), water diffuses from the collecting ducts into the hypertonic medullary interstitium. This makes the urine become progressively concentrated.

Also under the influence of ADH the collecting ducts, normally not permeable to urea, become highly permeable to urea. Urea diffuses from the collecting ducts into the medullary interstitial fluid. The urea trapped in the medullary interstitium extracts water from the descending limb of the loop of Henle and amplifies the effect of the counter-current multiplier. This permits the production of a more highly concentrated urine.

Hormones and the Kidneys

Many hormones influence various aspects of renal function. These are antidiuretic hormone, cortisol, aldosterone, parathyroid hormone, growth hormone, sex hormones, erythropoietin, prostaglandins and angiotensin II.

The autoregulation of renal blood flow maintains and regulates the GFR. Changes in the mean arterial pressure can induce changes in the opposite directions of afferent and efferent arteriolar resistances, resulting in near constancy of the GFR. For example, a reduction in systemic arterial pressure produces dilatation of afferent arterioles thus increasing the blood flow to the glomeruli and maintaining the perfusion pressure. However, if the efferent arterioles also dilate, the pressure will be transmitted to the post-glomerular capillary bed and GFR will decrease.

Vasoconstriction of the efferent arteriole is achieved by intrarenal generation of angiotensin II. The juxta-glomerular apparatus senses the perfusion pressure by means of stretch receptors in the afferent arteriole. A decrease in systemic arterial pressure releases renin from afferent arterioles.

In glomerular hyperfiltration, there is afferent arteriolar dilatation with increase of blood flow to the glomerulus. At the efferent arteriole, angiotensin II receptors induce vasoconstriction. The end result is increase in intraglomerular blood pressure (intraglomerular hypertension). This causes increase in single nephron GFR with increase in creatinine clearance and proteinuria. With time, however, the intra-glomerular hypertension induces glomerulosclerosis. Hyperfiltration occurs in any condition where some glomeruli are sclerosed. Hyperfiltration or hyperperfusion then occurs in the remnant glomeruli. This condition occurs in diabetic nephropathy and IgA nephritis.

Prostaglandins play an essential role in normal renal function, especially PGE_2, Prostaglandins are located in the renal medulla. They modify the adenylcyclase cyclic AMP system and also have a role in regulation of renal blood flow and of ADH secretion and actions. Prostaglandins have also been implicated in hypertension. This is based on observations that a reduction in the renal production of certain types of prostaglandins is associated with reduced natriuresis and hypertension in experimental animals.

Other hormones like antidiuretic hormone (vasopressin) regulates water excretion. Cortisol promotes sodium retention and potassium and hydrogen loss by the kidneys. Aldosterone enhances the reabsorption of sodium from the distal tubular fluid in exchange for potassium and hydrogen ions which have increased excretion.

Parathyroid hormone diminishes the urinary output of calcium and hydrogen ions and increases that of phosphate and potassium ions. Growth hormone has some sodium retaining properties. Oestrogens may lead to salt and water retention and to a rise in GFR and renal blood flow in pregnancy. Progesterone induces some sodium and water loss.

REFERENCES

1. Chung SD *et al.* Intrathoraxic kidney with right Bochdalek's hernia. *Kidney Int* 2009, **77**:166.
2. Giebisch G *et al.* Renal and extra renal regulation of potassium. *Kidney Int* 2007, **72**:397–410.

CHAPTER 2

Symptoms and Signs in Renal Medicine

HISTORY TAKING

1. **Pain:** Backache as a symptom of renal disease can be in the loin or over the lumbar spine. In renal colic due to renal stones the pain may start in the loin and radiate towards the groin and from there to the penis, sometimes even to the tip of the penis as in the case of a stone at the trigone of the urinary bladder. Suprapubic pain can be due to infection of the bladder (cystitis) or it could be due to a bladder stone. When pain is associated with fever or chills it is due to infection of the urinary tract.

2. **Swelling** due to oedema usually involves the extremities, i.e. the face, the ankles and legs. There can be associated swelling of the abdomen (ascites) as in the case of the nephrotic syndrome. When swelling becomes generalised there is collection of fluid in the abdominal, pleural and even the pericardial space. This is referred to as anarsarca.

3. **Haematuria** or the presence of blood in the urine is said to be gross when it is apparent to the naked eye. It is microscopic when there are more than 3 red blood cells per high power field on urine microscopy. Enquire into the relationship of haematuria to renal stones or nephritis as in the acute nephritic syndrome which usually is associated with what is described as smoky urine in the case of post infectious glomerulonephritis. Post infectious glomerulonephritis is also

associated with a history of preceding sore throat. If gross haematuria occurs with sorethroat at the same time it is referred to as synpharyngitic haematuria and in the Singapore context this is a useful clue to the diagnosis of IgA nephritis, the commonest form of nephritis seen here. Haematuria in IgA nephritis may also be precipitated by exercise. Another cause of exercise induced haematuria is stress haematuria. This has now been found to be due to trauma to the blood vessels at the base of the bladder brought on by exercise or jogging.

4. **Dysuria** or pain on passing urine is due to infection of the bladder or the urethra (urethritis). Tuberculous cystitis or a tumour in the bladder can also give rise to dysuria.

5. **Strangury** is also painful micturition but in this case only a few drops of urine are passed. This is due to a severe inflammation of the bladder.

6 **Double micturition** is when a patient, soon after emptying the bladder wants to do so again. This occurs in patients with vesicoureteric reflux as they have a large residual urine volume in the bladder.

7. **Frequency of micturition** is when the patient passes urine many times over his normal micturition habits. This is often due to urinary tract infection.

8. **Nocturia** is when the patient awakes to pass urine a few times at night when previously he may usually do so only once at night. This is due either to urinary infection or it could be an early sign of renal failure as renal concentration is one of the earliest functions to be impaired in renal failure.

9. **Oliguria** refers to a decrease in urine output when the patient passes less than 400 ml of urine. This is a sign of renal failure.

10. **Anuria** is when there is absolutely no urine output. In this case acute renal failure due to an obstruction in the urinary tract has to be excluded. If obstruction is excluded, consider bilateral renal infarction due to thrombosis of the renal arteries

or a descending dissecting aneurysm involving the renal arteries.

11. **Renal failure:** The patient may complain of tiredness, shortness of breath, itch which is often generalised, poor appetite or anorexia, nausea, vomiting, giddiness, headache and swelling of the face and legs and passing scanty urine.

12. **Woman:** In the case of a female patient, enquire about her previous pregnancies, whether there was a history of swelling during pregnancy, protein in the urine and hypertension as this may suggest toxaemia of pregnancy. In the case of a woman with symptoms of urinary infection, enquire about the relationship to sexual activity.

13. **Man:** In a male patient with urinary infection, enquire about exposure to venereal disease and think of prostatic infection.

14. **System review:** Ask for history of a rash, alopecia or joint pain as these may be clues to systemic lupus erythematosus. Does the patient have a cough or history of tuberculosis? This may be useful when suspecting renal tuberculosis. Fever together with weight loss may mean a cancer. Renal cell carcinoma is one of the causes of pyrexia of unknown origin. If the patient is an elderly lady with urinary infection and renal failure, one should perform a vaginal examination to exclude cancer of the cervix.

15. **Past and family history** of kidney disease, childhood nephritis and urinary infection. If the patient had a history of kidney disease what investigations were performed? Enquire about treatment and follow-up. Was there a family history of hypertension or diabetes mellitus?

16. **Finally:** Does the patient take **drugs** like analgesics (nonsteroidal anti-inflammatory drug or NSAID) or traditional *sin-seh's* (Chinese physician) medicine which may do harm to the kidneys? Was there a history of recent instrumentation like in the case of those with catheter fever? Occupational hazards: A sewage or farm worker may contract leptospirosis, lead or hydrocarbon exposure may cause nephritis.

PHYSICAL EXAMINATION OF THE RENAL MASS

The renal mass is felt in the loin and has a well defined rounded lower border. It is felt bimanually and can be pushed from one hand to the other, i.e. ballotable. The front hand should be pressed towards the hand at the loin immediately at the end of inspiration.

One may be able to get above it. This feature would exclude a splenic and hepatic mass.

The differential diagnosis of a renal mass are polycystic kidneys, hydronephrosis, amyloidosis and renal carcinoma.

As part of the examination one should auscultate for a renal bruit which is a clue to the presence of renal artery stenosis.

An Enlarged Kidney or a Spleen?

The spleen has a sharp edge as well as a splenic notch. The edge of a kidney is rounded and there is no notch.

The fingers can be passed between the upper end of the kidney swelling and the ribs. A renal mass is bimanually palpable.

There is a colonic resonance in front of the renal mass.

KIDNEY DISEASES IN SINGAPORE

1. **Glomerulonephritis** is one of the commonest causes of chronic renal failure. Chronic glomerulonephritis accounts for at least 25% of end stage renal disease.
2. **Diabetes mellitus** causes diabetic nephropathy, urinary tract infection and hypertension. Diabetic nephropathy is the commonest cause of chronic renal failure in Singapore, accounting for 54% of end stage renal failure.
3. **Leptospirosis** is a common cause of acute renal failure. The patient may have fever, jaundice, conjunctival suffusion and calf tenderness.

4. **Systemic Lupus Erythematosus** affects mainly young women. It causes lupus nephritis and presents as acute nephritic syndrome, nephrotic syndrome or asymptomatic urinary abnormalities. It is a cause of acute as well as chronic renal failure.

5. **Henoch-Schonlein purpura** causes nephritis and is associated with a purpuric rash over the buttocks and lower limbs.

6. **Urinary tract infection:** Acute and chronic pyelonephritis, cystitis, prostatitis, urethritis.

7. **Renal stones, hydronephrosis, medullary sponge kidneys, renal tubular acidosis.**

8. **Adult polycystic kidneys** usually bilateral; causes chronic renal failure in the older age group.

9. **Gout** causes joint pain, renal stones, urinary infection and hypertension.

10. **Hypertension:** Renal and essential hypertension are common. Kidney failure results from malignant and accelerated hypertension.

11. **Tuberculosis** is a cause of sterile pyuria with tuberculous pyelonephritis. It also presents with haematuria.

12. **Prostatic diseases:** Hypertrophy of the prostate is a cause of obstructive uropathy and urinary tract infection.

13. **Cancer:** Hypernephroma or renal cell carcinoma can present as a renal mass, painless haematuria or fever of unknown origin.

14. **Pregnancy:** Pre-eclampsia, pregnancy superimposed on pre-existing glomerulonephritis, urinary tract infection are all complications that could result in deterioration of renal function with renal failure as the outcome.

15. **Drugs:** Analgesics giving rise to analgesic kidney with renal failure; non-steroidal anti-inflammatory drugs (NSAID) like indomethacin, brufen, ponstan, rofecoxib (vioxx) etc. can all cause acute renal failure by inhibiting prostaglandin synthesis. Traditional *sin-seh's* medicine too is a cause of tubulo-toxic acute renal failure.

URINE EXAMINATION

The following should be noted, viz. colour, reaction (pH), specific gravity, sugar, albumin, blood, deposit (urine microscopy) — RBC, WBC, other cells, casts.

Further Remarks on Haematuria

Haematuria or the passage of bloody urine is a danger signal that cannot be ignored. Enquire about associated dysuria, vesical symptoms and whether there is blood throughout the urinary stream.

Exclude red urine after beets, laxatives, colouring agent rhodomine B in which case the urine would be translucent rather than opaque because of the absence of red blood cells. Haemoglobinuria due to the haemolysis of red blood cells also gives rise to red urine.

Symptoms and Diagnosis

1. Haematuria with renal colic could be due to a stone, clot colic or renal tumour.
2. Terminal haematuria could be due to tuberculosis of the bladder, bladder stone or prostatic bleeding.
3. A tumour of the bladder ulcerates and presents with infection and bleeding, i.e. cystitis with haematuria.
4. Prostatic hypertrophy may be associated with dilated veins at the bladder neck which rupture when the patient strains.
5. Haematuria without other symptoms or "silent" haematuria could be due to a tumour of the bladder or kidney. Bleeding may be intermittent and stop for months before recurring.
6. Staghorn calculus, polycystic kidneys, renal cyst may also cause haematuria.
7. Stress haematuria is caused by exertion, usually after jogging or running for a long distance. This is due to trauma of blood vessels at the base of the bladder.

8. Glomerulonephritis like IgA nephritis can also be associated with haematuria on exertion or haematuria can be precipitated by an upper respiratory infection, gastroenteritis or any fever. Urine phase contrast microscopy will show dysmorphic RBC in these cases. In contrast, bleeding due to a stone or vascular cause will show isomorphic RBC under the phase contrast microscope.

Time of Haematuria

Try to determine if haematuria occurs at the initial part of the micturition stream, terminally or throughout micturition in order to facilitate the localisation of the site of haematuria.

Haematuria occurring at the initial portion could be due to some cause at the anterior urethra (urethritis, urethral stricture or meatal stenosis). Terminal haematuria could be due to posterior urethritis or a lesion at the bladder neck or trigone (polyps or tumours). Haematuria present throughout micturition means that the lesion is above the urinary bladder and could be due to a stone, tumour, tuberculosis or nephritis.

Loin Pain Recurrent Haematuria Syndrome

See Chapter on Renal Stones.

Nutcracker Syndrome- an Overlooked Cause of Haematuria

1. This condition was first described in 1972. It is due to the compression of the left renal vein between the aorta and the superior mesenteric artery, hence the term "nutcracker". Obstruction to left renal vein outflow causes venous hypertension with formation of intrarenal and extrarenal collaterals with intrarenal and perirenal varicosities and development of

gonadal vein reflux. Haematuria results when the thin walled septum separating the vein from the collecting system ruptures.

2. The clinical presentation is mainly haematuria with or without loin pain. Exercise seems to aggravate the condition. Sometimes anemia may result from blood loss. Some patients may present with haematuria and proteinuria.

3. Investigations: Computed Tomography of the abdomen, angiography with venography, magnetic resonance angiography. A proper diagnosis would spare unnecessary investigations.

4. There is no clear agreement with regards to treatment. Some cases resolve spontaneously. One lady had intermittent haematuria 16 years apart. Another was detected in the course of investigation for hypertension as part of angiographic workup. Another, a renal donor was found to have pelvi-ureteric varices. One patient presented with anemia and gross haematuria and the condition disappeared spontaneously 14 months later. The best approach is to observe and wait for spontaneous resolution. However there was the case of a young man with haematuria and left flank pain which resolved after a successful renocaval reimplantation. In another case of a middle aged woman with pelvic congestion due to pelvic varices, the condition resolved after successful embolisation of the gonadal veins and pelvic collaterals [Rudloff U *et al.* Ann Vasc Surg 2006, 20:120–129].

REFERENCES

1. Dube GK *et al.* Loin pain haematuria syndrome. *Kidney Int* 2006, **70**:2152–2155.
2. Oteki T *et al.* Nutcracker Syndrome associated with severe anemia and mild Proteinuria. *Clinical Nephrol* 2004, **62**:62–65.
3. Rudloff U *et al.* Mesoaortic compression of the left renal vein (Nutcracker Syndrome): Case reports and review of literature. *Ann Vasc Surg* 2006, **20**:120–129.

CHAPTER 3

Renal Investigations

A proper evaluation of kidney functions consists of the following:

1. Urine examination
2. Quantitative measurement of proteinuria
3. Glomerular function
4. Tubular function

URINE EXAMINATION

Urinary Red Blood Cells (RBC)

Under bright field microscopy, normal urine contains not more than 3 red blood cells (RBC) or white blood cells (WBC) per high power field (hpf). Apart from hyaline casts, other types of casts like RBC casts, granular or broad waxy casts should be absent. However, exercise can increase the number of cells and casts excreted, even in normal individuals and occasionally, granular casts are also excreted.

In patients presenting with haematuria it is particularly important to determine whether the bleeding is from a glomerular or non-glomerular source. This is now possible using Phase Contrast Microscopy. In glomerular bleeding (due to glomerulonephritis) the urinary RBC have a dysmorphic pattern. There is a profusion of RBC of bizarre shapes and dissimilar sizes. Normal centrifuged urine contains up to 8000 dysmorphic RBC per ml of urine. Increased number of dysmorphic RBC suggests a diagnosis of glomerular disease. The presence of concomitant proteinuria is another clue which points to a diagnosis of glomerular disease.

In non-glomerular bleeding associated with urinary calculus, tumours and papillary necrosis, the RBC are of isomorphic (of uniform size and shape). A count as low as 4000 per ml is indicative of non-glomerular bleeding, and an intravenous pyelography (IVP) may be required to exclude a stone or a cystoscopy required to exclude a tumour in the bladder.

Sometimes in patients with IgA nephritis or lupus nephritis, the patient may have a mixed pattern, i.e. both glomerular and non-glomerular RBC.

Leukocytes

The presence of WBC (pyuria) indicates infection or interstitial nephritis. Look for associated squamous epithelial cells in a female patient. The presence of epithelial cells with WBC indicates contamination by vaginal secretions and not a true urinary infection.

Casts

RBC casts imply the presence of glomerular disease and WBC casts indicate pyelonephritis. Normal urine contains hyaline casts (<100/ml of urine). However, diuretic treatment can increase the number of hyaline casts in normal individuals (up to 20,000/ml of urine). Granular casts, oval fat bodies and broad waxy casts suggest an underlying renal lesion. In normal subjects, casts are composed of Tamm Horsfall protein but in diseased states, casts are found from different cellular elements. Triamterene, a diuretic, can induce the formation of large brown bizarre casts containing triamterene crystals which can be mistaken for granular casts. However, triamterene casts and crystals will polarise when examined under polarised light.

QUANTITATIVE MEASUREMENT OF PROTEINURIA

Absence of significant proteinuria is a sign of renal integrity and its presence indicates renal disease. In normal individuals the 24-hour urinary protein is less than 150 mg per day.

Proteinuria could be due to:

1. Increased glomerular filtration because of increased permeability of basement membrane.
2. Decreased reabsorption of proteins.
3. Addition of protein to urine (renal tubular cells, lymphatics, genitalia). In Bence Jones proteinuria, there are abnormal light chains which coagulate on heating at a temperature of 45° to 55°C and redissolve on boiling.

Protein selectivity refers to the ratio of the clearance of a large molecular weight protein like IgG to a smaller one like transferrin. Patients with the nephrotic syndrome with selective proteinuria tend to respond to therapy with steroids as opposed to those with non-selective proteinuria. In our experience, patients with Minimal Change nephrotic syndrome and those with mild diffuse mesangial proliferative glomerulonephritis tend to respond to prednisolone or cyclosporine A therapy when they have selective proteinuria.

Proteinuria is greater during the day than at night and increases during upright position and exercise.

A reduction of proteinuria may indicate an improvement of glomerular disease or it may mean increasing glomerulosclerosis allowing less protein to be filtered into the urine.

Intermittent proteinuria may signify developing or healing lesions.

Persisting proteinuria of less than 1 gm a day indicates a less benign glomerular lesion on renal biopsy.

Functional proteinuria can be due to exercise or fever, extreme heat or cold.

Postural proteinuria occurs in 3 to 5% of healthy individuals. It is mild during the upright position and disappears on recumbence. The upright posture with lordosis causes renal venous congestion with decreased renal blood flow and proteinuria.

GLOMERULAR FUNCTION

Clinical measurement of renal function for:

1. Detecting disease
2. Evaluating its severity
3. Following its progress
4. Safe and effective use of drugs excreted by the kidney

Blood Urea Level

Urea production is rapidly affected by protein intake. It fluctuates more widely than creatinine.

When protein catabolism is increased, urea rises rapidly as in haemorrhage in the bowels or body tissues, severe infections, burns, muscle injury, ingestion of steroids and tetracycline (except doxycycline). Urea level falls with a low protein diet, starvation and liver damage.

Factors Affecting Serum Creatinine

1. Increase
   — large muscle mass
   — diet rich in meat
   — ketones, drugs (cephalosporin, aldactone, aspirin, co-trimoxazole)
2. Decrease
   — reduced muscle mass

— severe renal failure causes decreased muscle mass, increased tubular secretion and intestinal destruction of creatinine

3. Variable — due to laboratory error

Glomerular Filtration Rate (GFR)

Renal blood flow (RBF) and GFR are maintained over a wide range of renal arterial pressures by altering the tone in afferent and efferent arterioles. The GFR is maintained by net filtration pressure and permeability of membrane.

GFR is the most widely used test of renal function. Ideally, it is measured using a substance which is:

1. eliminated only by the kidney
2. freely filtered
3. neither secreted nor absorbed by tubules
4. easily and accurately measured.

Fig. 3.1 shows the relationship between serum creatinine and GFR.

Measurement of GFR

Inulin Clearance

1. GFR as measured by inulin clearance is a research tool. Its accuracy is therefore a gold standard.
2. For the test, infuse inulin for 3 hours to ensure a steady concentration in the extracellular fluid (ECF).
3. Maintain a high fluid intake.
4. At equilibrium, the amount of inulin filtered by the glomerulus

(GFR × P) equals the amount excreted in the urine (U × V).

$$\text{GFR} = \frac{U \times V}{P} = \frac{U \times \text{Volume}}{P \times T \text{ (Time)}}$$

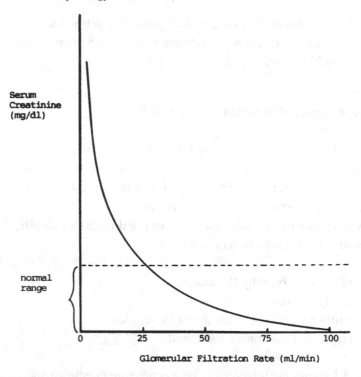

Fig. 3.1   Relationship between glomerular filtration rate and serum creatinine

Creatinine Clearance

1. The endogenous production of creatinine by muscle metabolism is constant and proportional to the muscle mass.
2. There is a slight amount secreted by the tubules but common methods slightly overestimate plasma concentration.
3. A 24-hour urine collection is necessary. This urine specimen is also useful for quantitation of urinary protein.
4. The GFR varies inversely with the plasma concentration.

Chromium^{51}-EDTA

1. There is a small extra renal clearance which slightly underestimates the GFR.

2. Clearance is obtained using an intravenous infusion and timed urine collection as for inulin.
3. A single intravenous injection is given which diffuses quickly into the ECF.
4. After the initial drop, plasma radioactivity falls exponentially. The slope is determined by the line of the GFR.
5. For calculation: slope of line multiplied by volume of distribution. The volume of distribution is determined by injected dose divided by plasma activity at zero time.

Estimation of GFR by Radiopharmaceuticals

1. Chromium^{51}-EDTA
2. Iodine^{125} sodium iothalamate
3. 99m technetium DTPA

These are gamma emitting isotopes. They are easily measured and there is no need for urine sample or collection.

Estimation of GFR Using Beta 2 Microglobulin

1. Beta 2 microglobulin is a surface constituent of most cells.
2. It is present in plasma in low concentration and is a low molecular weight protein of 11,800 daltons.
3. It is filtered freely at the glomerulus and is reabsorbed by cells of the proximal tubules.
4. B2m is produced at a constant rate and is not affected by muscle mass or diet.
5. It is measured by means of a radioimmunoassay.

eGFR or estimated Glomerular Filtration Rate

Nowadays, instead of using the 24 hours Creatinine Clearance test [CCT], the eGFR which is the estimated Glomerular Filtration Rate is employed. The eGFR is actually an estimated

Creatinine Clearance Rate. The serum creatinine which has been routinely used to measure renal function is often not a reliable index of renal function, especially among elderly people since the creatinine estimation is dependent on muscle mass. As a person grows older, he loses weight as his muscle mass gets less and the serum creatinine correspondingly becomes lower even though his true renal function may have decreased with age as estimated by the CCT. Hence, a 'normal' serum creatinine value in an elderly person may not mean he has normal renal function and the CCT or the eGFR may in fact be much lower indicating loss of renal function often related to aging. In practice, the CCT entails a 24 hour urine collection. This is cumbersome and often the urine collection is incomplete giving rise to inaccurate readings. The eGFR takes into account the age and the sex of the person and is therefore a better reflection of renal function.

The two formulae commonly employed to calculate the estimated Creatinine Clearance Rate to derive the eGFR are the Cockcroft-Gault formula and the Modification of Diet in Renal Disease [MDRD] formula.

The Cockroft-Gault formula is a commonly used surrogate marker for estimation of the Creatinine Clearance, which in turn estimates GFR, hence the terminology eGFR as calculated by the Cockroft Gault formula:

$$eC_{cr} = (140\text{-Age}) \times (\text{mass in kg})$$
$$\times [0.85 \text{ if } \textit{Female}] \textit{ divided by } 72$$
$$\times \text{ Serum Creatinine (in mg/dL)}$$

When Serum Creatinine is measured in μmol/L:

$$eC_{cr} = (140\text{-Age}) \times \text{Mass (in kg)}$$
$$\times \text{ Constant } \textit{divided by } \text{Serum}$$
$$\text{Creatinine (in } \mu\text{mol/L)}$$

where Constant is 1.23 for men and 1.04 for women.

The Cockroft-Gault equation shows how dependent the estimation of Creatinine Clearance is based on age. The age term is (140-age). This means that a 20 year old person (14–20) will have twice the Creatinine Clearance as an 80 year old (140–80) for the same level of creatinine (120 is twice as great as 60). The Cockroft-Cault equation also shows that a woman will have a 15% lower Creatinine Clearance than a man at the same level of serum creatinine.

Estimated GFR (eGFR) Using Modification of Diet in Renal Disease (MDRD) Formula

The most recently advocated formula for calculating the eGFR is the one developed by the Modification of Diet in Renal Disease Study Group. The most commonly used formula is the 4 variable MDRD which estimates GFR using 4 variables of serum creatinine, age, race and gender. This formula underestimates the GFR in healthy persons with GFRs over 60 ml/min.

For serum creatinine in mg/dL:

$$eGFR = 186 \times \text{Serum Creatinine}^{-1.154} \times ^{-0.203}$$
$$\times [1.210 \ if \ Black] \times [0.742 \ if \ Female]$$

For serum creatinine in μmol/L:

$$eGFR = 32788 \times \text{Serum Creatinine}^{-1.154} \times \text{age}^{-0.203}$$
$$\times [1.210 \ if \ Black] \times [0.742 \ if \ Female]$$

Since these formulae do not adjust for body mass, they [relative to the Cockroft-Gault Formula] underestimate eGFR for heavy people and overestimate it for underweight people.

The eGFR forms the basis for staging or classification for Chronic Kidney Disease (CKD) which is now widely used:

CKD 1: abnormal urinary findings with eGFR > 9 0 ml/min
CKD 2: eGFR 90 to 60 ml/min
CKD 3: eGFR 59 to 30 ml/min

CKD 4: eGFR 29 to 15 ml/min
CKD 5: eGFR <15 ml/min (end stage renal failure)

The CKD Classification is based on eGFR derived from the Cockroft–Gault or the MDRD formula.

However, there are concerns with the use of eGFR reporting as eGFR values above 60 ml/min are unreliable. Also eGFR less than 60 ml/min is based on the false premise that GFR is diet independent and conserved throughout life in healthy individuals. eGFR values decline with age, even in normal individuals and these values can be further reduced by a habitually low protein intake in otherwise healthy people [Glassock RJ and Winearls CG. Nature Clinical Practice Nephrology, 2008, 4(8):422–423]. Hence, many individuals age above 65 with eGFR < 60 ml/min, especially females do not have CKD. Glassock and Winearls have suggested that we should use percentile charts of eGFR by age and sex and only those with values of eGFR lower than the fifth percentile need referral to a nephrologist.

Serum Cystatin C

1. Serum Cystatin C is an endogenous 13 kilo Dalton protein filtered by the glomeruli and reabsorbed and catabolised by epithelial cells of the proximal tubule with only small amounts excreted by the urine. Cystatin is being considered as a potential replacement for serum creatinine because it appears to be less affected by muscle mass.

2. Some studies have shown a strong association of serum cystatin C with mortality and cardiovascular disease, especially in studies of older adults. There may be differential effects of factors other than GFR on levels of serum cystatin C and creatinine that are more prevalent in older adults [Stevens LA *et al.*, New Engl J Med 2005, 352:2122–2124]. In this study diabetes, higher C reactive protein, higher white blood cell count and lower serum albumin were associated

with higher serum cystatin C and lower serum creatinine. However, the associations of cystatin C with non GFR determinants are relatively small though statistically significant. Clinicians may have to use their knowledge of non GFR determinants of serum cystatin when interpreting serum cystatin C levels.

3. Cystatin C has promise as an alternative filtration marker to creatinine, but like creatinine is is also affected by factors other than GFR. The use of both markers may minimize the impact of physiological processes other than GFR that affect each marker. Further studies are required to define the use of both these two markers in the estimation of GFR.

4. In a recent study it was found that plasma cystatin C levels was well correlated with GFR in patients with anorexia nervosa [Delanaye P *et al.*, Nephron Clinical Practice, 2008, 110: 158–163]. Serum creatinine concentration was not correlated with GFR, but the reciprocal of the plasma cystatin C showed a strong correlation with GFR (r = 0.62, p < 0.001). detection of decreased GFR < 60 ml/min was achieved with greater sensitivity and specificity than by serum creatinine. Plasma cystatin was not affected by muscle mass and plasma cystatin seems a better marker of renal function than serum creatinine in patients with anorexia nervosa.

5. Studies have also shown that cystatin C is a better predictor of cardiovascular disease and mortality than serum creatinine based GFR (eGFR) [Fried LF. Creatinine and cystatin C: what are the values? Kidney Int 2009, 75:578–580].

REFERENCES

1. Stevens LA *et al*. Factors other than GFR affect serum cystatin C levels. *Kidney Int* 2009, **75**:652–660.
2. Delanaye P *et al*. Cystatin C or creatinine for detection of stage 3 CKD in anorexia nervosa. *Nephron Clinical Practice*, 2008, **110**:158–163.
3. Fried LF. Creatinine and cystatin C: what are the values? *Kidney Int* 2009, **75**:578–580.

TUBULAR FUNCTION

I.   Proximal tubular function is assessed by reabsorption of glucose, phosphate, urate and amino acids.
II. Distal tubular function is assessed by urine concentration, dilution and acidification.

Proximal Tubular Function

1.   Four functions are commonly assessed — reabsorption of glucose, phosphate, urate and amino acids.
2.   Urine glucose, plasma phosphate, plasma urate and urinary amino acids are measured.

Amino Acids

a.   Amino acids are freely filtered at the glomerulus and are almost completely reabsorbed by the proximal tubule.
b.   The commonest are cystine, ornithine, lysine and arginine.
c.   Proximal tubular lesions cause generalised or isolated amino acid leak.
d.   Two-dimensional chromatography can be used to detect the leak.
e.   In patients with cystinuria, the excretion of cystine is measured.

Urate

a.   If plasma urate (serum uric acid) concentration is low, perform simultaneous measurement of 24-hour urate and creatinine clearance.
b.   In the presence of low or normal plasma urate; a urate clearance:creatinine clearance ratio of over 10% indicates a tubular leak.

Phosphate

a. If plasma phosphate is consistently low or at the lower limit of the normal level, carry out simultaneous measurement of phosphate and creatinine clearance.
b. If the plasma phosphate is low and the phosphate clearance: creatinine clearance ratio is high (>20%), this is evidence of proximal tubular dysfunction.

Glycosuria

a. This is tested for in random urine samples throughout the day.
b. Simultaneous measurement of plasma glucose is performed if any urine sample contains glucose.
c. Glycosuria without hyperglycaemia indicates proximal tubular malfunction.

Urinary Concentration Ability

1. Specific gravity
   If the morning urine has a SG of 1.018 or more, no further test is necessary as it implies normal concentration ability.
2. Osmolality
   If the early morning urine has an osmolality >550 mOsmol/kg, no further test is necessary.

If the osmolality is <550 mOsmol/kg, further investigation is required.

Maximal Osmolar Concentration

1. After an overnight fast, give pitressin tannate 5 units subcutaneously or 20 μgm intranasally of desmopressin in each nostril.

2. Urine osmolality is measured hourly for 8 hours or until a sufficiently concentrated sample of urine is obtained before that.
3. An osmolality of 800 mOsmol/kg is accepted as normal.

Impaired Urinary Concentration

The following are possible causes:

1. high plasma calcium
2. low plasma potassium
3. protein malnutrition
4. prolonged high fluid intake
5. diabetes insipidus
6. drugs (e.g. lithium)

Dilution Test

This is a measure of tubular functional integrity. Usually, the ability of the kidneys to concentrate urine is lost before its diluting ability. Complaints about nocturia is a signal that there may be a defect in concentration. At this stage the patient has polyuria and passes a dilute urine. Later on with further renal damage and with decreased renal perfusion, the patient passes less urine (oliguria).

1. For the test, the patient drinks 1 litre of fluid over 30 minutes. Urine is collected over 3 hours.
2. A normal person should excrete more than 50% of the volume in 3 hours.
3. The SG in one of the urine samples should be less than 1.003.

Urinary Acidification

1. No test is required if the overnight urine pH is 5.3 or less.
2. A plasma bicarbonate of less than or equal to 20 mEq/l is sufficient stimulus to acidify the urine.

3. Urine pH should be 5.3 or less in the Ammonium Chloride Loading Test.

Short Test of Wrong and Davis

1. Ammonium chloride, 100 mg/kg body weight is given in capsules or in a flavoured mixture at breakfast.
2. The pH is measured in all urine samples collected over 8 hours.
3. Blood samples are taken at the start and the end of the test to confirm a significant fall in plasma bicarbonate. This is to check that patient has not vomited the ammonium chloride ingested.
4. At least one urine sample should have pH 5.3 or less.
5. Titratable acid and ammonium excretion are also measured at the same time.
6. Refer to chapter on Renal Tubular Acidosis for more details.

RENAL FUNCTION WITH INCREASING AGE

1. There is a gradual decrease in all aspects of renal function after the age of 40 years.
2. This is due to involution and renal vascular degeneration.
3. There is a reduction in GFR which is accompanied by a decrease in muscle mass with age. Hence there is little change in the serum creatinine. Therefore if the GFR is not simultaneously measured with the serum creatinine, it may be presumed that the person still has his normal renal reserve (normal GFR).
4. In this instance if the person is given the normal dose of digoxin or an aminoglycoside antibiotic without being aware that in fact his GFR is lower than presumed (in the presence of still normal serum creatinine), he will run the risk of drug toxicity as well as nephrotoxicity.
5. This explains why old patients with apparently normal serum creatinine who are given a dose of gentamicin 80 mg or 60 mg

three times a day often develop renal impairment (as evidenced by a rise in serum creatinine) soon after. It is therefore useful to remember that old people with apparently normal serum creatinine in fact do not have "normal" renal function.

REFERENCES

1.   Richard J Glassock, Christopher G Winearls. Routine reporting of estimated Glomerular Filtration Rate; Not ready for prime time. *Nature Clinical Practice Nephrology*, 2008, **4**(8):422–423.
2.   Richard J Glassock. Estimated glomerular filtration rate : Time for a performance review? *Kidney Int* 2009, **75**(10):1001–1003.
3.   Stevens LA *et al.* Factors other than GFR affect serum cystatin C levels. *Kidney Int* 2009, **75**:652–660.
4.   Delanaye P *et al.* Cystatin C or creatinine for detection of stage 3 CKD in anorexia nervosa. *Nephron Clinical Practice*, 2008, **110**:58–163.
5.   Fried LF. Creatinine and cystatin C: what are the values? *Kidney Int* 2009, **75**:578–580.

CHAPTER 4

Glomerulonephritis

The term glomerulonephritis refers to an inflammation of the kidneys.

The major clinical syndromes are:

1. Acute nephritic syndrome
2. Rapidly progressive glomerulonephritis
3. Persistent urinary abnormalities
4. Nephrotic syndrome
5. Nephritic nephrotic syndrome

Glomerulonephritis may be:

1. Primary or idiopathic
2. Secondary to multisystem diseases

Table 4.1 shows the histological distribution of Primary Glomerulonephritis (GN) in Singapore over 3 decades. Comparing the data, the commonest histopathological diagnosis was IgA Nephritis (IgA Nx), 42% in the first decade, 45% in the second decade and 40% in the third decade. The prevalence of IgA nephritis has remained the same. Mesangial Proliferative GN (Non IgA Nx) was the second commonest cause of primary GN in the first decade (32%) but has steadily declined to 17% in the second decade and only 7% in the third decade (p < 0.000001). The decrease in the 3rd decade of Mesangial Proliferative GN was accompanied by a significant increase in Minimal Change (p < 0.000001), Focal Segmental Glomerulosclerosis (FSGS) (p < 0.000001) and Membranous GN (p < 0.001) compared to the 1st and 2nd decade. The increase in both FSGS and Membranous

Table 4.1   Primary Glomerulonephritis : Histological Presentation over 3 decades

Histology	1st Decade [1976–1989]	2nd Decade [1990–1997]	3rd Decade [1998–2008]	p (χ^2) D1 vs D2 vs D3	p (χ^2) D2 vs D3
1 Minimal Change	97 (9%)	87 (13%)	151 (19%)	< 0.000001	< 0.002
2 Focal Global Sclerosis	72 (6%)	83 (12%)	31 (4%)	< 0.000001	< 0.000001
3 Mesangial Proliferative Glomerulonephritis	357 (32%)	112 (17%)	55 (7%)	< 0.000001	< 0.000001
4 IgA Nephritis	473 (42%)	300 (45%)	316 (40%)	0.17	0.07
5 Focal & Segmental Glomerulosclerosis (FSGS)	57 (5%)	41 (6%)	115 (15%)	< 0.000001	< 0.000001
6 Membranous Glomerulonephritis	38 (3%)	42 (6%)	90 (11%)	< 0.000001	< 0.001
7 Crescenteric Glomerulonephritis	5 (1%)	1 (1%)	8 (1%)	0.07	0.08
8 Others	28 (2%)	0	20 (3%)	< 0.0002	< 0.0001
Total	1127 (100%)	666 (100%)	786 (100%)		

GN in the 3rd decade had been 2 fold that of the 2nd decade; FSGS (6% versus 15%) and Membranous GN (6% versus 11%) in the 2nd and 3rd decade (p < 0.000001 and < 0.001 respectively).

Therefore, over the past 3 decades in Singapore the pattern of Glomerulonephritis has evolved from that of a third world country to that of a developed nation. In the first decade, Mesangial Proliferative Glomerulonephritis was the most common form of Primary Glomerulonephritis just as in the surrounding Asian countries. In the second decade the prevalence of Mesangial Proliferative Glomerulonephritis has decreased with a rise in Membranous Glomerulonephritis which is also seen in China and Thailand. In the third decade there is a dramatic increase in Focal Sclerosing Glomerulosclerosis. The rise in the prevalence of Focal Sclerosing Glomerulosclerosis reflects aging and obesity in keeping with more developed countries like Australia, India, Saudi Arabia, Thailand and the United States. Apart from geographical and genetic influence, other socio-economic factors play a significant role in the evolution of the renal biopsy pattern. Mesangial Proliferative Glomerulonephritis remains prevalent in many Asian countries but in Singapore the prevalence is decreasing just as in Japan, Korea and Malaysia. Worldwide, the prevalence of Focal Sclerosing Glomerulosclerosis continues to increase in many countries [Woo KT *et al.*, Global evolutionary trend of the prevalence of Primary Glomerulonephritis over the past three decades, Nephron Clinical Practice, 2010, 116: c337–c346] [Woo KT *et al.*, Changing pattern of Primary Glomerulonephritis in Singapore and Other Countries over the past three decades. Clinical Nephrology, 2010, 74(5):372–383].

ACUTE NEPHRITIC SYNDROME

The features are oedema with gross haematuria (smoky urine) and frequent association with hypertension. Sometimes the symptoms are complicated by encephalopathy and congestive heart failure. This condition may be caused by bacteria, parasites, viruses, systemic lupus erythematosus, Henoch-Schonlein purpura and Guillain-Barre syndrome.

Post streptococcal glomerulonephritis which classically presents as the nephritic syndrome is better referred to as Post Infectious Glomerulonephritis because apart from streptococci, other bacteria and viruses can be the causative agent. It affects children principally, but no age is exempt. There is usually a latent period of 10 to 21 days. The urine characteristically shows a rusty or smoky hue. Mild renal impairment is common. Serum Complements (CH50 and C3) are usually low but normalises after 6 to 8 weeks.

Renal biopsy in patients with post infectious glomerulonephritis shows diffuse endocapillary proliferative glomerulonephritis with exudation of polymorphonuclears (acute exudative glomerulonephritis) (see Fig. 4.1). Electron microscopy (EM) shows subepithelial humps. Immunofluorescence (IMF) shows IgG often with C3. Sometimes IgA and IgM may be present in smaller amounts.

Treatment is usually symptomatic: generally bed rest is recommended during the acute phase. Restrict fluids and salt if oedema

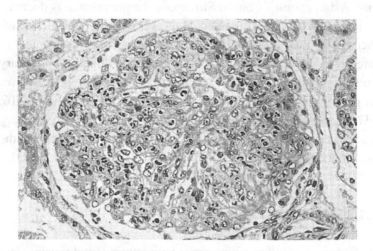

Fig. 4.1 Endocapillary glomerulonephritis. There is proliferation of endocapillary cells with polymorph infiltration. HE Stain original magnification 300X

is present. Treat accompanying hypertension and heart failure. A course of Penicillin is given if throat swab grows streptococci. Dialysis may be required in some instances to tide the patient over the acute renal failure which may complicate the course of a few patients.

For the majority of patients, this is a benign disease, with children faring better than adults. Glassock[1] reported a 99% 5-year and a 97% 10-year survival for children whereas adults have 95% 5-year and a 90% 10-year survival. Potter[2] in a series of 534 patients from Trinidad followed up for 12 to 17 years reported only 2 deaths from chronic renal failure. Both those patients had persistent urinary abnormalities. Of the surviving patients, 3.6% had urinary abnormalities and another 3.6% had hypertension. All had normal serum creatinine.

In a paper from Israel, Drachman[3] showed that 80% of an original group of 155 children followed up for 11 to 12 years had normal urinary findings and blood pressure. Singhal[4] however showed in his study from India that 25 out of 144 of his patients died within 2 years and another 6 had renal impairment. In the next 8 years, 6 others developed renal impairment and 3 end stage renal failure (ESRF).

The bad prognostic features in this disease are persistent nephrotic syndrome, hypertension, renal impairment and crescents. These bad prognostic features however, as we shall see later, are true for most forms of glomerulonephritis.

RAPIDLY PROGRESSIVE GLOMERULONEPHRITIS (CRESCENTERIC GLOMERULONEPHRITIS) (Fig. 4.2)

This is a clinical syndrome of rapid and progressive decline in renal function, usually resulting in end stage renal failure in weeks to months, where there is extensive and exuberant proliferation of epithelial cells of Bowman's space.

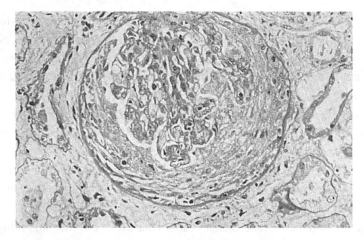

Fig. 4.2   Crescenteric glomerulonephritis. Crescent formation with compression of the glomerular tuft is seen. PAS Stain original magnification 300X

In clinical practice, this condition is diagnosed when a patient has a rapid decline in glomerular filtration rate (acute renal failure), usually with oliguria, haematuria, hypertension in the presence of normal sized or enlarged kidneys. A renal biopsy will show extensive crescents of more than 70%.

Preceding flu-like illness is found in 50% of patients. Hypertension is often mild. Urine microscopy shows many RBC with RBC casts. Serum complements (CH50, C3 and C1q) are often normal. Fibrin degradation products are often present and anti-streptolysin 0 titre is increased in 30% of patients.

Histology shows extensive extracapillary proliferation (crescents). IMF may show diffuse linear IgG, diffuse granular IgG, IgM and C3 or negative staining as in vasculitis. Fibrin related antigens are also present. Linear IgG with lung haemorrhage suggests Goodpasture's syndrome. Diffuse granular IgG indicates an immune complex glomerulonephritis like post streptococcal glomerulonephritis, systemic lupus erythematosus or nephritis due to subacute bacterial endocarditis.

Classify by absence or presence of glomerular Immune-Complexes (I.C)

(i) Linear anti GBM antibody — Goodpasture's Syndrome
(ii) Granular Immune Complexes — SLE, HSP, SBE, PSGN
(iii) Pauci-immune Complexes — Wegener's Granulomatosis, Microscopic Polyarteritis Nodosa (PAN), Idiopathic Crescenteric GN

Treatment consists of Pulse therapy with methylprednisolone of 0.5 gm IV daily for 3 days. In addition patients may require plasmapheresis with steroids and cyclophosphamide ideally administered prior to the onset of oliguria. A quadruple regimen with heparin, prednisolone, cyclophosphamide and anti-platelet agents (dipyridamole) has been used with success,[5] but caution should be exercised when using heparin. A low dose continuous heparin regimen during the acute phase to avoid haemorrhage and then switch over to warfarin therapy is safer. Nowadays heparin therapy is no longer practised because of the risk of haemorrhage. A better alternative is to use pulse therapy with methylprednisolone (0.5 gm I.V. daily for 6 days). Other measures include restriction of salt and water, treatment of hypertension and supportive dialysis.

This is a disease with a bad prognosis. The outlook for recovery is especially poor in the presence of:

1. circumferential crescents.
2. severe tubular atrophy and interstitial fibrosis.
3. extensive glomerular fibrosis and reorganisation of crescents, a late finding signifying irreversibility.
4. oliguria with a glomerular filtration rate of less than 5 ml per minute.

Patients with 50% to 80% crescents on biopsy have less than 30% 5-year and less than 10% 10-year survival. Those with 80% crescents have an 8% 5-year and less than 5% 10-year survival.

ASYMPTOMATIC HAEMATURIA AND PROTEINURIA

Asymptomatic haematuria and proteinuria is the most common presenting sign for a wide variety of glomerulonephritis. In the Singapore context, this is the usual presentation for IgA nephritis, the commonest form of glomerulonephritis occurring in Singapore. Patients with such urinary abnormalities are often referred by their general practitioners following a routine investigation for some unrelated complaints. Such cases are also detected on community health surveys or in the course of screening of national service registrants, for example at the Central Manpower Base as in the case of Singapore. Surgeons too, often refer patients with asymptomatic haematuria after they have been shown to have normal intravenous pyelogram and cystoscopic examination.

History

One should ascertain that the patient is truly asymptomatic. Enquire for a history of gross or macroscopic haematuria, dysuria or frequency of micturition which may point to a diagnosis of haemorrhagic cystitis. A history of nocturia, backache, passage of stones, oedema or recurrent sore throat may provide useful clues to the underlying basis of the urinary abnormalities.

If the patient has episodes of gross haematuria, determine if there is a relationship to upper respiratory tract infection, fever or exercise as IgA nephritis is associated with synpharyngitic haematuria, i.e. gross haematuria occurring simultaneously with sore throat.

Always ask for a history of systemic illness. Tuberculosis, Systemic Lupus Erythematosus and Henoch-Schonlein purpura may present with urinary abnormalities. A family history of nephritis, hypertension and diabetes mellitus may be important. In a married woman, enquire into a past history of pre-eclampsia.

Physical Examination

In the general examination look for pallor, sallowness, presence of oedema and the rash of Henoch-Schonlein purpura or Systemic Lupus Erythematosus. Examine the abdomen for ballotable kidneys or renal masses which may suggest polycystic kidneys or a renal tumour. Always check the blood pressure, examine the fundi and listen for a renal bruit.

In most cases with asymptomatic haematuria and proteinuria the physical examination is usually normal; nevertheless a complete physical examination is mandatory to exclude any obvious underlying cause for the urinary abnormality.

Investigations

1. A full blood count and erythrocyte sedimentation rate (ESR) may be the first clues to SLE and tuberculosis.
2. Urine Microscopy

    i. RBC count is usually variable and may be anything from 5–10 to 100–300 per high power field.
    ii. WBC count: if pyuria is present, exclude urinary tract infection by doing a urine culture. For sterile pyuria, tuberculosis has to be excluded.
    iii. Casts: RBC casts point to a glomerulonephritis. Granular casts associated with more than a gram of proteinuria per day denotes a more severe lesion.
    iv. Albumin may vary from trace to 3 plus.

3. Quantitation of total urinary protein (TUP) in 24 hours. Normally this should not exceed 0.15 gm. In our experience, a TUP of more than 1 gm generally denotes a more severe glomerular lesion on renal biopsy, i.e. the presence of glomerular scarring (glomerulosclerosis).
4. Blood urea, serum creatinine and creatinine clearance should be documented.

5. Lupus erythematosus (LE) cell and anti-nuclear factor (ANF) should be done when one suspects SLE together with Anti-DNA and Serum Complement.

Mild microscopic haematuria (< 20 RBC/high-power field (hpf)) in the absence of significant proteinuria is of little prognostic significance. In our experience, renal biopsies of this group of patients usually reveal only mild glomerulonephritis which generally has a good prognosis.

Sometimes on follow-up, patients may develop gross haematuria which may be precipitated by respiratory tract infections or exercise. Such patients on biopsy usually have IgA nephritis.

Proteinuria of 1 gm or more is an indication for a renal biopsy. Biopsy is performed under ultrasound guidance.

The intravenous pyelogram usually shows normal kidneys in patients with asymptomatic haematuria and proteinuria. If there is bilaterally symmetrical contracted kidneys it means that the patient probably has chronic glomerulonephritis. The presence of irregular scarring with calyceal distortion denotes chronic atrophic pyelonephritis due to vesico-ureteric reflux. Localised strictures of the calyces may be a clue to tuberculosis. The IVP may sometimes reveal polycystic kidneys, renal cysts or a renal tumour.

Indications for Renal Biopsy

Renal biopsy should be considered in patients with asymptomatic haematuria and proteinuria if they have:

1. Proteinuria of 1 gm or more.
2. Urine RBC persistently greater than 100 per hpf.
3. Gross haematuria on follow-up, associated with heavy proteinuria.
4. Presence of abnormal renal function or hypertension.

Renal Biopsy

Specimens are processed for light microscopy, immunofluorescence and electron microscopic studies.

1. IgA Nephritis the commonest GN in Singapore, comprised 42% (473/1127) of Primary GN in the 1st decade, 45% (300/666) in the 2nd decade and 40% (316/786) in the 3rd decade. The clinical and histopathological profile of the patients with IgA Nephritis over the past 3 decades is shown in Tables 4.2 and 4.3. A comparison of the clinical presentation showed that in the 3rd decade, more patients were biopsied when they presented with Nephrotic Syndrome (p < 0.00005). In the first 2 decades among patients with IgA Nephritis, those presenting with Nephrotic Syndrome accounted for 9% and 15% respectively. But in the 3rd decade Nephrotic Syndrome accounted for 25% presentation among IgA nephrotic patients (p < 0.002). However relatively less number of patients with IgA Nephritis presenting with Asymptomatic Haematuria and Proteinuria and Gross Haematuria were biopsied but the number of patients for these 2 groups were not significantly different between the 2nd and 3rd decades. Correspondingly there were more patients with IgA Nephritis presenting as chronic renal failure and hypertension in the 3rd decade compared to the 1st and 2nd decades (p < 0.0004 and 0.00005 respectively).

   In the 3rd decade, among patients presenting with IgA Nephritis, Mesangial Proliferative accounted for 74% of biopsies, by far the commonest histopathology, though a little less compared to the preceding 2 decades where Mesangial Proliferative GN accounted for 77% and 79% respectively. There was a dramatic increase in the number of patients with IgA Nephritis having Focal and Segmental Glomerulosclerosis (14%), compared to 8% and 7% in the 1st and 2nd decade respectively (p < 0.02). Crescentic GN among IgA Nephritic

Table 4.2   IgA Nephritis: Clinical Presentation over 3 decades

	Clinical Presentation	1st Decade [1976–1989]	2nd Decade [1990–1997]	3rd Decade [1998–2008]	p (χ^2) D1 vs D2 vs D3	p (χ^2) D2 vs D3
1	Hematuria & Proteinuria	296 (63%)	157 (52%)	154 (49%)	< 0.0002	0.37
2	Gross Hematuria	65 (14%)	17 (6%)	9 (3%)	< 0.00005	0.16
3	Nephrotic Syndrome	41 (9%)	45 (15%)	80 (25%)	< 0.00005	< 0.002
4	Acute Nephritis	4 (1%)	26 (9%)	7 (2%)	< 0.00005	0.0016
5	Chronic Renal Failure	25 (5%)	2 (1%)	20 (6%)	< 0.0004	< 0.00005
6	Hypertension	25 (5%)	45 (15%)	46 (15%)	< 0.00005	0.88
7	Others	17 (3%)	8 (2%)	0 (0%)	< 0.001	< 0.01
	Total	473 (100%)	300 (100%)	316 (100%)		

Table 4.3 IgA Nephritis: Histological Presentation over 3 decades

Histology	1st Decade [1976–1989]	2nd Decade [1990–1997]	3rd Decade [1998–2008]	p (χ^2) D1 vs D2 vs D3	p (χ^2) D2 vs D3
1 Minimal Change	12 (3%)	9 (3%)	16 (5%)	0.14	0.2
2 Focal Global Sclerosis	21 (4%)	17 (6%)	14 (4%)	0.75	0.76
3 Mesangial Proliferative Glomerulonephritis	365 (77%)	238 (79%)	232 (74%)	<0.00005	<0.00005
4 Focal & Segmental Glomerulosclerosis (FSGS)	36 (8%)	20 (7%)	45 (14%)	<0.002	<0.003
5 Crescenteric Glomerulonephritis	1 (<1%)	1 (<1%)	1 (<1%)	0.9	0.95
6 Others	38 (8%)	15 (5%)	8 (3%)	<0.004	0.1
Total	473 (100%)	300 (100%)	316 (100%)		

patients remains uncommon throughout the 3 decades. Minimal Change and Focal Global Sclerosis (FGS) remain low at 5% and 4% respectively, not significantly different from the preceding 2 decades.

2. A small proportion of patients with asymptomatic haematuria and proteinuria have Minimal Lesion which has an excellent prognosis.

3. Occasionally one may see Membranous GN and very rarely Mesangiocapillary GN. In both instances SLE has to be excluded. Full house immunoglobulins on IMF study is a clue to the diagnosis of SLE as the cause of the nephritis.

4. Focal and segmental glomerulosclerosis (FSGS) and diffuse sclerosing GN connote a bad prognosis.

Most patients with asymptomatic haematuria and proteinuria have a benign course as they are likely to have mesangial IgA nephritis which has a favourable prognosis in most cases. No treatment is required for most of these patients and all they require is reassurance. They could be followed up by their general practitioners and have their blood pressure, urine microscopy, serum creatinine and urinary protein checked once a year. It is important to treat any existing hypertension as uncontrolled hypertension often leads to renal impairment in patients with IgA nephritis.

In those patients with IgA nephritis with significant glomerulosclerosis especially in the presence of severe proteinuria, the prognosis is guarded. Patients with crescents on biopsy have a poorer long-term prognosis.

On long-term follow-up, some patients may develop gross haematuria precipitated by upper respiratory tract infections or exercise. They may have colicky loin pain due to clot colic. These patients require reassurance, rest and plenty of fluids as well as antibiotics for the respiratory tract infections.

Those who develop oedema or the nephrotic syndrome will require diuretic therapy. In those with mild diffuse mesangial proliferative GN with the nephrotic syndrome, a 12-week course of prednisolone therapy starting at 60 mg/day or 1 mg/kg body weight and tailing off by 12 weeks may induce a remission in about 50% of cases. These are patients with selective proteinuria. Hypertension when it occurs must be treated aggressively as uncontrolled hypertension can lead to rapid deterioration of renal function, culminating in ESRF.

On the whole, most patients with asymptomatic haematuria and proteinuria due to IgA nephritis run a benign course, except for about 30% (usually associated with glomerulosclerosis and heavy proteinuria) who develop renal failure over a period of 10 years. These patients would ultimately require renal transplantation or dialysis. In other words, IgA nephritis is not always a benign disease, especially in Singapore where we have large numbers of people with the disease. It is therefore an important cause of ESRF.

Factors Influencing the Progression of IgA Nephritis

In a study of 151 patients with IgA nephritis in our Department,[6] 76% had stable renal function, 12% had slow deterioration of renal function and 11 % progressed to end stage renal failure during a followup period of 65 ± 4.0 months (range 6 to 102 months). The cumulative renal survival at the end of 8 years is 82%.

Patients with IgA nephritis when they develop renal impairment run two different courses. One is a slowly progressive course over years which probably represents the natural history of deterioration in renal function due to the nephritis per se, resulting in a constant decline in renal function. The other course is a more rapid one, progressing to end stage renal failure within a few years, and where severe uncontrolled hypertension seems to be the major adverse factor.

A comparison of various factors which might have influenced the patients' clinical course showed that those with stable function had less proteinuria, crescents and a lower incidence of hypertension in contrast to patients who develop renal failure. The latter had more proteinuria, crescents and a higher incidence of hypertension. When proteinuria exceeded 1 gm, there was a higher incidence of renal failure as well as an increased incidence of crescents on renal biopsy. Heavier proteinuria seemed to be related to more severe histological lesions.

Our data showed that patients with crescents had a higher chance of developing end stage renal failure. Shirai found that patients who developed chronic renal failure at follow-up evaluation showed marked capsular adhesions, fibrocellular crescents and glomerular hyalinisation and sclerosis at the initial biopsy. Lawler believed that focal global sclerosis or capsular crescents adversely affected the course of the disease.

Hypertension[7] was present in 23% of the patients. It is a bad prognostic sign as 44% of those with hypertension developed chronic renal failure. Their histological lesions were also severe with 97% having associated glomerulosclerosis and 22% associated crescents.

The conclusion from our study was that IgA nephritis is not always a benign disease. It has a cumulative renal survival of 82% after 8 years. The data showed that renal deterioration in IgA nephritis is generally slowly progressive over a long period of time (average 7.7 years). The single most important intercurrent cause for accelerated deterioration to end stage renal failure (average 3.3 years) seems to be uncontrolled hypertension. The unfavourable long-term prognostic indices are proteinuria of more than 1 gm a day, hypertension, glomerulosclerosis exceeding 20%, presence of crescents, medial hyperplasia of blood vessels on renal biopsy. It would appear that control of hypertension is of paramount importance in preventing or delaying the onset of end stage renal failure.

In 1985 we studied 151 patients with biopsy proven IgA nephritis [IgAN]. After a mean follow up period of 5 years, 84% had stable renal function, 5% had renal impairment and 11% progressed to end stage renal failure [ESRF]. The unfavourable prognostic indices were proteinuria > 1 gm/day, hypertension, crescents on renal biopsy, glomerulosclerosis and medial hyperplasia of blood vessels. The cumulative renal survival was 89% at 5 years. Fifteen years later, in 2000, with data from the Singapore Renal Registry it was ascertained that 53 patients (35%) had developed ESRF. Using multivariate analysis by the Cox regression model, it was found that serum creatinine, protein selectivity, segmental glomerulosclerosis, crescents and medial hyperplasia were significant predictors of progression. It was also shown that the presence of low molecular weight (LMW) proteinuria is another index of poor prognosis. Cumulative renal survival of the 151 patients was 65% at 20 years [Woo KT *et al.*, IgA nephropathy: effect of clinical indices, ACEI/ATRA therapy and ACE gene polymorphism on disease progression. Nephrology, 2002,7:S166–S172].

In the recent Oxford Classification of IgA Nephropathy: rationale, clinopathological correlations and classification [A working group of the International IgA nephropathy Network and the Renal Pathology Society: Daniel C. Cattran *et al.*, Kidney International, 2009, 76; 534–556] the four independent histopathological features with reproducibility and predictive power were Mesangial cell hypercellularity, Segmental sclerosis or adhesion, Endocapillary hypercellularity* and Interstitial fibrosis/tubular atrophy. It was stated that multivariate analysis remains to be clarified which of these 4 lesions could predict effectiveness of treatment with RAS blockers and immunosuppressives. Endocapillary hypercellularity* based on univariate analysis, suggested responsiveness to immunosuppressants.

How Does Glomerulonephritis Come About?

Most forms of nephritis arise because of abnormal immunological mechanisms in the body. The immunological system defends our body against invasion by foreign organisms (bacteria, viruses, fungi, parasites). It does so by mobilising a certain group of white corpuscles called lymphocytes to attack and destroy the foreign organism. It can also cause these lymphocytes to produce antibodies which are directed against the foreign organism. To be specific, the antibodies are directed against the antigen on the surface of the organism. During this warfare, the antibody reacts with the antigen to form clumps or complexes (antigen-antibody complexes) and these circulate in the bloodstream.

As the blood containing these immune complexes passes through the body, the complexes are deposited in the glomeruli of the kidneys since the glomeruli filter all our blood. In the glomeruli an inflammatory reaction is triggered off and spreads to other glomerulus. This inflammation of the glomerulus leads to leakage of red blood cells and protein into the urine, hence explaining the presence of red blood cells and protein as an abnormal finding in patients suffering from glomerulonephritis. If the inflammatory reaction is temporary then the damage is negligible and healing occurs rapidly. If the inflammation continues, sometimes for years, more and more glomeruli become damaged. With time, the glomeruli die and appear as sclerosis in a renal biopsy. When sclerosis becomes severe (diffuse scierosing GN) renal failure occurs.

The above is a relatively simplistic explanation for what is in fact a very complexly orchestrated chain of inflammatory reactions which take place. In addition to the lymphocytes, other types of white corpuscles, platelets, clotting factors which induce a low grade intravascular coagulation and other forms of acute and chronic phase reactants including cytokines also take part in the inflammation.

We do not know why some people develop glomerulonephritis and others do not or why some have a mild disease while others develop renal failure. Research is being conducted here and abroad. One of the beliefs is that certain individuals have the ability to clear these antigen antibody complexes very rapidly and thus avoid nephritis. Others may have some deficiency in one or several aspects of the immune system resulting in poor clearance of the complexes and therefore develop nephritis.

Renal Biopsy

This is a procedure which enables the kidney specialist to obtain a sample of kidney tissue in order to determine the particular type of kidney disease the patient has. The patient is admitted into hospital. After the procedure he stays overnight and if there is no blood in the urine the next day the patient can be discharged.

For renal biopsy, the position of the kidney is first localised by means of intravenous pyelogram or ultrasound examination of the kidney. The patient lies prone on his or her abdomen and the position of the kidney is marked on the back. Local anaesthetic is administered to the skin down to the surface of the kidney. The biopsy needle is then introduced into the kidney and a core of kidney tissue taken out, usually about 1 mm wide and 10 to 20 mm long. The patient should feel no pain and after the biopsy he rests in bed until the next day. He is encouraged to drink about 3 litres of fluid to wash out the blood leaking from the puncture wound in the kidney. A few patients may pass blood in the urine but this will usually go off.

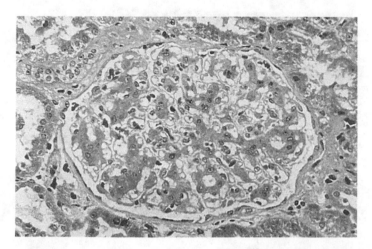

Fig. 4.3 IgA nephropathy. Increase in mesangial matrix and cells are seen. HE Stain original magnification 300X

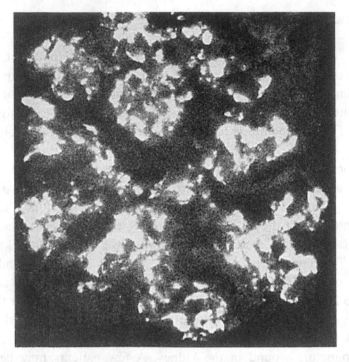

Fig. 4.4   IgA nephropathy. Deposits of IgA are seen on immunofluorescence. Original magnification 300X

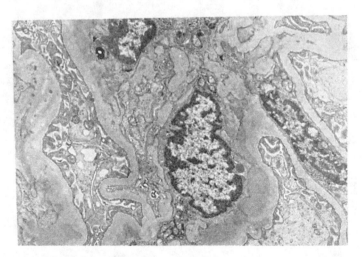

Fig. 4.5   IgA nephropathy. Electron dense deposits are present in the mesangium. Electron micrograph original magnification 13000X

The sample of kidney tissue is sent for light microscopy, immunofluorescence and electron microscopic examination. This will give a clue to the nature, type and severity of the kidney disease. It will therefore be of use for prognosis and planning of management of the renal disease.

What investigations are usually performed on a patient who is suspected of having Glomerulonephritis?

A fresh specimen of urine is examined for protein, red cells and casts. Nowadays, by using a phase contrast microscope, the type of red cells in the urine can be further characterised as to their site of origin. Red cells resulting from glomerulonephritis are usually distorted (dysmorphic) whereas those arising from some other source of non-glomerular bleeding (stone, tumour) are usually of normal shape (isomorphic).

Blood samples are taken to determine the level of creatinine to assess renal function. A 24-hour urine collection is usually requested for the estimation of creatinine clearance and protein loss in the urine. Further samples of blood are sent to exclude or confirm the diagnosis of various forms of kidney diseases, especially SLE causing lupus nephritis.

If it is decided after the above tests that the patient will require a renal biopsy then an intravenous pyelogram may be ordered prior to the renal biopsy. If the biopsy is to be performed under ultrasound guidance an IVP is usually not necessary.

Significance of Repeatedly Passing Blood in the Urine (Visible Blood or Gross Haematuria)

The repeated passing of red or brown urine, an indication of the presence of blood in the urine especially if associated with fever or sore throat or other respiratory tract infection, is likely to be a symptom of glomerulonephritis. Further examination may reveal that the patient is also passing protein in the urine. A kidney biopsy in these patients will usually show a particular type of glomerulonephritis called IgA nephritis. IgA means immunoglobulin A. The disease is so named because when the kidney biopsy specimen is examined under a special immunofluorescent technique, it stains strongly for IgA.

There are of course other causes for passing grossly blood-stained urine, one of which is a condition called stress haematuria. This occurs in some people after they have engaged in heavy exercise or after jogging for a few kilometres. The condition is due to trauma of blood vessels in the urinary bladder. The best way to confirm the diagnosis is to pass a tube called a cystoscope into the bladder and identify the source of the bleeding. Sometimes kidney stones or even a tumour in the bladder can also cause gross bleeding into the urine on exertion. If in doubt it is always wise to have an IVP to exclude a stone and a cystoscopy to exclude a tumour.

Significance of finding a small amount of blood and protein in the urine on routine medical examination

The medical term for this is asymptomatic haematuria and proteinuria. Many forms of glomerulonephritis present in this way with the patient well and healthy with absolutely no symptoms. In fact some patients start to experience symptoms after they have been told they have kidney disease. They become neurotic and require a lot of reassurance that this type of kidney condition does not cause backache.

Asymptomatic haematuria is usually discovered following pre-employment or life assurance screening. Such patients will need a microscopic examination of the urine, blood tests and 24-hour urine collection for creatinine clearance and protein estimation. Those found to have more severe abnormalities will require a renal biopsy. In the Singapore context, the majority of these patients will have IgA nephritis.

We shall first deal with those who have gross bleeding in the urine. If there is no accompanying loss of protein in the urine the outlook is good, though the presence of blood in the urine is alarming. The bleeding will clear up after one to two days but may return whenever the patient has fever or a sore throat. If he has a throat infection, he may require antibiotics. He should drink plenty of fluids to dilute the blood in the urine so that it can pass out easily without clotting and causing a clot colic. He should, of course, try to rest and refrain from heavy work. With the passage of years the episodes of bleeding gradually disappear.

In patients with more than 1 gm of protein loss in the urine the disease is more severe whether it is in a patient with gross bleeding or in one who has asymptomatic haematuria and proteinuria. A renal biopsy will usually show some scars and with time some will develop hypertension and renal failure.

It is a good policy to remind patients even with mild urinary abnormalities to see their general practitioner once a year to have the urine, serum creatinine and urinary protein as well as blood pressure checked as there will always be some patients with mild urinary abnormalities who may develop hypertension or have progression of their disease with worsening proteinuria. In such cases it is important that their blood pressure be controlled and renal biopsy performed to assess the renal status.

REFERENCES

1. Glassock RJ, Adler SG, Ward HJ, Cohen AH. Primary Glomerular Diseases. In: Brenner BM, Rector FC (eds.), The Kidney. Philadelphia: WB Saunders Company, 1991, 1182–1279.
2. Potter EV, Lipschultz SA, Abidh S *et al*. Twelve to seventeen year follow up of patients with poststreptococcal acute glomerulonephritis in Trinidad. *N Engl J Med* 1982, **307**:725–729.
3. Drachman R, Aladjem M, Vardy PA. Natural History of an acute glomerulonephritis epidemic in children: An 11 to 12 year follow up. *Israel J Med Sci* 1982, **18**:603–607.

4. Singhal PC, Malik GH, Narayan G, Khan AS, Bhusnurmath S, Datta BN, Chugh KS. Prognosis of Post-Streptococcal Glomerulonephritis: Chandigarh Study. *Ann Acad Med* Singapore 1982, **11**:36–41.

5. Kincaid-Smith P. Severe acute oliguric renal failure in glomerular and vascular disease. In: Kincaid-Smith P. The Kidney: A clinico-pathological study. Oxford: Blackwell Scientific Publications, 1975, 259–275.

6. Woo KT, Edmondson RPS, Wu AYT, Chiang GSC, Pwee HS, Lim CH. The Natural History of IgA Nephritis in Singapore. *Clin Nephrol* 1986, **25**:15–21.

7. Woo KT, Wong KS, Lau YK, GSC Chiang, CH Lim. Hypertension in IgA Nephropathy. *Ann Acad Med*, Singapore, 1988, **17**:583–588.

8. Woo KT, Lau YK, Choong HL, Zhao Y, Tan HB, Cheung WW, Yap HK, Chiang GSC. IgA nephropathy: effect of clinical indices, ACEI/ATRA therapy and ACE gene polymorphism on disease progression. *Nephrology*, 2002, **7**, S166–S172.

9. Woo KT, Glassock R, Lai KN. IgA nephropathy: Discovery of a distinct Glomerular disorder. Chap1 in: Monograph on IgA Nephropathy". Lai KN (Ed.), World Scientific Publication, Singapore; 2009, pg 1–7.

10. Woo KT, Chan CM, Chin YM, Choong HL, Tan HK, Foo Marjorie, Anantharaman Vathsala, Lee SL Grace, Chiang SC Gilbert, Tan PH, Lim CH, Tan CC, Lee JC Evan, Tan HB, Fook-Chong Stephanie, Lau YK and Wong KS. Global Evolutionary Trend of the Prevalence of Primary Glomerulonephritis over the past three decades. *Nephron Clinical Practice*, 2010, 116:c337–c346.

11. Woo KT, Chan CM, Chin YM, Choong HL, Tan HK, Marjorie Foo, Lee SL Grace, Anantharaman Vathsala, Lim CH, Tan CC, Lee JC Evan, Chiang SC Gilbert, Tan Ph, Tan HB, Fook-Chong Stephanie and Wong KS. Changing Pattern of Primary Glomerulonephritis in Singapore and Other Countries over the past three decades. *Clinical Nephrology*, 2010, 74(5):372–383.

CHAPTER 5

Nephrotic Syndrome

Nephrotic Syndrome is a clinical entity of multiple causes characterised by increased glomerular permeability manifested by massive proteinuria of more than 3 gm per day associated with oedema and hypoalbuminaemia of less than 30 gm. Very often, there is also associated hypercholesterolaemia and hypertriglyceridaemia and lipiduria. Any glomerular lesion may be associated, at least temporarily, with heavy proteinuria in the nephrotic range.

Table 5.1 shows the distribution of the histopathologial profile of the nephrotic syndrome over the past 3 decades. In the 1st decade, Mesangial Proliferative GN formed 33% of all primary nephrotic syndrome with Minimal Change (18%), FGS (14%), FSGS (10%) and Membranous GN (8%). In the 2nd and 3rd decade, Minimal Change Nephrotic Syndrome was the commonest GN compared to the 1st decade; 29% for the 2nd and 30% for the 3rd decade versus 18% in the 1st decade ($p < 0.0003$). Mesangial Proliferative GN in the 2nd and 3rd decade had also decreased significantly compared to the 1st decade, 33% in the 1st decade, 15% and 8% in the 2nd and 3rd decade ($p < 0.000001$).

However there was an increase in FSGS in the 3rd decade compared to the 1st and 2nd decade (13% in the 3rd decade versus 7% and 10% in the 1st and 2nd decade ($p < 0.05$). Similarly for Membranous GN there was also a significant increase in the 3rd decade compared to the 1st and 2nd decade (19% in the 3rd decade versus 8% and 12% in the 1st and 2nd decade) ($p < 0.0001$).

In many Western countries, Membranous GN is the commonest GN, accounting for about 35%. In Asian countries, Mesangial

Table 5.1   Nephrotic Syndrome: Histological Presentation Over 3 Decades

Histology	1st Decade [1976–1989]	2nd Decade [1990–1997]	3rd Decade [1998–2008]	p (χ^2) D1 vs D2 vs D3	p (χ^2) D2 vs D3
1 Minimal Change	65 (18%)	68 (29%)	107 (30%)	<0.0003	0.78
2 Focal Global Sclerosis	53 (14%)	45 (19%)	15 (4%)	<0.000001	<0.000001
3 Mesangial Proliferative Glomerulonephritis	120 (33%)	35 (15%)	29 (8%)	<0.000001	<0.02
4 IgA Nephritis	51 (14%)	40 (17%)	86 (24%)	<0.002	<0.05
5 Focal & Segmental Glomerulosclerosis (FSGS)	35 (10%)	16 (7%)	46 (13%)	<0.05	<0.03
6 Membranous Glomerulonephritis	30 (8%)	29 (12%)	68 (19%)	<0.0001	<0.04
7 Crescenteric Glomerulonephritis	2 (1%)	1 (<1%)	1 (<1%)	0.85	0.67
8 Others	7 (2%)	4 (1%)	5 (2%)	0.86	0.1
Total	363 (100%)	238 (100%)	357 (100%)		

Proliferative GN is the commonest (as was Singapore before the 1990's). The high incidence of Mesangial Proliferative GN was attributed to infection in these countries. IgA nephritis with Mesangial Proliferative GN is an uncommon cause of the Nephrotic Syndrome, accounting for about 25% of Nephrotics. However we are now seeing more patients with Minimal Change and Focal Global Sclerosis not responding to Steroids or Prednisolone, meaning that they have Focal and Segmental Glomerulosclerosis (FSGS) which is less responsive to therapy. What this implies is that the true incidence of FSGS is not at 7% but is probably closer to 13% or more. In other words, there is a rising incidence of FSGS in keeping with the incidence in other countries.[1] The incidence of Membranous GN has increased to 19%. Mesangio Capillary GN (MCGN) and Crescenteric GN are uncommon. About 20 years ago MCGN was common in the West and it was related to infection, now it is uncommon.

The epidemiology of GN follows a racial and geographical distribution which is influenced by the environment (infection) and the foodstuff we ingest (allergens) or the air we breathe in which contains many types of industrial and other allergens.

1. MINIMAL CHANGE DISEASE

This is referred to as Lipoid Nephrosis. The renal biopsy shows normal findings on light microscopy (LM) (Fig. 5.1), but there is foot process fusion on electron microscopy (EM) (Fig. 5.2). Immunofluorescence (IMF) studies may show IgE but usually there is no immunoglobulin staining on IMF.

Young children are especially affected with a peak from 2 to 4 years. Minimal Change accounts for 60 to 70% of all idiopathic nephrotic syndrome in children and 10 to 30% in adults. In Singapore this is also the commonest lesion in adults (30%). Hypertension and renal impairment are uncommon complications and microscopic haematuria is rare. Shaloub[2] considers this disease a disorder in T cell function with abnormal lymphokine

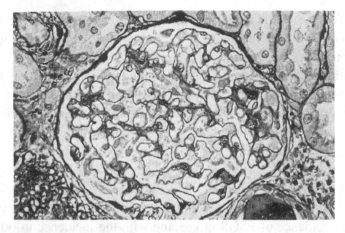

Fig. 5.1   Minimal lesion. The glomerulus is normal on light microscopy. PAS Stain original magnification 400×

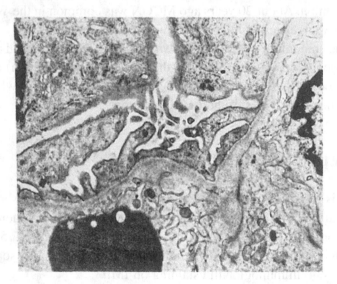

Fig. 5.2   Fusion of foot processes is seen along the glomerular basement membrane. Electron micrography original magnification 13000×

production. Focal Global Sclerosis (FGS) accounts for only 4% of Nephrotics in adults in Singapore. Clinically FGS behaves like Minimal Change, is steroid responsive and has a good prognosis.

Treatment consists of a three months' course of prednisolone. In those who fail to respond or where they have frequent relapses, cyclophosphamide for three months may induce long lasting remissions. Cyclosporine A [CyA] is a good alternative to cyclophosphamide especially among the younger patients as it does not have the side effect of sterility among males or infertility among females unlike cyclophosphamide. It can be given in a dose of 5 mg/kg BW for 3 months, then reduce to 4 mg /kg BW at 4th month, then at 3 mg at 5th month and at 2 mg at 6th month and maintain for a year. For those patients who relapse or if proteinuria increases on decreasing the dose of CyA the dose of CyA will have to be increased and these patients may have to continue CyA at 2 mg/kg BW until 2 years [Woo KT *et al*., Case reports of low dose Cyclosporine A therapy in Adult Minimal Change Nephrotic Syndrome, Ann Acad Med, Singapore, 2001, **30**(4):430–435]. CyA is useful for patients who are steroid dependent or who are frequent relapsers. However compared to Cyclophosphamide it is expensive. CyA is also useful for pregnant women with Nephrotic Syndrome and they can take CyA safely throughout pregnancy.

This is a disease with a good prognosis even though the relapse rates are high. Depending on a patient's response to prednisolone and his frequency of relapses various categories have been described. Thirty eight per cent are primary responders, non-relapsers. If a patient has less than 2 relapses in the first 6 months of the initial response he is a primary responder, infrequent relapser (19%). If he had 2 or more relapses in 6 months he is a primary responder, frequent relapser (42%). Five per cent of patients do not respond to steroids following an initial response (secondary non-responder).[3]

If there is no response to initial treatment but response after completion of treatment the patient is said to be a primary non-responder, late responder (7%). A continuing non-responder shows no response at any time (30% of primary non-responders). Spontaneous remission without treatment refers to the group of spontaneous responders. Relapse may occur after treatment is withdrawn or during reduction of steroids (steroid dependent responder).

White[4] reported lasting remission in 7% and Habib[5] in 18% of patients. Arneil[6] found that 40% were free of disease 5 to 10 years after a single course with no relapse. The frequency of relapse decreases after 10 years.

In a study among adults, Cameron[7] showed that 18% responded with early loss of proteinuria but 70% of them relapsed, 63% repeatedly. A small number, after repeated relapse and remission acquired steroid unresponsiveness. They displayed focal glomerulosclerosis on renal biopsy. The use of cytotoxics is recommended in this group. Fifty to 60% of adults with Minimal Lesion will remit for 5 years or more. Those who fail to respond to Cyclophosphamide can be given a course of Cyclosporine A and if they do not respond to CyA then we should consider the use of Mycophenolate Mofetil [MMF].

Of 49 adults followed up by Cameron for 19 years, 9 had died but only one from uraemia and 3 from complications of treatment. Twenty-nine of the original 49 were well and on no treatment. In Habib's series,[8] 14 of 209 followed up from 1 to 10 years had died, only 3 from CRF 5 to 8 years from onset (steroid resistant). The survival rates in Cameron's series was 98% at 5 years and 97% at 10 years.

A patient with Minimal Lesion has an excellent long-term prognosis if he has minimal glomerular lesion on light microscopy, foot process fusion on electron microscopy, absence of immunoglobulins on immunofluorescence (IMF), and complete remission following a course of steroids. Even so, multiple relapses will still occur.

2. FOCAL & SEGMENTAL GLOMERULOSCLEROSIS (FSGS) (FIG. 5.3)

Rich in 1957 first described focal sclerosis of the glomeruli especially at the juxtamedullary zones of the cortex. The disease is due

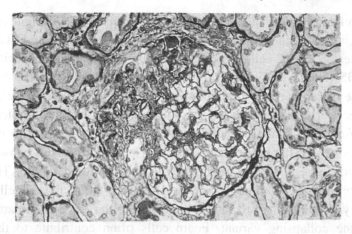

Fig. 5.3 Focal segmental sclerosis. A segment of the glomerulus is sclerotic. PAS Stain original magnification 300×

to an Abnormal T cell function with lymphokine inducing a proteinuric factor. The frequent recurrence of this disease is caused by a circulating factor secreted by an abnormal clone of T cells causing podocyte injury. This is thought to be a circulating factor bound to protein A with molecular weight of 50 kDalton. The permeability factor induces redistribution and loss of nephrin as well as reduced expression of podocin giving rise to massive proteinuria.

There is a slight preponderance of males with a peak at 20 to 30 years accounting for 10 to 20% of idiopathic nephrotic syndrome. The incidence of FSGS is rising in most countries.[1] In Singapore it is now about 15%.

About 70–90% present as the Nephrotic Syndrome; hypertension may be an associated feature.

Light microscopy shows segmental hyaline sclerosis with an increase in mesangial matrix, spreading from the hilus with no proliferation or necrosis. There is subsequent progression to global sclerosis. EM shows foot process fusion with subendothelial and mesangial electron dense deposits and sclerosis. IMF shows IgM and C3 staining.

Based on the character and glomerular distribution of lesions, 5 major structural variants of FSGS have been recognised that

correlate with the outcome and may be caused by different etiologies and pathogenic mechanisms. The 5 are: collapsing FSGS,
tip lesion FSGS, cellular FSGS, perihilar FSGS and non specific
FSGS (NOS). (i) Collapsing FSGS has segmental to global collapse of capillaries with obliteration of lumen. Visceral epithelial
cells overlying the collapsed segments have resorption droplets.
HIV and heroin abusers have this type as do those cases of recurrent disease after renal transplant. (ii) The tip variant has consolidation of segments contiguous with the proximal tubule. The
lesion may be sclerotic or cellular. However, the increased cellularity is within the tuft unlike the extracapillary hypercellularity
of the collapsing variant. Foam cells often contribute to this
hypercellularity. (iii) The Cellular Variant as defined by D'Agati
has lesions resembling the cellular lesion for the tip variant but
they are distributed throughout the glomerular tuft. (iv) The perihilar lesion is characterised by lesions in the perihilar accompanied often by hyalinosis. (V) NOS variant is one which does not
fit into any of the other 4 variants.

The majority of patients with this form of nephritis experience
a progressive decline in GFR; hypertension and persistent proteinuria. Initially patients present with asymptomatic proteinuria
but often they ultimately become nephrotic. Initial studies reported
little benefit with treatment. Nowadays with treatment, response
range from 30% to 50% (include partial response). High dose
Prednisolone (1 mg/kg BW a day) for first 2 months, then 30 mg
for 3rd month and thereafter reduce gradually to 10 mg and maintain till end of 6 months. Those who do not respond to prednisolone should have Cyclosphosphamide at 2 mg/kg BW a
day together with Prednisolone (30 mg/day) for 3 months, then
reduce and maintain for another 3 months. In those who fail
Cyclophosphamide they could be given Cyclosporine A at
5 mg/kg BW a day for 3 months, than 4 mg at 4th month, then
3 mg at 5th month and 2 mg at 6th month and maintain for 1 year.
For those who fail to respond to CyA, one would have to consider
the use of Mycophenolate Mofetil [MMF] in a dose of 0.5 gm
twice daily to 1 gm twice daily for 6 months. Be careful of

infections, as patients on MMF are more prone to sepsis. The studies of MMF in FSGS have the same shortcomings as those in the Minimal Change Disease trials, being small, uncontrolled and using multiple immunosuppressives at the same time [Alice S Appel and Gerald B Appel, An update on the use of MMF in lupus nephritis and other primary glomerular diseases, Nature Clinical Practice Nephrology, 2009 (5)3:132–142]. There may be a potential role for Tacrolimus [FK 506] at a dose of 0.1 to 0.2 mg/kg BW a day but again the evidence is still inconclusive.

The 5-year and 10-year survival according to Cameron's series[7] are 70% and 50% respectively. The presence of nephrotic syndrome affects the prognosis. Beaufils[9] reported a 90% 10-year survival in non-nephrotic patients and a 45% survival in those who were nephrotic.

Rydel *et al.*[10] reported a renal survival at 10 years for 100% of responders, 39% for non-responders and 47% for untreated nephrotics while Banfi[11] reported survival of 98% for responders and 30% for non-responders.

Thirty per cent of renal allografts in patients with FSGS as the original disease experience a recurrence of the disease. Pregnant patients with FSGS do poorly as there is a high incidence of pre-eclampsia and renal impairment.

Among children with this disease, 30 to 40% respond to steroids. If FSGS develops later on a background of Minimal Change Lesion, patients remain steroid responsive. However if FSGS develops on a background of Mesangial Proliferative Lesion, the prognosis is poorer.

After a renal transplantation, proteinuria will herald the development of recurrent FSGS. If proteinuria exceeds 2 gm/day, plasmapheresis should be commenced, 2 to 3 exchanges a week for 2 weeks, followed by 1 to 2 per week. If proteinuria persists, plasmapheresis will have to be continued up to even 6 months or more but at reduced frequency, once a week or fortnitely. Administer high dose ARB as well as statins. If there is no response to plasmapheresis, one would have to consider the use of Rituximab which is an anti-tumour necrosis factor alpha agent.

This is given in a dose of 375 mg/m^2 every week for 4 weeks to 1 gm given 2 weeks apart, repeated at 6 months [Claudio Ponticelli, Recurrence of FSGS after renal transplantation, Nephrol and Dial Transplant, 2010, 25: 25–31].

There have been recent reports of **Anabolic Steroid Abuse leading to FSGS** [Herlitz LC *et al*., Development of FSGS after anabolic steroid abuse. *J Amer Soc Nephrol* 2010, **21**:163–172]. Anabolic steroid abuse is known to have adverse effects on the endocrine system including testicular atrophy, decreased fertility, gynecomastia, abnormal blood lipids, hepatotoxicity, neuropsychiatric disorders. In addition a report of 10 patients (Nine body builders and one strongman) with renal biopsy of FSGS in 9 and 1 with glomerulopathy, presenting as proteinuria and renal impairment, all with history of long term anabolic abuse, with follow up duration of 2.2 years. They were treated with ARB , 1 progressed to ESRF while the others improved. All had stopped steroid abuse. However, 1 patient resumed body building and steroid abuse again and the condition recurred, hence this relapse provided proof of the etiology. The etiology here is likely to be multifactorial, involving overworked kidneys and raised BMI and resulting glomerular hyperfiltration.

Obesity Related Renal Damage

Obesity has been recognised as a risk factor for development of ESRF. The mechanism invoked is related to **glomerular hyperfiltration** as in the world wide setting of type 2 diabetes. The eGFR of obese patients is higher and is associated with proteinuria and **secondary FSGS**. Studies have shown that a protein load markedly increases GFR and continuous intake of a high protein diet can exacerbate glomerular hyperfiltration and is harmful in obesity related kidney disease. Dietary protein alone however does not explain fully obesity related elevation of GFR and proteinuria. Morales [Morales E *et al*., *Amer J Kid Disease* 2003, **41**: 319–327] reported a prospective randomised study in overweight or obese patients with proteinuria >1gm/day, assigned to follow a low calorie diet or to maintain their usual diet for 5 months. The low calorie diet group was given an energy reduction of 500 kcal with respect to their usual diet with a protein content of 1–1.2 kg/day. After 5 months, they had lost $4.1 \pm 3\%$ of their baseline weight, and mean body mass index decreased from 33 ± 3.5 to 31.6 ± 3.2 kg/m^2. Despite this rather modest weight loss and even though protein intake were unchanged, mean proteinuria showed a significant decrease from 2.8 ± 1.4 to 1.9 ± 1.4 g/day, equivalent to a $31.2 \pm 37\%$ reduction in baseline values. But this reduction in proteinuria was achieved only after a month of hypocaloric diet, when patients had lost only $2.8 \pm 2.1\%$ of the baseline weight. The pathophysiologic mechanisms responsible for such early influences warrant further investigations.

Recent studies have shown that lower adiponectin and higher fetuin A serum levels are associated with obesity, the metabolic syndrome and albuminuria [Ix JH *et al.*, Mechanisms linking obesity, CKD, and liver disease; the roles of fetuin A, adiponectin and AMPK. J Amer Soc of Nephrol, 2010, **21**:406–412]. Both proteins could orchestrate the cross talk among fat, kidney and liver. Inhibition of the energy sensor 5′-AMP-activated protein kinase (AMPK) mainly through lack of adiponectin stimulation could play a harmful role for renal and liver parenchyma. Caloric restriction would induce a decline in serum fetuin A, an increase in adiponectin levels and a stimulation of AMPK. The effects of dietary modifications on the secretion of oxidised polyunsaturated fatty acids and on the enhanced aldosterone signalling that frequently accompanies obesity are other fields of study relevant to solving the problem of the epidemic of obesity related renal disease.

REFERENCE

Praga M and Morales E. Obesity related renal damage: changing diet to avoid progression. *Kidney Int* 2010, **78**:633–635.

3. MESANGIAL PROLIFERATIVE GLOMERULONEPHRITIS (FIG. 5.4)

Histologically there is increase in mesangial cells and matrix with no capillary wall thickening. IMF is negative staining in the majority (44%) whilst others have shown IgM, IgA either predominantly or with other Ig in equal or lesser strength. In those with negative IMF the EM also show no electron dense deposits (EDD).

It occurs in about 8% of idiopathic nephrotic syndrome among adults in Singapore but appears to be a much less common cause of nephrotic syndrome in Western countries. IgA nephritis accounts for about 24% of nephrotic syndrome seen in Singapore and is therefore a common cause of nephrotic syndrome.

The long-term evolution of this type of nephritis is not well understood. This discussion excludes IgA nephritis which has been dealt with earlier but it includes IgM nephropathy, IgG and the IMF negative group.

Patients with this lesion who become nephrotic and develop focal and segmental sclerosis have a higher incidence of developing

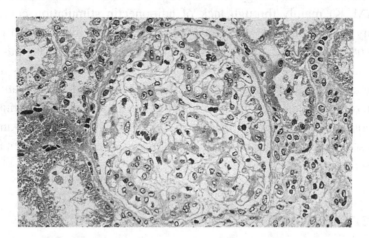

Fig. 5.4 Mesangial proliferative glomerulonephritis. The glomerulus shows an increase in mesangial matrix and cells. HE Stain original magnification 300×

chronic renal failure (CRF). Only 30% of those with nephrotic syndrome experience complete remissions with steroid. They are usually the ones with mild mesangial proliferation with no focal and segmental sclerosis.

In those patients therefore who have mild proliferation of the mesangium with no evidence of focal and segmental sclerosis and negative immunoglobulin staining on IMF, a trial of steroid therapy should be offered as they have a good chance of achieving remission. Habib[8] in fact considered such patients as part of the spectrum of Minimal Change GN. Waldher[12] reported that more than 50% of patients with Mesangial Proliferative GN were steroid resistant, 70% with associated focal and segmental sclerosis. There is a need for controlled therapeutic trials in patients with this form of nephritis. In our experience those with selective proteinuria tend to respond to steroids and failing that cyclophosphamide.

Those who fail cyclophosphamide can be offerred Cyclosporine A or Mycophenolate Mofetil [MMF] as for patients with Minimal Change Disease [MCD].

4. MEMBRANOUS GLOMERULONEPHRITIS (FIGS. 5.5 AND 5.6)

Patients with Membranous Glomerulonephritis usually present as Nephrotic Syndrome. Characteristically there is thickening of glomerular capillary wall on LM. EM shows electron dense deposits (EDD) in a subepithelial location. IMF shows linear "granular" IgG. Majority of patients are above 40 years of age at diagnosis with a peak around 40 to 50 years. Males are more commonly affected than females. This used to be the most common form of GN in the West constiutiong 35% of all nephrotic syndrome but in Singapore it is present in about 19% of all idiopathic nephrotic syndrome.

Hypertension and azotaemia are late features of the disease. Microscopic haematuria is common but gross haematuria is a rare

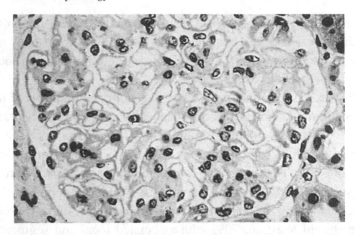

Fig. 5.5   Membranous glomerulonephritis. There is diffuse thickening of the glomerular basement membrane. HE Stain original magnification 500×

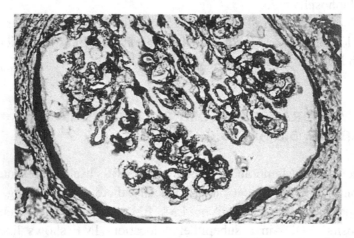

Fig. 5.6   Membranous glomerulonephritis. Well formed spikes are seen along the glomerular basement membrane using the silver stain. PAAg-MT Stain original magnification 400×

feature. Renal vein thrombosis is secondary to the glomerulopathy rather than the cause of it.

This disease runs an indolent and slowly progressive course with remissions and exacerbations of the nephrotic syndrome.

Children have a better prognosis with less than 5% CRF after 5 years and a 90% 10 year survival. Adults however have a less benign course; 25% achieve spontaneous remission with another 25% spontaneous partial remission (less than 2 gm proteinuria). Cameron's series[13] had a 75% 5-year and 50% 10-year survival. Even patients with partial remission have a better outlook than those who have no response at all.

In a patient with Membranous GN who develops progressive renal failure within a few months, the following should be considered:

1. Hypersensitivity interstitial nephritis
2. Superimposed crescents
3. Renal vein thrombosis
4. Profound hypovolaemia from proteinuria

A controlled trial with high dose alternate-day prednisolone in the USA has reported a reduction in proteinuria and progression of CRF.[14] However, if there is already abnormal GFR, steroid therapy is not of much use. We would offer a 3 months course of prednisolone therapy and failing that cyclophosphamide. There is a potential role for other agents like Chlorambucil (0.15–0.2 mg/kg BW/day),[23] Cyclosporine A (5 mg/kg BW/day), Mycophenolate Mofetil [MMF] (0.5 gm twice daily to 1 gm twice daily) and FK 506 (0.1–0.2 mg/kg BW/day up to 1 year).[24]

Patients with membranous GN can be graded based on the degree of Proteinuria: <3 gm/day, 3–6 gm/day and >6 gm/day. Those with <3 gm/day may be put on supportive therapy with ACEI/ARB and statins. Those in between (3–6 gm/day) could be treated with a combination of steroids and cyclophosphamide or chlorambucil in alternate monthly pulses (Ponticelli regime) or steroids plus low dose CyA 2–4 mg/Kg BW for 6 months and maintain at 2 mg for up to 1 year. Patients with >6 gm/day Proteinuria could be given high dose CyA at 5 to 6 mg/Kg BW or MMF in a dose of 500 mg to 1000 mg twice daily for 6 months followed by a lower dose for another 6 months.

CyA has been shown to induce more complete or partial remissions in these patients. More remissions occurred with CyA therapy than with those on cytotoxics (85% versus 55%) but relapses occurred more frequently among the CyA treated patients (4!% versus 29%). CyA patients are generally treated for 1 to 2 years whereas those on cytotoxics are on for about 6 months.

Ponticelli advocates a 6 month regimen consisting of corticosteroids and alkylating agent alternating monthly. On months 1, 3 and 5 patients are given IV methylprednisolone 1 gm for 3 days followed by oral prednisolone 0.5 gm/kg BW for 27 days. On months 2, 4 and 6 chlorambucil 0.2 mg/kg BW per day is given. Ponticelli found a remission rate of 76% for treated patients compared to 36% for those on no treatment. The 10 year survival is from 60% to 92% for treated patients. Substitution of cyclophosphamide produces the same results. Oral Cyclophosphamide can be given in a dose of 2 mg/kg BW/day [Ponticelli C *et al*. Kidney Int 1995, **48**:1600–1604].

MMF has been useful in some patients in uncontrolled trials. Chan *et al*. [Chan TM *et al*., Nephrology, Carlton, 2007, **12**:576–581] in patients with TUP >3 g/day treated for 6 months [20 patients] randomized to either MMF plus prednisolone or a regimen of chlorambucil alternating monthly with prednisolone achieved remission rates of 65% with MMF suggesting that MMF in conjunction with steroids have the same efficacy as the Ponticelli regime. Azathioprine has also been tried. But in the light of popularity with MMF, azathioprine is seldom used nowadays. Sirolimus has also been tried but there were many side effects like pneumonitis, other infections and poor response with uremia and early trials have been abandoned.

Tacrolimus has been evaluated by several investigators. It is as effective as CyA and rate of complete remission greater. But relapses were frequent, occurring in about 50% of treated patients within 4 months of discontinuation of Tacrolimus.[26]

Personally, in my own practice, those patients with proteinuria <3 gm with normal serum albumin and have no edema or other symptoms, I would treat with ARB, Aliskiren (renin inhibitor) and statins. If they worsen with increasing proteinuria and lowering of serum albumin and development of edema, we would treat with a small dose of prednisolone, 15 to 20 mg a day plus CyA at a dose of 5 to 6 mg/Kg BW for 3 months. If there is no response, we can increase the dose of CyA up to 8 mg/Kg BW for another 1 to 2 months. If at the end of these 2 months there is still no response, we would reduce CyA to 4 mg and continue for another 3 months and stop CyA and gradually withdraw steroids over the next 1 to 2 months. So far, in our experience, most of the patients respond quite well to this regime. For those who respond, after 6 months we would reduce CyA to about 4 mg/Kg BW and after another 3 months maintain at about 2 mg/Kg BW for another 3 months and then stop CyA. If patients have a relapse then we increase the dose of CyA to the previous dose and continue for another 3 to 6 months. Check CyA levels and monitor serum creatinine and eGFR for CyA nephrotoxicity. For those who fail this therapy, then we go on to the next drug, using MMF in a dose of 500 mg to 1000 mg twice daily over 6 months. For those who respond after 6 months, reduce dose of MMF from 1000 mg twice daily to 500 mg twice a day or for those on 500 mg twice daily we can reduce to 250 mg twice daily and stop after another 6 months. Patients below 50 kg BW can be on 500 mg twice daily and those above 50 kg BW can be on 1000 mg twice daily. Beware of sepsis, especially pneumonia which could be lethal in the immunocompromised patient. This is the big disadvantage of using MMF. In this sense CyA is much preferred.

Rituximab is a chimeric monoclonal antibody that targets the CD20 antigen of B cells and was used for the treatment of B cell proliferative disorders. The decrease of B cells from the circulation may be rapid, after 1 dose of Rituximab, but the decrease in proteinuria may take much longer. In a small study[27] involving 8 high risk patients, given 4 weekly doses of 375 mg/m^2, mean proteinuria was decreased by 51% after 3 months and 66% after 1 year.

In another study of 15 patients[28] all failed previous immunosuppressive treatment, proteinuria 8–14 gm/day, given 1 gm

Rituximab on days 1 and 15, 27% or 4 patients had partial remission after 6 months and after 1 year, 2 (14%) patients had complete remission and 6 (43%) had partial remission. Five patients showed no response and 5 patients had progressed to ESRD.

Infusion reactions with Rituximab are often mild and manageable, more potentially fatal reactions have occurred (acute respiratory distress syndrome, bronchospasm, angioedema, shock and myocardial infarction). There are also potentially fatal mucocutaneous reactions like Steven–Johnson syndrome and toxic epidermal necrolysis. Severe infections are uncommom, 1–2%. Of great concern are rare cases of multifocal leukoencephalopathy which have been reported with the use of Rituximab.

Rituximab therefore cannot be recommended for routine use. Adequately powered, randomised controlled trials with data from prolonged follow up, rates of relapse, dosing regimens, used as monotherapy or in combination with other drugs, as well as effects on renal survival are necessary before it can be recommended.

REFERENCE

Waldman M, Austin HA, Controversies in the treatment of idiopathic membranous nephropathy. *Nature Reviews Nephrology*, 2009, 5(8): 469–479.

5. MESANGIOCAPILLARY GLOMERULONEPHRITIS (MCGN) (FIG. 5.7)

The presence of prominent increase in mesangial cellularity and their extension into peripheral capillary wall leads to the appearance of thickened and reduplicated capillary wall on LM. EM of Type I MCGN shows electron dense subendothelial deposits. In Type II MCGN or what is referred to as Dense Deposit Disease (DDD), EDD is found within the substance of the glomerular basement membrane proper. IMF of Type I shows irregular C3 in a granular distribution along the capillary walls with IgG and/or

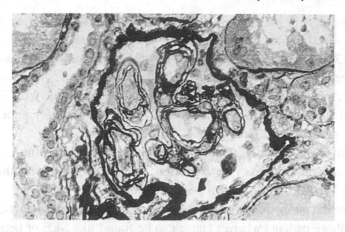

Fig. 5.7 Mesangiocapillary glomerulonephritis. A double contour glomerular basement membrane is seen. PAAg-MT Stain original magnification 500×

IgM in about 50%. In Type II MCGN only C3 is found in the mesangium.

Complement: In Type I MCGN, 70% have prolonged depression of C3. C1q and C4 may be low when C3 is low. In Type II MCGN there is persistent low C3 (persistent hypocomplementemic GN). C3Nef, a gamma-globulin that cleaves C3 is also present. The values of C1q and C4 are normal.

All age groups are involved, especially those aged 5 to 15 years. It occurs in 5 to 10% of children with the nephrotic syndrome. Fifty per cent have associated upper respiratory tract infection and 40% have high anti-streptolysin 0 titre (ASOT).

Half of patients with MCGN present as the nephrotic syndrome, 30% as asymptomatic haematuria and proteinuria, and the remaining 20% as acute nephritic syndrome. Hypertension is present in 33%. About 50% develop renal impairment. If the patient is nephrotic and crescents are present on renal biopsy the prognosis is worse. Idiopathic MCGN occurs uncommonly in Singapore.

This type of nephritis has a relentless but slowly progressive course. The bad prognostic features are low GFR, hypertension, persistent nephrotic syndrome and the presence of diffuse crescents on renal biopsy.

For Type I MCGN (Subendothelial Deposits) the 5-year and 10-year survival are 80% and 60% respectively. For Type II MCGN (Dense Deposit Disease) the respective survival rates are poorer, 60% and 45% at 5 and 10 years. Other series reported a poorer prognosis in the presence of nephrotic syndrome with 40% survival at 10 years, compared to 85% at 10 years for patients with no nephrotic syndrome.

But even in the patients with nephrotic syndrome the occasional remission has been reported. In general, however, those with Type II disease have a poorer outlook.

For the moment there is no clearly established form of treatment. For those patients where a cause can be found like SLE or hepatitis, treatment should be that of the underlying cause as for hepatitis C or for lupus nephritis or for that matter as in those with croyoglobulinemia, treatment should be that of the underlying cause. For the majority, usually treatment for the idiopathic variety is directed towards Type I MCGN as there is no treatment for Type II or DDD. For Type I MCGN, McEnery[15] reported the beneficial effects of continuous low dose prednisolone whereas Kincaid-Smith[16] reported 3-year survival of 82% using a combination regimen of cyclophosphamide, persantin and warfarin (Melbourne Cocktail) in an uncontrolled trial. We would advocate a 3 months course of prednisolone and failing that Cyclosporine A or Mycophenolate Mofetil [MMF]. Among those patients who respond to therapy, they should continue at a reduced dose for another 3 months followed by a low maintainance dose for another 6 months, total duration of 1 year therapy. In addition, patients should have maximum doses of Angiotensin Receptor Blockers [ARB], statins to control hypercholesterolaemia with BP control as well.

6. HEREDITARY NEPHRITIS AND DEAFNESS (ALPORT'S SYNDROME)

This is often discovered in childhood or young adult life. Males are affected in an autosomal dominant fashion. Females are unaffected but may sometimes present with hypertension and thrombocytopenia and anemia.

Patients have gross or recurrent microscopic haematuria which is worsened by respiratory infections. Some may have occasional loin pain.

Sensory neural deafness (high frequency sound) occurs in 30 to 50% and is usually associated with thrombocytopathia. Ocular features are also present in the form of spherophakia, lenticonus, myopia, retinitis pigmentosa and amaurosis.

Renal failure is usual before 40 years.

Pathology

Light microscopy shows endocapillary proliferation which is focal or diffuse associated with focal sclerosis and tubulo-interstitial lesions with presence of foam cells. Electron microscopy shows irregularly thickened and attenuated basement membrane with pronounced splitting and lamination of the lamina densa. The splits enclose electron-lucent areas. Immunofiuorescence studies usually show negative staining with occasional C3.

This condition is due to a disorder of basement membrane synthesis involving the X chromosome with a defect in the structural gene.

The course is one of slowly progressive renal failure.

CLINICAL ASPECTS OF THE NEPHROTIC SYNDROME

The term "Syndrome" implies "A Symptom Complex". It comprises:

1. Oedema
2. Proteinuria of 3 gm or more
3. Hypoproteinaemia, i.e. serum albumin of less than 30 gm
4. Hypercholesterolaemia is often an associated feature.

Oedema

i. The degree of oedema is proportional to the serum albumin concentration.
ii. Reduction of plasma oncotic pressure leads to a reduction in plasma volume (20 to 30%).
iii. Hypovolaemia stimulates renin which in turn causes aldosteronism with resulting Na^+ retention and K^+ excretion.
iv. When oedema fluid accumulates, the urine Na^+ may be nil (norrnal is 80 to 150 mEq/day).

Renal Function

1. The kidney excretes urea and creatinine normally but retains Na^+. There is increased excretion of K^+ and protein.
2. Blood urea alone as a test of renal function is falsely low as patients are in negative nitrogen balance.
3. Pre-renal failure may occur because of glomerular hypoperfusion.

Symptoms

1. Frothy urine accompanies proteinuria.
2. Patients complain that their legs are heavy, swollen, cold and numb.
3. They feel lethargic and tired because of negative nitrogen balance and anaemia.
4. Anorexia and diarrhoea may result from oedema of the gut.

SIGNS OF NEPHROTIC SYNDROME

1. Oedema may be present periorbitally, in the abdominal wall, genitalia, knee joints, ascites, pleural effusion, conjunctival

oedema and retinal oedema. Long standing oedema causes pale striae in the distended skin.

2. Pallor may simulate anaemia. The nephrotic facies is often characteristic.
3. Muscle wasting is due to loss of skeletal muscle. In addition, steroid therapy causes proximal myopathy.
4. Nails may show transverse white bands called Muerchke's Bands due to low serum albumin.
5. Hypertension if it is due to nephritis may augur badly for the patient as it usually indicates a more severe histological lesion. Steroids too can cause hypertension.

Infections

1. Pneumococcal peritonitis is a well-known complication of the nephrotic syndrome.
2. Patients are prone to lung and skin infections.
3. In the Nephrotic Crisis the patient presents with severe abdominal pain with vomiting and tenderness. At laparotomy sterile fluid with fibrin strands is found. The differential diagnosis for this condition includes primary peritonitis, perforated appendicitis, perforated gastric ulcer and "cramps" due to excess diuretics.

COMPLICATIONS OF NEPHROTIC SYNDROME

1. Subnutritional state.
2. Infections.
3. Clotting tendency due to increased clotting factors (V, VIII, Fibrinogen), increased platelet aggregation and low anti-thrombin III.

   This leads to spontaneous thrombosis involving veins and arteries.

4. Atheroma formation giving rise to ischaemic heart disease and renal artery stenosis and renal vein thrombosis.
5. Hypovolaemic collapse.
6. Complications of treatment, e.g. side effects of steroids and cytotoxic drugs.

CAUSES OF NEPHROTIC SYNDROME

— 80% due to glomerulonephritis
— 20% due to miscellaneous causes

1. Diabetes mellitus
2. Amyloidosis
3. Precipitating causes of renal vein thrombosis (RVT)

   i. Nephrotic syndrome (hypercoagulable state)
   ii. Renal arnyloid gives rise to thrombosis of intrarenal veins
   iii. Hypernephroma gives rise to obstruction and RVT
   iv. Trauma of renal veins
   v. Severe dehydration especially in infants suffering from gastroenteritis

   RVT is a complication of Nephrotic Syndrome and not a cause of Nephrotic Syndrome.
4. Malignancy: Hodgkin's Disease, bronchogenic carcinoma, cancer of the breast, bowel, leukaemias, myeloma
5. Infections: Hepatitis B and C, Malaria, syphilis, leprosy
6. Drugs: Trimethadione, penicillamine, phenindione, gold, mercury, bismuth, captopril [ACE inhibitors], NSAIDS.
7. Autoimmune Disease, SLE, Cryoglobulinemia, Thyrotoxicosis.
8. Congenital Nephrotic Syndrome
   Causes: Congenital syphilis, cytomegalovirus infection, mercury poisoning, maternal tuberculosis.

9. Miscellaneous: Prophylactic inoculation (smallpox, polio, tetanus), bee stings, pollen allergy.

MANAGEMENT OF NEPHROTIC SYNDROME

I. General Treatment

1. Diuretic Treatment
    These are the major agents in treatment:

    i.   Frusemide can be used alone. Increase the dose till diuresis occurs. K^+ supplements are required.
    ii. Spironolactone should be avoided if serum K^+ is high or patient has renal impairment.
    iii. Chlortride has a synergistic action with frusemide and spironolactone.

    We usually use a combination regimen of all 3 diuretics as they have synergistic actions (see chapter on Diuretics).
2. Treatment of hypertension.
3. Use Angiotensin Receptor Blockers [ARB] to reduce Glomerular Hyperfiltration Proteinuria.
4. Treatment of infections. Use the appropriate antibiotics.
5. Diet: The patient requires a high protein, low salt diet with fluid restriction.
6. Infusion of Na^+ free albumin induces diuresis but its benefit is evanescent.
7. Since these patients tend to have a hypercoagulable state it would be useful to put patients with Nephrotic syndrome on a low dose warfarin regime to prevent thrombosis.

II. Specific Treatment

1. Investigate and try to elucidate the cause of Nephrotic Syndrome and if possible remove or treat it.

2. Check through list of causes and investigate accordingly. In all patients always exclude SLE.

    Do anti-nuclear factor (ANF), anti-DNA, and serum complement. A patient with membranous glomerulonephritis should be screened for hepatitis B and C antigen and antibody.

III. Treatment with Steroids and Cytotoxic Agents

Primary Treatment to induce remission.

1. Minimal change GN and lupus nephritis respond well to a course of prednisolone starting at 60 mg or 1 mg/kg BW/day and reducing gradually over a period of 3 months. For those who fail to respond to prednisolone or who are frequent relapsers, cyclophosphamide (2 mg/kg BW) for 3 months is advocated. Those who fail cyclophosphamide can be given a course of Cyclosporine A [CyA] at 5 mg/kg BW for 3 months with reduction over the next 3 months and maintain at 2 mg/kg BW up to a year.

    Mycophenolate Mofetil [MMF] can be used for those who do not respond to CyA. MMF can be given in a dose of 0.5 to 1 gm twice daily for 3 months followed by another 3 months at a reduced dose.
2. Mild diffuse mesangial proliferative GN may respond to prednisolone, failing that try Cyclophosphamide, CyA or MMF.
3. Membranous GN may respond to a course of prednisolone for a period of 3 months, failing that try cyclophosphamide, CyA, MMF and Tacrolimus in that order.
4. Focal and Segmental Glomerulosclerosis may respond to Prednisolone or Cyclophosphamide If no response, try CyA, MMF and Tacrolimus.

5. The newer agents include Mycophenolate Mofetil (MMF) (0.5–1 gm twice daily)[25] for 3 months and Tacrolimus [FK 506] (0.1–0.2 mg/kg BW/day).[24]

IV. Persantin and Warfarin Plus Regimen (P and W + regimen)

All patients who fail to respond to Steroids and Cytotoxics should be offerred P and W + regimen which would help to retard progression to ESRF.

1. Persantin (Dipyridamole) — anti-platelet and anti-PDGF, 75 mg tds with low dose Warfarin (anti-thrombotic), 1 to 2 mg (INR <2.0).
2. Treat Hypertension
3. Angiotensin Receptor Blockers or ARBs to reduce intraglomerular Hypertension and retard progression of renal failure
4. Restricted Protein Diet (0.8 gm/kg BW) to decrease afferent arteriolar vasodilation
6. Treat raised Lipids as Cholesterol is toxic to mesangial cells and can cause renal injury.

Note: Nowadays, with the availability of newer and more potent therapy, especially with the advent of the ARBs like Losartan and Telmisartan including the use of Aliskiren, the new anti-renin agent, even if patients do not respond to immunosuppressants and require only empiric therapy, Persantin and Warfarin are seldom used as first line therapy since the ARBs can do a fairly good job of inducing a significant decrease of proteinuria though not to the extent of a complete remission which can be achieved only with steroids or other immunosuppressive drugs. However, one should be mindful that, as long and so long as a patient is in the Nephrotic State he is at great risk of developing arterial or venous thrombosis of the limbs and organs and it makes good sense to put such patients on prophylaxis with persantin and low dose warfarin.

THERAPEUTIC CONCEPTS OF PROTEINURIA AND INTRA-GLOMERULAR HYPERTENSION

Proteinuria is the hallmark of renal disease.[17] Proteinuria can also be used as a prognostic marker. In patients with glomerulonephritis, those with more than 1 gm of protein excretion per day in the urine are more likely to have glomerulosclerosis or scarring of the kidneys on renal biopsy and those exceeding 2 gms a day a higher incidence of developing renal failure on long term follow up.[18] Hitherto if was believed that proteinuria is the result of damage to the kidneys but recently, evidence suggest that the converse is also true, that proteinuria can also directly cause renal damage.

When there is excessive leakage of protein in the renal tubules, the proximal tubular cells (PTC) become overloaded with protein. Lysosomes present in the PTC when they engulf excessive proteins would swell and rupture and release injurious lysosomal enzymes which cause tubulointerstitial damage and fibrosis and with time give rise to renal failure. In the second mechanism, protein overload of the PTC also triggers the release of certain growth factors such as platelet-derived growth factor (PDGF) and transforming growth factor-beta (TGF-β) which are mitogenic to the PTC. They cause excessive production of collagen as well as interstitial cell proliferation eventually leading to fibrosis and renal failure. Finally, protein overloading of the PTC causes the activation of transcriptase genes which in turn trigger genes encoding vasoactive and inflammatory mediators, the release of these lead to vasoconstriction and inflammation of the renal tissue with injury and renal failure.[19]

Therapeutic reduction of proteinuria in kidney disease is now considered as important as the reduction of BP in hypertensive patients as both are important in the preservation of renal function. Normally the two kidneys in our body excrete less than 150 mg of protein in the urine a day. We must try to reduce proteinuria to as low a level in our patients, if possible to a level below 0.5 gm a day. One of the best strategies to protect the kidneys against damage due to proteinuria is the use of Angiotensin Receptor Blockers [ARB]. In many renal conditions associated with proteinuria there exists a phenomenon known as Glomerular Hyperfiltration (HF)[21] which induces proteinuria apart from the direct immunological effect of the glomerulonephritis (GN) which also causes renal damage with leakage of protein into the urine. HF is a condition which occurs whenever some of the glomeruli are diseased or sclerosed. The surrounding glomeruli which are normal are then subject to excessive blood flow with vasodilatation of the afferent glomerular arteriole. In the efferent glomerular arteriole there is associated Angiotensin II (ATII) mediated vasoconstriction. Therefore with increase in blood flow at the inlet and reduction of blood flow at the outlet there is excessive amount of blood in the glomeruli which is subject to HF with the result that there is raised intraglomerular (IG) blood pressure or IG HPT. IG HPT is associated initially with increase in single nephron Glomerular Filtration Rate (GFR) with leakage of protein in the urine. With time as a consequence of IG HPT there is renal damage with glomerular sclerosis and eventually renal failure. ARBs by blocking the action of ATII on the efferent glomerular arteriole will cause vasodilatation thereby reducing IG HPT and preserving renal function of the affected glomeruli.

ARB competes with the receptor for angiotensin and therefore inhibits the action of angiotensin. It is effective in the reduction of proteinuria and preservation of renal function. When using an ARB one should initially target for a 50% reduction of proteinuria with eventual reduction to <0.5 gm proteinuria a day. In other words, the dose of ARB should be increased gradually if necessary to its maximum dose for effective reduction of proteinuria. If the standard dose of an ARB is not effective, one can use a high dose ARB regime [e.g. Losartan 100 mg twice daily where the daily dose is 100 mg daily or in the case of telmisartan from 80 mg daily to 80 mg twice daily. If there is no response despite high dose therapy, Aliskiren, an anti-renin drug could be employed. Aliskiren is a new renal protective agent that inhibits renin, the rate limiting step in the renin angiotensin aldosterone system [RAAS]. In both healthy volunteers and disease states, aliskiren reduces angiotensin II levels and plasma renin activity [PRA], without stimulating compensatory increases in PRA, angiotensin I and angiotensin II as seen with ACEI and ARB. Aliskiren allows for total blockade of the renin angiotensin system and its beneficial effect is independent of BP control.[29] Aliskiren can be given in a dose of 150 mg to 300 mg daily.

RECOMMENDED PRACTICE

In the light of present evidence as well as fear of long term therapy with ACEI and ARBs causing renal fibrosis, one may consider using Alisikeren as the drug of first choice failing which one may then resort to the use of ARBs plus Aliskiren. For patients who have responded to high dose ARB therapy, it may be wiser to reduce to the standard dose of ARB and continue therapy with Aliskiren. When the proteinuria is well controlled, one could then consider removal of ARB and continue on Aliskiren alone. After another year, if there is no proteinuria and renal function is normalised one may stop Aliskiren altogether.

Salt restriction is important. For those who cannot restrict salt, 12.5 mg of hydrochlorothiazide daily can potentiate the effect of ATRA but be careful in the case of elderly patients and those with reduced eGFR as diuretics, even in small doses can worsen renal function due to shrinkage of ECF volume.

In summary, recent studies have highlighted the important contribution of filtered urinary protein to deterioration of renal function. In depth analysis of proteinuria may assess the degree of glomerular and tubular involvement and help in prognostication of an individual patient with proteinuria. One should consider not only the quantity but also the quality of the urinary protein.

This is especially so if there is presence of significant amounts of low molecular weight (LMW) proteins in the urine. In this respect, Woo *et al.*[22] reported that the presence of LMW proteins in the proteinuric SDS-PAGE patterns of patients with IgA nephritis was significantly associated with higher rates of chronic renal failure after 6 years of follow up. There was a significant correlation between the LMW patterns and tubular atrophy and tubulointerstitial lesions. This work has since been confirmed by other workers and today the presence of LMW proteinuria has been established as an adverse prognostic factor.

Caution on the use of ACEI and ARB: At this stage, based on what information we have available, many patients for years now have been prescribed ACE inhibitors and ARBs, including the newer anti-renin inhibitors. The cause for concern is that all these agents may be indirectly inducing the excessive amounts of 'blocked' renin to cause glomerular and tubular interstitial fibrosis, something long suspected of ACE inhibitor usage to explain why despite the number of patients prescribed ACEI for years, yet the number of patients eventually reaching ESRF does not seem to be abating. The same criticism could be directed to the use of ARBs. Both ACEI and ARB will induce the phenomenon of "Aldosterone Breakthrough" with deleterious consequences. This explains why patients who do well initially after a period gradually develop worsening proteinuria again with declining eGFR.

Aldosterone Escape versus Breakthrough

[Schrier RW. Editiorial. Nature Reviews Nephrology, 2010, 6:61]

Administration of large doses of aldosterone initially causes an initial decrease in urinary sodium excretion which leads to sodium retention. However, urinary sodium excretion subsequently increases to balance sodium intake before detectable edema develops. This phenomenon is referred to as "aldosterone escape" and explains why edema formation is not a feature of primary hyperaldosteronism.

"Aldosterone breakthrough" is a different phenomenon. ACEI and ARB inhibit the action of type 1 angiotensin II receptors with a resultant decrease in aldosterone. However, **since Angtensin II inhibits renin release, a large increase in plasma renin activity occurs** with the administration of either ACEI or ARB. Also after some weeks of treatment with ACEI or ARB, plasma aldosterone level returns to pretreatment level in 30 to 40% of patients. This phenomenon is termed **"aldosterone breakthrough"**. Patents who develop aldosterone breakthrough have a worse prognosis because the increased aldosterone causes inflammation with renal fibrosis and oxidant injury.

The Way Forward

Direct renin inhibition with Aliskiren, does not increase plasma renin activity [PRA] and therefore may not be associated with aldosterone breakthrough. **Direct renin inhibitors affect the enzymatic action of renin**, but not its production or interaction with the renin receptor. In other words, Drugs like Aliskiren are catalytic or catalyses renin. **Aliskiren, because it catalyses renin therefore prevents the profibrotic action of renin**. The effect of renin on the renin receptor is profibrotic [Nguyen G *et al*. J Clin Invest, 2002, **109**:1417–1427]. The newer VIT D like VDR Paricalcitriol has also been shown to be anti fibrotic. Hopefully, using Aliskiren and or Paricalcitriol may the way to counter the deleterious effects of ACEI and ARB as well as protect the cardiovascular system since Paricalcitriol has been shown to prevent calcification of the blood vessels of the heart and thereby decrease the CVS morbidity and death in patients with CKD.

Are Vitamin D Receptor Agonists (VDRa) like ACEI Without Side Effects?

Agarwal R. Kidney Int 2010, **77**:943–945

1. **VDRa inhibit RAS and reduce podocyte loss and fibrosis over and above RAS blockade**. Studies have shown that VDRa are antiproteinuric and can delay progression of renal disease.

2. **Vit D suppresses renin expression** independent of its effects on calcium metabolism as well as the volume and salt sensing mechanisms and the angiotensin II feedback regulation. The mechanism of renoprotection appears to be by protection of the podocyte and blockade of TGFα system in the glomerulus. TGFα activates interstitial fibrosis and induces epithelial to mesenchymal transition. By blocking TGFα, VDRa has the potential to abrogate tubulointerstitial fibrosis.

3. Alborzi *et al.* reported 24 patients with CKD stage 3 randomly allocated to receive 0,1, or 2 μg paricalcitriol, a VDRa, orally for 1 month and showed that those had improvement in PCR and albuminuria.

4. Szeto CC *et al.* from Hong Kong {Szeto CC *et al.* Oral calcitriol for the treatment of persistent Proteinuria in IgA nephropathy. Am J Kidney Dis 2008, 51:724–731] in a trial of 10 patients with persistent Proteinuria despite RAS blockade, given 0.5 μg calcitriol twice weekly for 12 weeks, reported a decrease of PCR from 1.98+/–0.74 to 1.48+/–0.81 ($p < 0.007$) during the first 6 weeks which persisted throughout the trial duration. There was an associated decrease in TGFα which was correlated with the Proteinuria ($r = 0.643$, $p < 0.02$).

5. Fishbane [Fishbane s *et al.* Oral paricalcitriol in the treatment of patients with CKD and proteinuria: a randomised trial. *Am J Kidney Dis* 2009, **54**:647–652] in a controlled trial of 61 patients with CKD and Proteinuria >400 mg/d, assigned to either placebo or paricalcitriol 1 μg/day over a period of 6 months. At baseline the Protein Creatinine Ratio (PCR) was 2.6 and 2.8 gm/gm creatinine in the placebo and paricalcitriol group. But at end of study it was 2.7 and 2.3 gm/gm creatinine respectively ($p < 0.04$).

6. The largest study is the Selective Vit D Receptor activator for Albuminuria Lowering (VITAL) study which tests whether

paricalcitriol persistently reduces albuminuria in 281 patients with Type 2 Diabetes randomized equally to 1 or 2 μg paricalcitriol per day or placebo. The results of this trial are yet to be published.

REFERENCES

1. Haas M, Spargo BH, Conventry S. Increasing incidence of focal-segmental glomerulosclerosis among adult nephropathies: A 20-year renal biopsy study. *Am J Kidney Dis* 1995, **26**:740–750.
2. Shalhoub RJ. Pathogenesis of lipoid nephrosis: A disorder of T cell function. *Lancet* 1974, **2**:556–560.
3. Cameron JS. The long-term outcome of glomerular diseases. In: Diseases of the kidney, (2nd edn.), (ed. RN Schrier and CW Gottschalk). *Little Brown, Boston* 1992, 1895–1958.
4. White RHR, Glasgow EF, Mills RJ. Clinicopathological syndrome in children. *Lancet*, 1970, **1**:1353–1359.
5. Habib R, Kleinknecht C, Gubler MD. The Nephrotic Syndrome. In: Royer P, Mathieu H, Broyer M, Walsh A (eds.), Paediatric Nephrology. Philadelphia, W B Saunders Company, 1974, 258.
6. Arneil GC, Lam C. Long term assessment of steroid therapy in childhood nephrosis. *Lancet*, 1966, **2**:819–821.
7. Cameron JS. The problem of focal segmental glomerulosclerosis. In: Kincaid-Smith P, d'Apice AJF, Atkins R (eds.), Progress in Glomerulonephritis. New York, John Wiley and Sons, 1979, 209–228.
8. Habib R, Levy M, Gubler MC. Clinicopathological correlation in the nephrotic syndrome. *Paediatrician*, 1979, **8**:325.
9. Beaufils H, Alphonse JC, Guedon J, Legain M. Focal global sclerosis: Natural history and treatment. A report of 70 cases. *Nephron*, 1978, **21**:75–85.
10. Rydel JJ, Korbet SM, Borok RZ, Schwartz MM. Focal segmental glomerular sclerosis in adults: Presentation, course, and response to treatment. *AM J Kidney Dis* 1995, **25**:534–542.
11. Banfi G, Moriggi M, Sabadini E, Fellin G, D'Amico G, Ponticelli C. The impact of prolonged immunosuppression on the outcome of idiopathic focal-segmental glomerulosclerosis with nephrotic syndrome in adults. A collaborative retrospective study. *Clin Nephrol* 1991, **36**:53–59.

12. Waldher R, Gubler MC, Levy M, Broyer M, Habib R. The significance of pure diffuse mesangial proliferation in idiopathic nephrotic syndrome. *Clini Nephrol*, 1978, 10:171–179.
13. Cameron JS. The natural history of glomerulonephritis. In: Black D and Jones NF (eds.), Renal Disease. London: Blackwell Scientific Publishers, 1979, 329–382.
14. Collaborative Study of the Adult Idiopathic Nephrotic Syndrome. A controlled study of short term prednisolone treatment in adults with membranous nephropathy. *N Engl J Med*, 1979, **301**:1301–1306.
15. McEnery PT, McAdams AJ, West CD. Membranoproliferative Glomerulonephritis: Improved survival with alternate day prednisolone therapy. *Clin Nephrol*, 1980, **13**:117–124.
16. Kincaid-Smith P. The natural history and treatment of mesangiocapillary glomerulonephritis. In: Kincaid-Smith P, Mathew TH, Becker EC (eds.), Glomerulonephritis. Morphology, Natural History and Treatment. Part I. New York: John Wiley and Sons, 1973, 591–609.
17. Woo KT. Proteinuria in Renal Disease. Proc 11th Asian Colloquium in Nephrology, Singapore, 1996, 383–391.
18. Woo KT, Lau YK, Yap HK, Lee GSL, Chiang GSC, Lim CH. Protein selectivity: A prognostic index in IgA nephritis. *Nephron*, 1989, **52**:300–306.
19. Remuzzi G, Ruggenenti P, Benigni A. Understanding the nature of renal disease progression. *Kidney Int*. 1997, **51**:2–15.
20. Lewis EJ, Hunsicker LG, Bain RP, Rohde RD. For the collaborative study group: The effect of angiotensin coverting enzyme inhibition on Diabetic Nephropathy. *New Engl J Med*. 1993, **329**:456–462.
21. Brenner BM, Meyer TW, Hostetter TH. Dietary protein and the progressive nature of kidney disease. *New Engl J Med*. 1982, **307**:652–659.
22. Woo KT, Lau YK, Lee GSL, Wei SS, Lim CH. Pattern of proteinuria in IgA nephritis by SDS-PAGE: Clinical significance. *Clin Nephrol*, 1991, **36**:6–11.
23. Ponticelli C, Zucchelli P, Passerini P, Cesana B, Locatelli F, Pasquali S *et al*. A 10 year follow-up of a randomized study with methylprednisolone and chlorambucil in membranous nephropathy. *Kidney Int*, 1995, **48**:1600–1604.
24. MC Cauley J, Shapiro R, Ellis D, Igdal H, T Zakis A, Starzl TE. Pilot trial of FK 506 in the management of steroid resistant nephrotic syndrome. Nephrology, Dialysis and Transplantation, 1993, **8**:1286–1290.

25. Briggs WA, Choi MJ, Scheel PJ Jr. Successful Mycophenolate Mofetil Treatment of Glomerular Disease. *Amer J Kidney Disease.* 1998, **31**:213–217.
26. Waldman M, Austin HA. Controversies in the treatment of idiopathic membranous nephropathy. *Nature Reviews Nephrology,* 2009, **5**(8):469–479.
27. Ruggenenti P *et al.* Rituximab in idiopathic membranous nephropathy: A 1 year prospective study. *J Am. Soc. Nephrol,* 2003, **14**:1851–1857.
28. Fervenza FC. Rituximab treatment of idiopathic membranous nephropathy. *Kidney Int,* 2008, **73**:117–125.
29. Woo KT, Wong KS, Chan CM. Clinical Trials of the Past Decade in the Management of Chronic Kidney Disease. *Reviews on Clinical Trials,* 2009,4:159–162.
30. Alice S Appel and Gerald B Appel. An update on the use of MMF in lupus nephritis and other primary glomerular diseases. *Nature Clinical Practice Nephrology,* 2009, **5**(3):132–142.
31. Herlitz LC *et al.* Development of FSGS after anabolic steroid abuse. *J Amer Soc Nephrol* 2010, **21**:163–172.
32. Agarwal R. Are Vitamin D Receptor Agonists (VDRa) like ACEI without side effects? *Kidney Int* 2010, **77**:943–945.
33. Finkelstein FO and Finkelstein SH. Reassessment of the care of the patient with CKD. *Kidney Int* 2010, **77**:945–947.

CHAPTER 6

IgA Nephropathy: Discovery of a Distinct Glomerular Disorder

K.T. Woo, R.J. Glassock, K.N. Lai

INTRODUCTION

IgA nephropathy (IgAN) is the commonest form of primary glomerulonephritis in the developed world and it is an important cause of end stage kidney failure.[1,2] Epidemiologic studies have shown that IgAN is nearly universally distributed around the world but the frequency with which it is diagnosed varies, mostly according to local policies regarding the indications for renal biopsy. Prevalence appears highest in Asia (Singapore, Japan, and Hong Kong), Australia, Finland, and southern Europe (20 to 40 percent of cases of primary glomerulonephritis). In the United Kingdom, Canada, and the United States, prevalence rates are much lower (reviewed by Schena[3]). This chapter will focus on the early events which preceded and surrounded the discovery of IgAN by Berger and Hinglais more than four decades ago.

I. HISTORY OF IGA NEPHROPATHY (BERGER'S DISEASE)

It was the use of the techniques of immunohistochemistry and renal biopsy which led Berger to discover IgAN. The idea of using fluorescent-labelled specific antibodies to detect proteins in tissue was introduced by Coons and Kaplan[4] in 1950 and was first used for evaluation of disease renal tissue by Mellors and Ortega[5] in 1957. Percutaneous renal biopsy was initially described as a technique to diagnose kidney disease by Iverson and Brun in 1951.[6] By 1960, there were still only a relatively few sites where percutaneous renal biopsies were performed and even fewer laboratories skilled in the use of the immunofluorescenct technique and the antisera used were of poor specificity. In 1963, antibodies against class specific epitopes of the immunoglobulin light chains became commercially available so IgG, IgA and IgM could be identified separately. Tomasi *et al.*[7] had discovered the IgA immune system in 1965. Thus two techniques, immunofluorescent tagging of antibodies to detect antigens in tissues and percutaneous renal biopsy, along the discovery of an new immunoglobulin present in serum and in tissue secretions (IgA) all collided to prepare the way for the seminal observations, beginning in 1967 of Jean Berger and Nicole Hinglais at the Necker Hospital in Paris, France concerning a new entity they subsequently called mesangial IgA/IgG deposition. They described their novel observations in a brief paper published in 1968 which described predominant IgA mesangial deposition in some renal biopsies where the immunostaining of IgA strongly outshone the IgG reagent. This was the birth of IgA nephropathy, also subsequently called Berger's disease.[8] In the following year in 1969, Berger published another paper "IgA glomerular deposits in renal disease" in the Transplantation Proceedings.[9] This was a new journal in its first year. Fifty-five patients with various forms of glomerular morphology were described, mostly "focal glomerulonephritis". These patients had minor proteinuria, but all had microscopic hematuria, of whom 22 had one or more bouts of gross hematuria. It was also already known then that IgA could also be found in patients with nephritis associated with Henoch-Schonlein purpura as well as lupus nephritis. The nephrology world was still sceptical about the "new disease entity". In 1972, Levy and colleagues[10] used in print for the first time the term "Berger's Disease". It was recorded that Jean Berger was somewhat

Table 6.1.   Different Nomenclature of IgA Nephropathy

Nephropathy with mesangial IgA-IgG deposits
Les glomerulopathies primitives a depots mesangiaux d'IgA et d'IgG
Diffuse intra- und extrakapillare Glomerulonephritis mit IgA-Depots
IgA-IgG-Nephropathie
Glomerulites a depots d'IgA diffuse dan le mesangium
IgA-associated glomerulonephritis
IgA nephropathy
IgA-IgG deposits nephritis
Immunoglobulin A glomerulonephritis
Primary glomerulonephritis with mesangial deposits of IgA
Benign hematuria-loin pain syndrome

embarrassed, as one knows he is indeed a very modest man, following appearance of this paper in USA, UK, Netherlands, Japan and Australia.[11] By 1975, "Berger's Disease" became an established glomerular entity: a condition with moderate proliferative glomerular changes, usually mesangial but often focal or segmental in distribution; associated with microscopic hematuria and about 15% to 20% with macroscopic hematuria. Serum IgA levels were also shown to be elevated in some patients. It was a slowly progressive renal disease with increasing proteinuria, hypertension and renal failure in ~30% of patients over 25–30 years. The different nomenclature of "Berger's Disease" is shown in Table 6.1. When such patients were transplanted, Berger showed that about 50% had a recurrence, though not all grafts failed because of recurrent diease.[9]

II.   FIRST DESCRIPTION OF THE BROADER CLINICAL FEATURES OF "BERGER'S DISEASE"

Clarkson *et al.*[12], in an impressive collection of cases with "Berger's Disease" emphasized that "Berger's Disease" was a syndrome of uniform morphology, diverse clinical features and uncertain prognosis. It is now fully recognized that Berger's

Disease (henceforth called IgA nephropathy) is not always a benign disease. It has a cumulative renal survival of 89% after 5 years, 81% after 10 years and 65% after 20 years.[13,14] The data showed that renal deterioration in IgAN is generally slow and progressive over a long period of time (average: 7.7 years). The unfavorable long-term prognostic indices are proteinuria of more than 1 g/day, hypertension, glomerulosclerosis exceeding 20%, presence of crescents, and medial hyperplasia of blood vessels on renal biopsy. A smaller group of patients run a more rapid clinical course progressing to end-stage renal failure within a few years, in which severe uncontrolled hypertension seems to be the major adverse factor.

As in the time of Berger, the cause remains unknown in the majority of IgAN. However, cases of familial IgAN and secondary IgAN have been reported and these have provided insights into underlying genetic and environmental triggers for this common glomerular disease. Secondary IgAN is seen most commonly in patients with liver disease or mucosal inflammation, in particular affecting the gastrointestinal tract. A number of dietary and microbial antigens have been identified in circulating IgA immune complexes and mesangial IgA deposits, suggesting that environmental factors may play a role in the pathogenesis of IgAN.[15] Whether these reports represent chance associations or genuine shared pathophysiology remain to be confirmed.

III. THE RECOGNITION OF DISEASE PROGRESSION AND PROTEINURIA

At the time of its discovery, IgAN was believed to be a "benign" disorder. We now recognize that the majority of cases will progress to renal failure although at a widely varying rate. A small subset of patients with heavy proteinuria behaves clinically like minimal change disease. Their proteinuria responds to steroid and this subset was recognized as "an overlapping syndrome of

IgA nephropathy and lipoid nephrosis".[16] Otherwise, severe nephrotic-range proteinuria is not common in IgAN, but nephrotic-range proteinuria in the absence of minimal change disease is associated with poor prognosis.

IV. EVOLUTION OF BELIEFS REGARDING TREATMENT OF IgAN

Initially, IgAN was not thought to require any treatment. However, upon recognition that progression to renal failure was not uncommon, interest in attempting therapy become of significant importance. However, early attempts were reported mainly as anecdotes, small prospective, uncontrolled trials or retrospective observational analyses. This, whether truly beneficial and safe forms of therapy for IgAN existed was quite uncertain. The paucity of controlled clinical trials of therapy for IgAN during the past three decades contrasts with the number of recent reviews, illustrating frustrations in obtaining new, reliable long-term data on treatment for IgAN. Scrutiny and evaluation of other regimens can only be good for patients, but current recommendations are polarized and sometimes changeable, supporting or denying use of corticosteroids when proteinuria exceeds 1 g/24 h. The quality of randomized, controlled trials is substantially influenced by design parameters, so retrospective interpretation using a mathematically insufficient approach is a likely source of discrepancy between reviews. Recent commentaries address how disparate opinion may have risen and quantify existing data to balance recommendations.[17,18]

In sum, the paucity of good clinical trials highlights the remaining uncertainty persisting from the early 1970's concerning what is best treatment and for how long must treatment be continued. History has taught us that good clinical trials are difficult to conduct in IgAN because of the slow progressive nature of the disease, diverse clinical features, different biopsy criteria for determining prognosis, and selection of end-points.

V. CONCLUSION

It is now four decades since Berger's observation and description of this distinct clinico-pathological entity first called Berger's Disease and now called IgA nephropathy. The coalescence of immunohistochemistry, percutaneous renal biopsy and discovery of the IgA molecule in 1950–1965 set the stage for this discovery. We now know that IgAN is characterised immunologically by the presence of IgA immune complexes deposition in the mesangium in the clinical setting of diverse clinical features, but primarily asymptomatic hematuria and proteinuria. Histologically, most patients have a diffuse mesangial proliferative glomerulonephritis, whilst others have focal proliferative lesions and a very small minority develop acute renal failure with crescents as in "malignant" lgAN. We now recognise, not well understood in the initial years following the discovery of IgAN, that in the majority of patients, IgAN is a smouldering disease of a slowly progressive nature. Up to the present, there is no universally agreed-upon definitive therapy for IgAN, though renin-angiotensin system blockade can slow the progression to end stage renal failure.[19] Ever since Berger, investigators in the field of IgAN have pursued the underlying mechanisms responsible for the disease with a view to seeking a cure, yet the gap between the bench and the patient's bedside does not seem to be closing very rapidly. Slow progress has been made, particularly in the understanding of the abnormalities of the IgA molecule itself in subjects with IgAN (reviewed in Chapter 12). Seekers of the Holy Grail or the final chapter of the IgAN story which began in Paris so many years ago will have to continue to persevere and hopefully one day harness a solution for the commonest form of primary glomerulonephritis worldwide.

REFERENCES

1. D'Amico G. Natural History of idiopathic IgA nephropathy and factors mediative of disease outcome. *Semin Nephrol* 2004, **24**: 179–196.

2. Woo KT, Lau YK. Factors associated with progression of IgA nephropathy. *Clin Nephrol* 2003, **59**: 481–482.
3. Schena FP. A retrospective analysis of the natural history of primary IgA nephropathy worldwide. *Am J Med* 1990, **89**: 209–215.
4. Coons AH, Kaplan MH. Localization of antigen in tissue cells; improvements in a method for the detection of antigen by means of fluorescent antibody. *J Exp Med* 1950, **91**:1–13.
5. Mellors RC, Ortega LG, Holman HR. Role of gamma globulins in the renal lesions of systemic lupus erythematosus and chronic membranous glomerulonephritis, with an observation on the lupus erythematosus cell reaction. *J Exp Med* 1957, **106**: 191–201.
6. Iverson P, Brun C. Aspiration biopsy of the kidney. *Am J Med* 1951, **11**: 324–330.
7. Tomasi TB Jr, Tan EM, Solomon A, Prendergast RA. Characteristics of an immune system common to certain external secretions. *J Exp Med* 1965, **121**: 101–124.
8. Berger J, Hinglais N. Les depots intercapillaires d'IgA-IgG. *J Urol Nephrol* 1968, **74**: 694–695.
9. Berger J. IgA glomerular deposits in renal disease. *Transplant Proc* 1969, **1**: 939–944.
10. Levy M, Beaufils H, Gubler MC, Habib R. Idiopathic recurrent macroscopic hematuria and mesangial IgA-IgG deposits in children (Berger's disease). *Clin Nephrol* 1972, **1**: 63–69.
11. Cameron JS. History of Berger's Disease before Berger. The International IgA Nephropathy Network: http://www.iga-world.org/bergercameron.htm
12. Clarkson AR, Seymour AE, Thompson AJ, *et al.* IgA nephropathy: a syndrome of uniform morphology, diverse clinical features and uncertain prognosis. *Clin Nephrol* 1977, **8**: 459–471.
13. Woo KT, Edmondson RPS, Wu AYT, *et al.* The natural history of IgA nephritis in Singapore. *Clin Nephrol* 1986, **25**:15–21.
14. Woo KT, Lau YK, Choong HL, *et al.* IgA nephropathy: effect of clinical indices, ACEI/ATRA therapy and ACE gene polymorphism on disease progression. *Nephrology,* 2002, **7**: S166–S172.
15. Pouria S, Baratt J. Secondary IgA nephropathy. *Semin Nephrol* 2008, **28**: 27–37.
16. Lai KN, Lai FM, Chan KW, *et al.* An overlapping syndrome of IgA nephropathy and lipoid nephrosis. *Am J Clin Pathol* 1986, **86**: 716–723.
17. Ballardie FW. Quantitative appraisal of treatment options for IgA nephropathy. *J Am Soc Nephrol* 2007, **18**: 2806–2809.

18. Tumlin JA, Madaio MP, Hennigar R. Idiopathic IgA nephropathy: pathogenesis, histopathology, and therapeutic options. *Clin Am J Nephrol* 2007, **2**: 1054–1061.
19. Woo KT, Lau YK, Wong KS, Chiang GSC. ACEI/ATRA therapy decreases proteinuria by improving glomerular permselectivity in IgA nephritis. *Kidney Int* 2000, **58**: 2485–2491.

CHAPTER 7

Pathogenesis and Therapy of IgA Nephritis

INTRODUCTION

IgA nephritis (IgA Nx) is the commonest form of glomerulonephritis in Singapore accounting for 40% of all primary glomerulonephritis and is therefore a very important cause of end stage kidney failure.[1] Forty nine percent of patients present with asymptomatic haematuria and proteinuria, 23% with gross or visible haematuria, 25% with the nephrotic syndrome, 15% with hypertension, 6% with chronic renal failure and 2% with acute renal failure associated with crescents on renal biopsy. In IgA Nx there is an immunological defect, likely to be genetic in origin which causes the B lymphocytes of the patient to secrete increased IgA in response to an environmental antigen (microbial or otherwise). The presence of an abnormal T suppressor cell function and augmented T helper cell function results in increased B cells bearing surface IgA and T cells bearing receptors for Fc region of IgA.

PATHOGENESIS

In the pathogenesis of IgA Nx, four requisites must be present for glomerulonephritis to develop. There must be a propensity for IgA immune complexes (IgAIC) to be deposited in the kidneys. There must be a defective clearance of IgAIC by the kidneys. The mesangial cells of the kidneys must respond by producing certain cytokines

105

capable of eliciting a noxious response which are detrimental to the kidneys. As a result of the noxious response, inflammation or glomerulonephritis occurs, giving rise to haematuria and proteinuria.

Defective Clearance of Immune Complexes

Patients with IgA Nx have defective clearance of IgA coated particles, heat aggregated IgA or IgA-IgG by the liver and spleen.[2] They have a general defect in removal of immune complexes. An individual can have IgAIC within the circulation which is filtered by the kidneys, but as long as the kidneys can get rid of these IgAIC the person will not develop glomerulonephritis. It is only in certain individuals with the disease susceptible gene which makes the kidneys unable to clear these IgAIC that IgA Nx will develop. In addition, IgA binds complements poorly and inhibits complement activation by IgA immune complexes. Complement normally helps to solubulise IC but since the action of complements is inhibited, glomerular deposition of IC is enhanced in IgA Nx.

ROLE OF CYTOKINES

Recently, cytokines have been found to play an important role in IgA Nx.[3] Interlukin-5 (IL-5) has been shown to selectively increase IgA positive cells which is increased in IgA Nx. IL-6 too is elevated in IgA Nx. Transgenic mice with high IL-6 levels have elevated serum IgA and mesangial proliferative glomerulonephritis (GN) with IgA deposits. IL-6 is mitogenic for mesangial cells. In the presence of IL-6, mesangial cells would undergo proliferation, giving rise to mesangial proliferative glomerulonephritis typical of IgA Nx.

The Propensity for IgA Deposition in IgA Nx

Molecular weight (MW) of IgA, especially polymeric IgA favours deposition in the mesangium because of its larger size. IgA molecules are poorly solubilized by the complement system and allows its deposition in the kidney. IgA is also more anionic than IgG and M and therefore are preferentially deposited in the mesangium which attracts anionic or negatively charged molecules.[3] The mesangial cells bear cationic or positive charges. The IgA eluted from mesangial deposits is also more "anionic" than serum IgA.[4] Urinary albumin in IgA Nx patients too are "anionic".[4] Finally, serum IgA, circulating macromolecular IgA, all have an affinity for the mesangial matrix components like fibronectin and laminin which bear cationic charges.

It is postulated that in patients with IgA Nx there is a defect both in the "sera" (existence of IgAIC) and in the "renal tissue" (abnormal mesangial cells) This would explain the disappearance of IgA Nx from some donated kidneys after transplantation (these kidneys with IgA Nx were inadvertently transplanted), and the recurrence of IgA Nx in those receiving kidneys from living related donors, less so from cadavers.[5] These were patients with IgA Nx as the original disease but the transplanted kidneys did not have IgA Nx at the time of transplantation. In those patients where there is a recurrence of IgA in the kidney without any renal detriment, it would support the theory that lack of genetically mediated mesangial reactivity towards IgA Nx prevents the clinical and histological manifestations of IgA Nx.

Mechanism by Which Mesangial Deposits Initiate Glomerular Injury

The binding of IgA deposits to mesangial cells induces certain changes within the mesangial cells causing the secretion of cytokines associated with a decrease in prostaglandin E2 synthesis and increase in thromboxane A2 production promoting mesangial cell proliferation. Elicitation of Angiotensin II also induces mesangial cell contraction and efferent arteriolar vasoconstriction.[6]

IgAIC deposited in the mesangium then bind to mesangial cells and exert their nephritogenic effect through the stimulation of release of cytokines from mesangial cells. Cytokines exert noxious effects causing proliferation of mesangial cells and inflammatory injury which results in glomerulonephritis manifesting as haematuria and proteinuria. Macromolecules which are unable to bind to mesangial cells cannot exert nephritogenicity. The IgA antibody in the IgAIC concentrates and aggregates the antigen into the mesangium, but it is the antigen which is the critical pathogenic component in the equation of nephritogenecity.

Therapeutic Strategies

Various types of food antigen (soya bean protein, gliadin, bovine serum albumin) and infective agents (streptoccous, Sendai virus) have been implicated in patients with IgA Nx. It can occur in a sporadic or familial fashion. Currently, it is believed that a disease susceptible gene is involved but no gene has as yet been identified. Some suspect that it is a heterogenous disease with mulfactorial etiology.

Any form of therapy must be rational as well as practical. Based on the foregoing discussion on pathogenesis, the ideal therapeutic strategy should attempt to limit the amount of mesangial deposits as well as reduction of noxious glomerular responses to the deposits.[7]

Ways to Limit Amounts of Mesangial Deposits

1. **Reduction of antigen load**

   Gluten-free diet could be recommended for IgA Nx patients who have high levels of IgA directed against gliadin to reduce generation of gliadin/anti-gliadin complexes.[8]

2. **Tonsillectomy**

   This could be considered in patients with chronic tonsillitis because long term follow-up of patients with IgA Nx who have had tonsillectomy have shown that tonsillectomy blunts the progression of IgA Nx.[9]

3. **Lymphokines**

   In view of the significant role played by lymphokines in the pathogenesis of IgA Nx, various forms of therapy could be formulated to downregulate the effects of various lymphokines. The prospect to correct pathogenic immunologic defect induced by lymphokines is challenging. This will be discussed later.

4. **Enzymes**

   Systemically administered enzymes (Dextranase and Protease) have been used to remove glomerular immune deposits in rodents.[10] This has not been tried in patients but the prospects of such a therapy sounds promising.

A Pathophysiologic Approach

The focus for such an approach should be on the mesangial cell responses to immune complexes, complements, cytokines and vasoactive mediators.

1. **Immunomodulators**

   Steroids,[11] Cyclophosphamide,[12] Cyclosporine A [CyA][13] and Mycophenolate Mofetil [MMF] [Sydney C.W. Tang *et al.*, Long term study of MMF in IgA nephritis. Kidney Int 2010, 77(6): 543–549] have been used with varying success in patients with IgA Nx. These agents, since they are immunosuppressants, would attenuate lymphocyte function and serve to downregulate the effects of cytokines in the glomeruli but their toxicity and necessity for continuity limits their applicability. Proteinuria in patients rebounds on stopping the medication.

2. **Anti-platelet and anti-thrombotic Therapy**
    Patients with IgA Nx have evidence of platelet involvement and low grade intravascular coagulation with a tendency for increased thrombogenecity within the kidneys. Use of Dipyridamole (anti-platelet and anti-PDGF agent) and Warfarin (anti-thrombotic agent) have been successful in two separate trials[12,14] in patients with IgA Nx. The relative freedom from side effects and their low cost allow long-term treatment in these patients.

3. **Angiotensin Receptor Blocker and ACE inhibitors**
    In IgA Nx, glomerular hyperfiltration injury as evidenced by presence of late onset phase of proteinuria or increasing proteinuria is accompanied by intra-glomerular hypertension due to local hyperactivity of the renin angiotensin system and angiotensin II mediated efferent arteriolar vasoconstriction. The use of ACE inhibitor and ARB have been shown to be of benefit in reducing proteinuria and preservation of renal function.[15] In our study we also showed that ARB is as effective as ACEI in decreasing proteinuria and preservation of renal function[1] [Woo KT, Lau YK, Wong KS, Chiang GSC. ACE/ATRA therapy decreases proteinuria by improving glomerular permselectivity in IgA nephritis: Kidney Int 2000, 58:2485–2491].

    However there is a problem of renal fibrosis in patients on long term ACE inhibitors and ARBs, though preferable at this point in time, may also cause the same problem in the long term. We have also shown that High Dose ARBs [Eg. Losartan given in a dose of 100 mg twice daily may be better at preservation of renal function and for those patients who have been on long term ARBs, after 5 years some patients have improvement of their eGFR. The belief is that ARBs can in the long term contribute to improvement of renal function by causing regression of glomerulosclerosis. See Chapter on Nephrotic Syndrome [Woo KT *et al.*, Beneficial effects of high dose Losartan in IgA nephritis, Clinical Nephrol 2009,

71:617–624]. [Woo KT *et al.*, High dose losartan and ACE gene polymorphism in IgA nephritis. Genomics Medicine, 2009, 2:83–91].

4. **Anti-Renin Agent**

Aliskiren is a new renal protective agent that inhibits renin, the rate limiting step in the renin angiotensin aldosterone system [RAAS]. Aliskiren allows for total blockade of the renin angiotensin system and its beneficial effect is independent of BP control.[29] In addition, Aliskiren has the ability to catalyse renin and in so doing reduce the ability of renin to promote renal fibrosis. The use of ACEI and/or ARBs will cause an elevation of plasma renin activity (PRA). This increased plasma renin will promote renofibrosis. If Aliskiren is given together with an ARB, the Aliskiren can lower the PRA induced by the ARB and is therefore renoprotective. Patients who do not respond to ARBs can be given Aliskiren in addition in a dose of 150 mg to 300 mg daily. In the previous Chapter, I have alluded to the wisdom of starting therapy with Aliskiren as the first line and using ARBs only when one cannot control proteinuria or improve renal function depending on the need of the patient.

5. **Anti-platelet and anti-thrombotic Therapy**

Patients with IgA Nx have evidence of platelet involvement and low grade intravascular coagulation with a tendency for increased thrombogenecity within the kidneys. Use of Dipyridamole (anti-platelet and anti-PDGF agent) and Warfarin (anti-thrombotic agent) have been successful in two separate trials[12,14] in patients with IgA Nx. The relative freedom from side effects and their low cost allow long-term treatment in these patients. The point to note is that with the availability of ARBs which seem so much more potent compared to persantin and warfarin, many doctors are no longer prescribing P and W. However, long before ARBs became available, the use of P and W had already been retarding progression of disease in patients with renal impairment, helping them retard the progression to ESRF by as long as up to 20 years and beyond. Unfortunately, except for a very few patients now, we do not have much data documenting reno-protection up to 30 years and beyond.

6. **Low protein diet**

   A low protein diet (0.8 gm/kg bw/day) would reduce macro-molecular flux and afferent arteriolar vasodilation contributing to glomerular hyperfiltration. This would also help to retard progression of renal failure. However it is important to ensure that the patient has a minimum intake of 0.8 gm/kg BW of protein a day in order to prevent malnutrition. Patients with protein calorie malnutrition (PCM) will have a more rapid progression of renal failure. Also PCM itself will cause an increase in CVD with increase in deaths due to CVD. It is therefore not a good idea for renal patients to become vegetarians.

Future Therapeutic Strategies

1. **Inhibitors of mediators and cytokines**

   Drugs like platelet derived growth factor (PDGF) antagonists, tumour necrosis factor (TNF) inhibitor, platelet activating and thromboxane receptor antagonist have not been employed in clinical trials for IgA Nx but they appear to be rational and practical approaches from the pathophysiologic viewpoint. These therapeutic approaches would be directed to inhibit effects of mediators and cytokines involved in IgA Nx.

2. **Gene therapy**

   Gene therapy would offer the ideal therapeutic approach. Modulation of transduction by intracellular signal upon DNA transcription or translation of mRNA may prove effective. One could modulate a specific signal leading to abnormal response to mesangial cells. Another novel approach utilizes "antisense nucleotides". Gene expression in cells is normally regulated by DNA binding proteins, repressors and activators. It was found that complementary nucleic acids could also modulate gene expression. Antisense RNA complementary to regions of mRNA was demonstrated to suppress translation and hence gene expression. Hence there is a possibility of using synthetic oligonucleotides to regulate gene expression.[16]

In principle, one identifies a unique target sequence in the gene of interest and prepare a complementary oligonucleotide against the target sequence. Antisense DNAs were first utilised against Rous sarcoma virus by Zamecnik and Stephenson in 1978.[17] In IgA Nx, antisense nucleotides could arrest transcription or trans-duction of a specific mRNA which gives rise to mesangial cell proliferation. Another nucleotide could perhaps switch off the message leading to mesangial cell contraction. It is mesangial cell contraction, following mesangial cell proliferation which leads to mesangial sclerosis, with eventual global glomerulosclerosis with death of that particular glomerulus. It is hoped that therapy in the future may involve antisense nucleotides to modulate abnormal mesangial cell response.

This is the Genomic Era. The human genome project has been completed for 10 years now but in terms of delivery of genomic therapy, the post man is still a far cry away from the door bell of the nephrologist, This is because the postman may be redundant now with the use of e-mail. From the grapevine we know that more than 200 noxious and non noxious proteins have been identified genomically in various GN. They have been tagged with their genomic codes. The work in progress is to decipher the codes which categorise the noxious proteins causing glomerular and tubulointerstitial injury and then block these genetic codes so that these noxious proteins are not produced. This is especially important for the therapy of diabetic nephropathy where patients with heavy proteinuria do not seem to be responding well unlike proteinuria in other types of renal disease. At this point in time, the ultimate solution for protein-uria induced renal damage is to prevent the proteinuria from doing harm. For the other catrgory of patients with CKD who progress to renal failure in the absence of significant protein-uria, the task is even more daunting as we do not know where the culprit is hiding. Meanwhile many more patients are pro-gressing and heading towards dialysis, especially for the many elderly ones [with CKD Stage 3B with eGFR <45 ml/min] without much proteinuria. In some of these, the use of ARBs and Aliskiren seem to retard the progression to ESRF but for others no therapy is in sight.

Clinical Trials in IgA Nephritis:

There have been few randomised controlled trials with IgA nephritis as there is as yet no specific therapy for IgA nephritis.

1. Fish Oil
    Donadio [Donadio *et al.*, J Am Soc Nephrol 1999, 331: 1194–1199] in a randomised controlled trial [RCT] showed the benefits of fish oil. There were fewer patients with 50% increase in serum creatinine and they had slower decline of GFR. However, a more recent trial by Hogg [Hogg *et al.*, J Am Soc Nephrol 2003, 14:751] showed no benefits after 2 years. Pettersson [Pettersson *et al*, Clin Nephrol 1994, 41:183–190] in another trial also showed no renoprotective effect and fish oil actually led to further decline compared to placebo. The results of Fish Oil have therefore been contradictory.
2. Corticosteroids
    Pozzi [Pozzi C *et al.*, J Am Soc Nephrol 2004, 15:157–163] in a RCT from Italy on 56 patients with mean serum creati-nine of 1.5 mg/dl and proteinuria of 1.35 gm/day treated with pulse steroids at beginning followed by 6 months oral Prednisolone showed that the renal survival was better in the Steroid group compared to placebo. However the study was not controlled for BP and use of ACE inhibitors.

3. Cyclosporine A

   Ballardie FW [Ballardie FW *et al.*, J Am Soc Nephrol 2002, 13: 142–148] in 38 patients designated high risk patients with serum creatinine rising by 15% a year before entry with end stage renal failure [ESRF] predicted within 5 years, were randomised to either oral Cyclosporine A (CyA) in a dose of 1.5 mg/Kg BW per day for 3 months, plus steroids followed by Azathioprine (1.5 mg/kg BW/day for 2 years). The renal survival was 72% in the treatment group versus 6% in the Control group. However BP control was suboptimal, insufficient use of ARB/ACEI, small number of patients in the trial and unusually poor renal survival rate in the Control group.

4. Mycophenolate Mofetil [MMF]

   MMF has been evaluated in several trials.

   (i)   Chen X [Chen X *et al.*, Zhonghua Yi Xue Zhi 2002, 82:796–801] in an RCT involving 62 pateints with proteinuria >2 gms/day, showed that the MMF group did better with the Control group having higher serum creatinine at 72 weeks.

   (ii) Tang [Tang *et al.*, Kid International, 2005, 68:802–812] showed that MMF alleviated persistent proteinuria in IgA nephritis. There was greater reduction in proteinuria in the MMF group compared to placebo but no difference in the serum creatinine between the 2 groups.

   (iii) Maes [Maes *et al.*, Kid International, 2004, 65: 1442–1449] in a trial consisting of 34 patients with mean serum creatinine of 1.4 mg/dl and proteinuria of 1.6 gm/day treated with MMF 2 gm/day, showed no difference in serum creatinine or proteinuria after 3 years follow up.

   (iv) Frisch and Appel [Frisch and Appel *et al.*, Nephrol Dial Transpl 2005, 20:2139–2145] in a RCT of 40 patients with mean serum creatinine 2.4 mg.dl and proteinuria 2.7 gm/day were randomized to MMF or placebo. All

patients had optimum BP control with ACEI. The trial
was prematurely terminated after enrolling 40 patients
as there was a high rate of progression in both arms.

(v)   Tang [Tang SCW *et al.*, Long term study of MMF in IgA
nephropathy, Kidney Int 2010, 77:543–549] reported that
in his study of 40 patients with IgA nephritis, half of
whom were randomized to receive MMF for 6 months,
after 6 years, 11 patients required dialysis (2 from MMF
and 9 from the control group). Only 3 treated (as compared to 10 controls) patients reached the composite end
point of serum creatinine doubling or end stage renal
disease. The yearly decline in eGFR was less in the
MMF treated group (1.1 ml/min in MMF group compared to 3.8 ml/min in the Control group, p = 0.021). The
urinary protein excretion Albumin/Creatinine Ratio was
lower in the MMF group during the first 24 months compared to the control group, after this there was no difference. All patients were maintained on ACEI/ARB but
more patients in the MMF group received combination
therapy with ACEI and ARB.

5.   Angiotensin Receptor Blockers (ARB) and Renin inhibitors

(i)   In the recent Ongoing Telmisartan Alone and in
Combination with Ramipril Global End-point Trial
(ONTARGET) [Mann JF *et al.* Renal outcomes with
telmisartan, ramipril, or both, in people at high vascular
risk (the ONTARGET Study). A multicentre, randomized,
double-blind, controlled trial. Lancet 2008, 372:547–553].
The trial randomly assigned 25, 620 patients with established atherosclerotic vascular disease or diabetes with
end organ damage to ARB telmisartan, ACE Inhibitor
Ramipril or a combination of the two. Over a period of
56 months, even though the incidence of cardiac deaths
were the same in all 3 groups, the incidence of doubling
of serum creatinine, dialysis, renal transplantation
occurred more frequently among those on combined

ACEI/ARB compared to those on ACEI alone or ARB alone. Elderly patients (>50 years old) with cardio-vascular disease and without proteinuria should not be subjected to Dual RAS blockade. Such combination therapy has no clinically proven benefits on renal out-come and might even be harmful.

(ii) There may also be a problem of renal fibrosis in patients on long term ACE inhibitors and ARBs may be preferable. In proteinuric rats, the combination of ACE inhibitor and a low salt diet elicited pronounced renal interstitial damage, despite a significant reduction of proteinuria. ACEI induce renal fibrosis despite reduc-tion of proteinuria. The long term renoprotective effect of ACEI should not be taken for granted [Hamming I *et al.* ACE-inhibitor has adverse renal effects during dietary sodium restriction in proteinuric and healthy rats. J Pathology 2006, 209: 129–139.

(iii) We have shown that High Dose ARBs [Eg. Losartan given in a dose of 100 mg twice daily may be better at preservation of renal function and for those patients who have been on long term ARBs, after 5 years some patients have improvement of their eGFR. The belief is that ARBs can in the long term contribute to improve-ment of renal function by causing regression of glomeru-losclerosis. See Chapter on Nephrotic Syndrome [Woo KT *et al.*, Beneficial effects of high dose Losartan in IgA nephritis, Clinical Nephrol 2009, 71:617–624]. [Woo KT *et al.*, High dose Losartan and ACE gene polymorphism in IgA nephritis. Genomics Medicine, 2009, 2:83–91]. But the long term problem will still be one of renal fibrosis whether it is ACEI, ARBs or renin inhibitors, though among the three, renin inhibitors like Aliskiren seems better in terms of renal fibrosis. But Aliskiren is still new in the market and we do not have long term data as yet.

(iv)   Aliskiren as I stated, is a new renal protective agent that inhibits renin, the rate limiting step in the renin angiotensin aldosterone system [RAAS]. Aliskiren allows for total blockade of the renin angiotensin system and its beneficial effect is independent of BP control [Wigging KJ *et al.*, Aliskiren: a novel renoprotective agent or simply an alternative to ACE inhibitors? Kid International, 2009, 76:23–31]. Patients who do not respond to ARBs can be given Aliskiren in addition in a dose of 150 mg to 300 mg daily.

Beneficial Effects of High Dose ARB

Woo *et al.* [Woo KT *et al.*, Beneficial effects of high dose Losartan in IgA nephritis, Clinical Nephrol 2009, 71:617–624] performed a randomized controlled clinical trial comparing the effects of high dose ARB (Losartan 200 mg/day) versus normal dose of ARB (Losartan 100 mg/day), normal dose of ACEI (Enalapril 20 mg/day) and low dose ACEI (Enalapril 10 mg/day) in 207 patients with IgA nephritis over a 6 year period. Patients on high dose ARB had significantly higher eGFR and lower levels of proteinuria compared to the other 3 groups at the end of the trial. The more efficacious high dose of ARB probably translated into a much lower level of proteinuria in the patients and hence better renoprotection compared to patients on ACEI (Enalapril 20 mg/day and 10 mg/day) and normal dose ARB (Losartan 100 mg/day). In the long term (trial duration of 6 years) the high dose ARB patients have less decline of eGFR per year and lower incidence of ESRF. There were no significant differences between patients on the other 3 drug groups.

The results of multivariate analysis showed that the effect of high dose ARB on preservation of eGFR and proteinuria reduction was due to the effect of the increased dose of ARB (200 mg) employed in the study and independent of other covariates including both systolic and diastolic BP.

At year 5 there was a gain in the eGFR for patients on high dose ARB. This gain however was less significant in year 6 because the other groups also had some gain in eGFR though less than those in the high dose ARB group. The effect of the various agents on yearly changes of TUP was not significantly different. However, the slope corresponding to the decline in TUP from baseline to year 5 was significantly steeper for the high dose ARB group compared to the other groups. This coincided with the gain in eGFR found in year 5 in the high dose ARB group.

It is possible to have a favourable effect of the drug on eGFR without effecting the degree of proteinuria. In most instances anti-proteinuria effect occurred before eGFR improvement, sometimes at the same time. We have in this cohort at least 10 patients whose eGFR improved without any change in the degree of proteinuria. In a previous publication [Woo *et al.* 2000] we showed that even though the degree of proteinuria remains the same, the quality of proteinuria may have improved since ARB/ACEI can convert non selective to selective proteinuria which is less noxious to the kidneys.

Recovery or regression of glomerulosclerosis has been reported by various workers [Remuzzi *et al.* 2006, Fogo *et al.* 2006]. In the early 1990s, Marinides [Marinides *et al.* 1990] had reported reversal of proteinuria and glomerulosclerosis by combining a low protein diet with an ACE inhibitor in the puromycin aminoglycoside rat model. Adamazak [Adamczak *et al.* 2004] documented reversal of glomerulosclerosis after high dose enalapril treatment in subtotally nephrectomized rats. In a recent study, Ma [Ma *et al.* 2005] employing ACEI and or ARB in rats with subtotal nephrectomy showed decrease of glomerulosclerosis. Treatment was initiated 8 weeks after inducing renal injury. Four weeks later, sclerotic lesions were shown to decrease on autopsy.

In human disease, early on, Ruggenenti reported that prolonged therapy with ACEI can induce remission in CKD [Ruggenenti *et al.* 2001]. In the Ramipril Efficacy in Nephropathy (REIN) study [Ruggenenti *et al*. 1999], among 78 patients treated with ACEI, 10% had improvement in GFR after 6 years therapy indicating functional regression of disease. Remuzzi stressed the importance of using maximum tolerated dose of ACEI and ARB to achieve better remission [Remuzzi *et al*. 2005]. In this respect, Fogo's view is that super high doses of either ACEI or ARB are necessary to achieve regression of glomerulosclerosis [Fogo *et al*. 2006]. High dose therapy had the additional beneficial effects of decreasing renal inflammation and restoring glomerular and interstitial injury to pretreatment levels.

This study suggests that high dose ARB therapy is more efficacious in reducing proteinuria and preserving renal function when compared with normal dose ARB or normal dose ACEI. Our data on high dose Losartan are similar to those on Irbesartan [Rossing *et al*. 2005], Valsartan [Hollenburg *et al*. 2007] and Telmisartan [Aranda *et al*. 2005]. The safety profile of high dose therapy is not an issue for concern. All these ARBs help to further enhance reduction of proteinuria and stabilise or improve declining GFR in these patients. Another feature of our study which we share with the DETAIL study [Barnett *et al*. 2006] is the long duration of follow up, where we could show a sustained gain in eGFR from Year 5. This feature of gain in eGFR also occurs in patients on normal dose ARB Losartan (100 mg/day) and normal dose ACEI Enalapril (20 mg/day) but in both instances the gain in eGFR was significantly less than in the high dose Losartan group. These data may suggest better chances of recovery of renal function for patients on long term high dose ARB therapy. However, the effect of Enalapril at 40 mg/day or even at ultrahigh dose remains to be determined. Perhaps, a comparison study using ultrahigh dose of an ARB versus ACEI may be useful in the future.

In conclusion, the present data suggest that adequate blockage of the renin angiotensin system without resorting to the use of immunosuppresssants could achieve significant benefits for patients with IgA nephritis without the risks of immunosuppressive therapy, a view also expressed by Ballardie [Ballardie 2007].

Any form of renin angiotensin blockade would be effective as such benefits are not confined to the use of only ARB, since other workers have also shown that significant benefits could also be achieved by ACEI alone [Ruggenenti *et al.* 1999, Praga *et al.* 2003]. We belief that most patients may benefit from high dose ARB therapy irrespective of ACE gene I/D polymorphism as preliminary data from our unpublished studies suggest that high dose ARB could override the genomic effects of the ACE gene on their response to ACEI/ARB therapy. [References for this Section will be listed after References for Chapter on Pathogenesis and Treatment of IgA Nephritis].

Therapy of IgA Nephritis: Dept of Renal Medicine, Singapore General Hospital

1. **Intraglomerular effect of dipyridamole**

   Since 1979, Woo *et al.*[12] have used dipyridamole as an anti-platelet agent. Their[18] earlier work on platelet involvement in IgA Nx suppported a rationale for its use in combination with low dose warfarin. But relative importance of glomerular platelet infiltration versus direct intraglomerular effect of dipyridamole is not clear. Its anti-platelet effect within the glomerulus may be only one aspect of its effects within the glomerulus.

   Dipyridamole has been shown to have an anti-proliferative effect on mesangial cells.[19] It has also been demonstrated to have anti-proliferative effect on smooth muscle endothelial cells.[20] This anti-proliferative effect may be mediated through inhibition of PDGF, a cytokine produced by the mesangial cell and is a potent growth factor for mesangial cells.[21, 22] Further work is in progress to determine if dipyridamole also inhibits mesangial cell contractility.

2. **Effects of low dose warfarin**

   Intraglomerular coagulation has been proposed as one of the factors causing glomerular injury in IgA Nx. Yamebe *et al.*[23]

demonstrated the presence of Hagmann factor in 68% of 31 patients with IgA Nx using a polyclonal antibody against Factor XII. They postulated that local activation of the contact coagulation factors in the glomeruli initiated intra-glomerular coagulation via the intrinsic coagulation systems as well as activating other mediators of inflammation such as kinins and plasmin. In another study by Tan and Woo,[24] plasma concentration of Hagemann factor, pre-kallikrein and high molecular weight kininogen were measured in 24 patients with IgA Nx and 123 normal controls. The plasma titres of all 3 factors measured were significantly lower in IgA Nx compared to controls suggesting activation of the contact coagulation system in IgA Nx.

In IgA Nx, 30% of patients have fibrin deposits within the glomeruli.[25] The above studies by Yamabe,[23] Tan and Woo,[24] and Woo *et al*'s previous documentation of high plasma anti-thrombin III levels in IgA Nx,[26] suggest local intra-vascular coagulation and endothelial cell injury. Warfarin, used in low dose for its anti-thrombotic effect may ameliorate this injury. Lee has also recently demonstrated that warfarin inhibits proliferation of mesangial cells in culture.

Lee and Woo have published the results of a controlled trial using dipyridamole and low dose warfarin in patients with IgA Nx and have shown that such treatment significantly retarded the progression of patients to ESRF.[14] There were 11 patients on treatment and 9 controls, all with renal impairment with serum creatinine ranging from 1.6 mg/dl to 3.0 mg/dl. At 10 months the serum creatinine was higher in the control group but not in the treatment group. At 3 years the findings were similar but 4 from the control group were in end stage renal failure with one in the treatment group. Proteinuria was decreased in the treatment group at 10 months but not in the control group. There was no difference in proteinuria at the end of the trial at 3 years in both groups. This trial has supported the rationale for therapy of patients with IgA Nx and confirmed the findings of an earlier controlled trial by Woo *et al*.[12]

In the earlier trial,[12] there were 27 patients on treatment and 21 controls. The treatment group was administered cyclophosphamide 1.5 mg/kg bw for 6 months, dipyridamole 300 mg/day and anti-thrombotic dose of warfarin (thrombotest 30% to 50% or INR of about 1.2 to 1.5) for 3 years. In the treatment group, serum creatinine remained unchanged and proteinuria decreased significantly, but in the control group, serum creatinine worsened significantly and proteinuria remained unchanged. Repeat renal biopsies after 3 years showed a worsening in the control group.[27] Both groups were followed up for another 5 years. Those still on treatment with dipyridamole and low dose warfarin (13 patients) had small rises in serum creatinine, but 6 among those who stopped therapy (14 patients) were in end stage renal failure with none in the group still on treatment.[12] It would appear that life long therapy is required to retard progression to end stage renal failure.

In the past, dipyridamole and low dose warfarin would be indicated for any of the following parameters: proteinuria >1 gm/day; hypertension; renal impairment; glomerulosclerosis >20% on renal biopsy; presence of even a single crescent; medial hyperplasia of blood vessels on biopsy. However, today with the advent of ARBs and anti-renin agents like Aliskiren, drugs such as dipyridamole and low dose warfarin would only be used if ARBs and anti-renin agents are not effective. Use of immunosuppressants like Prednisolone, CyA or MMF are indicated if patients have the Nephrotic Syndrome or develop crescents or present with Rapidly Progressive IgA nephritis or Malignant IgA nephritis.

Our department's guidelines for treatment of patients with IgA Nx with asymptomatic haematuria and proteinuria consist of control of systemic hypertension to BP of 130/80 mmHg and below, **use of ARBs for glomerular hyperfiltration, anti-renin agents like Aliskiren to block renin angiotensin system**, restricted protein diet (0.8 gm/Kg BW/day) to reduce macromolecular flux of high protein diet as well as to reduce afferent vasodilation in glomerular hyperfiltration, and control of serum cholesterol to prevent lipid induced glomerulosclerosis. A low salt diet is important for good BP control and also for effectivity of ARBs. Dipyridamole and low dose warfarin are useful in those who do not respond to ARBs and anti-renin agents.

With the view that in the long term, ARBs can also induce renofibrosis, one should combine the use of ARBs with Aliskiren to reduce the PRA and thereby remove the increased renin activity induced by the ARBs. Alternatively, one may start with 150 mg of Aliskiren and increase to 300 mg if necessary if proteinuria or renal dysfunction does not improve. ARB is added if Aliskiren does not control the situation. For those who have responded to ARBs and where proteinuria is minimal and renal function stable, one should consider withdrawal of ARBs and maintain only on Aliskiren. This will address the problem of ARBs inducing renofibrosis in the long term.

Diet induced hypercholesterolaemia may be the initiating factor for endothelial cell injury, especially low density lipoprotein (LDL) and very low density lipoprotein (VLDL). Lipoprotein can pass through damaged glomerular filter into the mesangium thereby enhancing the flux of macromolecules and giving rise to hyperperfusion injury.[28] In Japan where IgA nephritis is very common, a similar clinical guideline very close to the one that we are practising has been implemented nationwide in 1995 by a joint committee of the Ministry of Health and Welfare of Japan and the Japanese Society of Nephrology.[29]

For those patients with IgA Nx who have the Nephrotic Syndrome with selective proteinuria, they should be treated with prednisolone in a dose of 1 mg/kg BW for a month and then gradually tapering and tailing off by the end on 3 months. Those who do not respond to steroids can be given a course of cyclophosphamide at 2 mg/Kg BW. The above rationale for therapy is based on our studies on proteinuria involving protein selectivity[30] and iso-electric focussing[31] which showed that although the majority of patients with IgA Nx have diffuse mesangial proliferative glomerulonephritis, as long as they have selective proteinuria they will still respond to steroids. Other agents which are useful include CyA and Mycophenolate Mofetil.

Those patients who present with acute renal failure associated with more than 20% of crescents on renal biopsy should be offered pulse therapy with methyl prednisolone 0.5 gm daily for 3 successive days or 0.5 gm daily every other day for 6 doses over 12 days. After this, oral prednisolone is prescribed at 1 mg/kg BW with oral Cyclophosphamide or Cyclosporine A [CyA]. Prednisolone dosage should be reduced gradually over 6 months and stopped and Cyclophosphamide or CyA maintained at the same dose for 6 months and then stopped. Patients with rapidly progressive glomerulonephritis (more than 50% crescents on renal biopsy) should in addition have plasmapheresis during the first 3 to 4 weeks of therapy.

About 13% of our patients with IgA Nx have predominantly tubular interstitital lesions out of proportion to the degree of glomerular sclerosis. These patients should be treated with a low dose steroid regimen, 30 mg/day of prednisolone for two months, with gradual dose reduction to 10 mg/day by six months and then long term maintenance of 5 to 10 mg/day. This is to retard ischemic renal damage induced by fibrosis of the post capillary vessel of the glomerulus due to fibrosis of the adjacent tubulo-interstitium.

CONCLUSION

IgA nephritis as a vasculitides has similarities to diabetic nephropathy in that both diseases have mesangial proliferation and sclerosis and glomerular hyperfiltration injury which contribute to progressive disease. The current treatment protocol and strategies for both diseases are therefore very similar. Whilst there is no cure for both these types of kidney disease, such therapeutic measures serve to retard the progression to end stage renal failure. Future therapeutic strategies lie in immunomodulation using inhibitors of cytokines and possibly gene therapy.

Pathogenesis and Treatment of IgA Nephritis 62

REFERENCES FOR PATHOGENESIS
AND TREATMENT OF IGA NEPHRITIS:

1. Woo KT, Edmondson RPS, Wu AYT, Chiang GSC, Pwee HS, Lim CH. The natural history of IgA nephritis in Singapore. *Clin Nephrol* 1986, **25**:15–21.

2. Rocatello D, Picciotto G, Coppo R, Piccoli G, Molino A, Cacace G *et al.* Clearance of polymeric IgA aggregates in humans. *Am J Kidney Disease*, 1989, **14**:354–60.

3. Gallo GR, Caulin-Glaser T, Emancipator SN, Lamm SE. Nephritogenecity and differential distribution of glomerular immune complexes are related to immunogen charge. *Lab Invest* 1983; **48**: 353–361.

4. Woo KT, Lau YK, Lee GSL, Wong KS, Chin YM, Chiang GSC, Lim CH. Isoelectric focussing and protein selectivity index as predictors of response to therapy in IgA nephrotic syndrome. *Nephron* 1994, **67**:408–413.

5. Brensilver JN, Mallat S, Scholes J, Mc Cabe R. Recurrent IgA nephropathy in living related donor transplantation: recurrence or transmission of familial disease? *Am J Kidney Dis* 1988; **2**:147–151.

6. Rifai A, Chen A, Imai H. Complement activation in experimental IgA nephropathy: An antigen mediated process. *Kidney Int* 1987, **32**:838–844.

7. Clarkson AR, Woodroffe AJ, Aarons IA, Thompson T, Hale GM. Therapeutic options in IgA nephropathy. *Am J Kidney Dis* 1988, **12**:443–448.

8. Coppo R, Rocatello D, Amore A, Quattrocchio G, Molino A, Gianoglio B *et al.* Effects of gluten-free diet in primary IgA nephropathy. *Clin Nephrol* 1990, **33**:72–86.

9. Bene MC, De Ligny GH, Kessler M, Faure G. Confirmation by tonsillar anomalies in IgA nephropathy: a multicenter study. *Nephron*, 1991, **58**: 425–428.

10. Gesualdo L, Ricanati S, Hassan MO, Emancipator SN, Lamm ME. Enzymolysis of glomerular immune deposits in vivo with dextranase/protease ameliorates proteinuria, hematuria and mesangial proliferation in murine experimental IgA nephropathy. *J Clin Invest* 1990, **86**: 715–722.

11. Kobayashi Y, Yoshiyuki H, Kazufumi F, Kurokawa A, Tateno S. IgA nephropathy: Heterogenous clinical picture and steroid therapy in progressive cases. *Semin Nephrol* 1987, **7**: 382–385.

12. Woo KT, Lee GSL, Lau YK, Chiang GSC, Lim CH. Effects of triple therapy in IgA nephritis: A follow up study 5 years later. *Clin Nephrol* 1991, **36**: 60–66.

13. Lai KN, Lai FM. Short term controlled trial of cyclosporine A in IgA nephritis. Abstract, Second International Symposium on IgA Nephritis, Bari, Italy, 1987, pg 34.

14. Lee GSL, Woo KT, Lim CH. Controlled trial of dipyridamole and low dose warfarin in patients with IgA nephritis with renal impairment. *Clin Nephrol* 1989; **31**:276.

15. Woo KT, Lau YK, Wong KS, Chiang GSC. ACE/ATRA therapy decrease proteinuria by improving glomerular permselectivity in IgA nephritis. *Kidney Int* 2000, **58**:2485–2491.

16. Agrawal G. Antisense oligonucleotides: A possible approach for chemotherapy of AIDS. In: Eric Wichstrom, editor. Prospects for Antisense Nucleic Acid Therapy of Cancer and AIDS. New York, USA: Wiler-Liss, 1991:143–158.

17. Zamecnik PC, Stephenson ML. Inhibition of rous-sarcoma virus replication and cell transformation by a specific oligodeoxyribonucleotide. *Proc Nat Acad Sci USA* 1978; **75**:280–284.

18. Woo KT, Tan YO, Yap HK, Lau YK, Lim CH. Beta-thromboglobulin in mesangial IgA nephritis. *Thromb Res* 1981; **24**:259–262.

19. Lee GSL, Woo KT, Tan HB, Lim CH. Effects of Dipyridamole in Mesangial Cell Proliferation and Collagen Synthesis in Cultures of Rat Mesangial Cells. 28th Singapore-Malaysian Congress of Medicine, 1994, Abstract, pg 67(b).

20. Choong HL, Tan HB, Woo KT. Proliferation of vascular smooth muscle cells is attenuated by dipyridamole. 28th Singapore-Malaysian Congress of Medicine, 1994, Abstract, pg 67(a).

21. Silver BJ, Jaffer FE, Abboud HE. Platelet derived growth factor synthesis in mesangial cells: Induction by multiple peptide mitogens. *Proc Natl Acad Sci USA* 1989, **86**:1056.

22. Abboud HE: Resident glomerular cells in glomerular injury: Mesangial cells. *Semin Nephrol* 1991, **11**:304–310.

23. Yamabe H, Sugawara N, Ozawa K, Kubota H, Fukushi K, Kikuchi K, Onodera K. Glomerular deposition of Hagmann Factor in IgA nephritis. *Nephron* 1984 **37**:62–63.

24. Tan CC, Woo KT. Plasma contact coagulation factors in IgA nephritis. *Ann Acad Med S'pore* 1996, **25**: 218–221.

25. Woo KT, Chiang GSC, Lau YK, Lim CH. IgA nephritis in Singapore: Clinical, prognostic indices and therapy. *Semin Nephrol* 1987, **7**:379–381.
26. Woo KT, Lee EJC, Lau YK, Lim CH. Anti-thrombin III in mesangial IgA nephritis. *Thromb Res* 1985, **40**:483–487.
27. Woo KT, GSC Chiang, Lim CH. Follow up renal biopsies in IgA nephritic patients on triple therapy. *Clin Nephrol* 1987, **28**: 304–305.
28. Diamond JR, Karnovsky MJ. Focal and segmental glomerulosclerosis: Analogies to atherosclerosis. *Kidney Int* **1988**, 33:917–924.
29. Sakai H, Abe K, Kobayashi Y, Koyama A, Shigematsu H, Harada T *et al*. Clinical guidelines of IgA nephropathy. *Japanese J of Nephrol* 1995, **37**: 417–421.
30. Woo KT, Lau YK, Yap HK, Lee GSL, Chiang GSC, Lim CH. Protein selectivity: a prognostic index in IgA nephritis. *Nephron* 1989, **52**: 300–306.
31. Woo KT, Lau YK, Wong KS, Lee GSL, Chin YM, Chiang GSC, Lim CH. Iso electric focussing and selectivity index in IgA nephrotic syndrome. *Nephron* 1994, **67**: 408–413.
32. Woo KT, Lee GSL, Pall AA. Dipyridamole and low dose warfarin without cyclophosphamide in the management of IgA nephropathy. *Kidney Int* 2000, **57**:348–349.
33. KT Woo, CM Chan, HK Tan, HL Choong, M Foo, A Vathsala, EJC Lee, CC Tan, GSL Lee, SH Tan, CH Lim, GSC Chiang, S Fook-Chong, KS Wong Beneficial effects of high dose Losartan in IgA nephritis *Clinical Nephrol* 2009, **71**: 617–624.
34. KT Woo, CM Chan, HL Choong, HK Tan, M Foo, EJC Lee, CC Tan, GSL Lee, SH Tan, A Vathsala, CH Lim, GSC Chiang, S Fook-Chong, Y Zhao, HB Tan, KS Wong High dose Losartan and ACE gene polymorphism in IgA nephritis. *Genomics Medicine*, 2009, **2**:83–91.

REFERENCES FOR BENEFICIAL EFFECTS OF HIGH DOSE ARB:

1. Ruggenenti P, Perna A, Remuzzi G. ACE inhibitors to prevent end-stage renal disease: When to start and why possibly never to stop: A post hoc analysis of the REIN trial results. Ramipril Efficacy in Nephropathy. *J Am Soc Nephrol* 2001, **12**:2832–2837.
2. Parving HH, Lehnert H, Brochner-Mortensen J *et al*. The effect of irbesartan on the development of diabetic nephropathy in patients with type 2 diabetes. *N Engl J Med* 2001, **345**:870–878.

3. Remuzzi G, Remuzzi A. Is Regression of Chronic Nephropathies a Therapeutic Target? *J Am Soc Nephrol* 2005, **16**:840–842.

4. Rossing K, Schjoedt KJ, Jensen BR *et al.* Enhanced renoprotective effects of ultrahigh doses of irbesartan in patients with type 2 diabetes and microalbuminuria. *Kidney Int* 2005, **68**:1190–1198.

5. Mahmood J, Khan F, Okada S *et al.* Local delivery of angiotensin receptor blocker into the kidney ameliorates progression of experimental glomerulonephritis. *Kidney Int* 2006, **70**:1591–1959.

6. Hollenberg NK, Parving HH, Viberti G *et al.* Albuminuria response to very high-dose valsartan in type 2 diabetes mellitus. *Journal of Hypertension*, 2007, **25**:1921–1926.

7. Woo KT, Lau YK, Wong KS *et al.* ACEI/ATRA therapy decreases proteinuria by improving glomerular permselectivity in IgA nephritis. *Kidney Int* 2000, **58**:2485–2491.

8. Woo KT, Lau YK, Chan CM *et al.* ATRA therapy restores normal renal function and renal reserve and prevents renal failure. *Ann Acad Med S'pore* 2005, **34**:52–59.

9. Barnett A. Prevention of loss of renal function over time in patients with diabetic nephropathy. *Am J of Med* 2006, 119(5A), 405–475.

10. Remuzzi A, Gagliardini E *et al.* ACE inhibition reduces glomerulosclerosis and regenerates glomerular tissue in a model of progressive renal disease. *Kidney Int* 2006, **69**: 1124–1130.

11. Fogo AB. Can glomerulosclerosis be reversed? *Nature Clinical Practice Nephrology*, 2006, **2**(6):290–291.

12 Marinides GN, Groggel GC, Cohen AH *et al.* Enalapril and low protein reverse chronic puromycin amino-nucleoside nephropathy. *Kidney Int* 1990, **37**:749–757.

13. Adamczak M, Gross ML, Amann K *et al.* Reversal of glomerular lesions involves coordinated restructuring of glomerular microvasculature. *J Am Soc Nephrol* 2004, **15**:3063–3072.

14. Ma LJ, Nakamura S, Aldigier JC *et al.* Regression of glomerulosclerosis with high-dose angiotension inhibition is linked to decreased plaminogen activator inhibitor-1. *J Am Soc Nephrol* 2005; **16**:966–976.

15. Ruggenenti P, Perna A, Benini R *et al.* In chronic nephropathies prolonged ACE inhibition can induce remission: dynamics of time-dependent changes in GFR. Investigators of the GISEN Group. Gruppo Italiano Studi Epidemiologici in Nefrologia. *J Am Soc Nephrol* 1999, **10**:997–1006.

16. Aranda P, Segura J, Ruilope LM *et al*. Long term renoprotective effects of standard versus high doses of telmisartan in hypertensive nondiabetic nephropathies. *Am J Kidney Dis* 2005, **46**:1074–1079.
17. Ballardie FW. Quantitative appraisal of treatment options for IgA nephropathy. *J Am Soc Nephrol* 2007, **18**(11): 2806–2809.
18. Praga M, Gutierrez E, Gonzalez E *et al*. Treatment of IgA nephritis with ACE inhibitors: A ramdomised and controlled trial. *J Am Soc nephrol* 2003, **14**: 1578–1583.

CHAPTER 8

The Geography and Evolution of Glomerulonephritis

This chapter on the Evolutionary Geography of Glomerulonephritis compares the changing prevalence of Primary Glomerulonephritis (GN) in Singapore over 3 decades with that of other countries in Asia and other parts of the world. It traces the evolution of the pattern of GN in Singapore as its economy develops over the past 30 years from 1976 to 2008, growing from a third world country to a more developed nation. In third world countries most forms of GN are related to exposure to microbial, parasitic and viral infections, in contrast to more developed countries where the antigenic exposure may be related to the diet, allergens and other industrial agents.[1-3]

We had previously reported in the 1st decade that the commonest form of GN was Mesangial Proliferative GN.[3] This was related to infection: bacterial, parasitic and viral. In the 2nd decade, the pattern had evolved to one where the commonest GN was still related to an infective agent though to a lesser extent and this would explain the decreased incidence of Mesangial Proliferative GN. Minimal Change Disease unlike in the West[4] was still very common but there was a rising incidence of Membranous GN in keeping with preponderance of Membranous GN in the West. In this chapter, with data for the 3rd decade, we can compare the changing trends in Mesangial Proliferative GN, IgA Nephritis (IgA Nx), Membranous GN and Focal and Segmental Glomerulosclerosis (FSGS) and in particular, evaluate whether the overall trend is in keeping with that observed in the Asian countries and the more

131

developed Western countries, especially with regards to Focal and Segmental Glomerular Sclerosis (FSGS) which is fast becoming a very common form of GN among the developed nations.[5] We also attempt to document whether the Asian pattern of GN in Singapore, derived from a common origin in this part of the world is still present despite recent economic and social development in the surrounding countries.

This chapter describes the evolving pattern of Primary GN in a population not affected by any significant immigration or change in racial make-up over the past 30 years. A Renal Biopsy Registry was established 30 years ago. Since then we have documented 3 decades of changes over the 1st, 2nd and 3rd decade (1978–1988, 1988–1998, 1998–2008) which parallel the development of the nation from the days of early independence where a significant proportion of the population was housed in wooden (attap) and zinc roofed homes. With the introduction of urbanized living in Housing Development Board Apartments, 3 decades ago, the transition from a rural to semi-urban and totally urbanized living today, the pattern of Primary GN has undergone much transformation in synchrony with improvement in socio-economic conditions. As the country becomes a developed nation with modern amenities compared to its earlier 3rd world environment the pattern of GN has also evolved in keeping with other forms of diseases prevalent in modern city living.

RENAL BIOPSY REGISTRY

The renal biopsy procedure was performed using a modified Vim Silverman needle and from 1987 using a Tru-Cut biopsy needle with ultrasound guidance. Specimens were prepared for light microscopy (L/M) and immunofluorescence (IMF) and where sufficient material was available electron microscopy (E/M) studies were performed. Specimens containing less than 5 glomeruli were not included in the study.

The Classification of GN (World Health Organisation, Collaborating Centre for the Histological Classification of Renal Diseases) used in this paper is similar to that adopted by Renal Biopsy Registries worldwide and this has not changed significantly during the past 3 decades and will allow ease of comparison of biopsy data among various countries.[6]

The present data do not purport to be an incidence study as our statistics are an underestimate of the true incidence of GN in the population since we do not have a population screening programme to detect silent cases of GN. This chapter only documents the prevalence of various subsets of Primary GN in Singapore. The population of Singapore was 2.7 millions in 1986, 3.7 millions in 1997 and 4.8 millions in 2008. Allowing for the lowest incidence of Primary GN in Singapore, the annual incidence of Primary GN in Singapore is 4.6 in 100,000/year (1976–1986), 1.7 in 100,000/year (1987–1997) and 1.6 in 100,000/year (1998–2008). There was a marked decline in the renal biopsy incidence rates between the 1st decade and the 2nd and 3rd decades due to a change in the indications for renal biopsies. In the 1st decade, patients with urine RBC persistently greater than 20 per high power field and or those with proteinuria of more than 0.2 gram a day were biopsied. But a review of these patients revealed that majority of them had very mild glomerular lesions with no significant glomerulosclerosis. So from the 2nd decade onwards the renal biopsy criteria were changed to include only those with urine RBC persistently greater than 100 per high-power field and or proteinuria more than 1 gram a day.

These indications have since not changed over the past 2 decades but the change in biopsy policy from the 2nd decade onwards accounted for the decreased number of biopsies done in the 2nd and 3rd decade. Even though the majority of patients affected would be those with IgA nephritis who presented with asymptomatic haematuria and proteinuria, the prevalence of IgA nephritis remained at 42%, 45% and 40% during the 1st, 2nd and 3rd decade respectively. Perhaps the prevalence of IgA nephritis may have shown an increase in the subsequent 2nd and 3rd decade if the biopsy criteria were the same throughout the 3 decades. Another category which could be affected were those patients with Mesangial Proliferative GN where the prevalence was 32%, 17% and 7% during the 1st, 2nd and 3rd decade respectively. But since the indication for biopsy in the 2nd and 3rd decade were the same, the decrease from 17% to 7% represented a true decrease in the prevalence of Mesangial Proliferative GN.

During the period 1976 to 2008 spanning a period of 32 years, 2586 renal biopsies were performed. To enable us to observe whether the pattern of GN had changed, patients were divided into 3 decades from 1976 to 1986 (1st decade, D1) comprising 1286 patients; from 1987 to 1997 (2nd decade, D2) comprising 816 patients and from 1998 to 2008 (3rd decade, D3) comprising 1195 patients.

Among the 1286 patients in the 1st decade, 1127 (88%) had primary GN and 159 (12%) had secondary GN. In the 2nd decade, among 816 patients, 666 (82%) had primary GN and 150 (18%) had secondary GN. In the 3rd decade, among 1195 patients in the 3rd decade, 786 (65%) had primary GN and 409 (35%) had secondary GN. The indications for biopsy for secondary GN have also changed in the 3rd decade as there are now more patients with lupus nephritis who were biopsied prior to therapy with the newer immunomodulating drugs like cyclosporine A and mycophenolic acid mofetil. Patients with diabetic nephropathy were also biopsied if they had associated microscopic haematuria in order to exclude other forms of concommittant GN which could be amenable to therapy. These would explain why more patients with secondary GN were biopsied in the 3rd decade compared to the earlier two decades.

RENAL BIOPSY DATA FROM SINGAPORE

Table 1 shows that the commonest histopathological diagnosis was IgA Nephritis, 42% in the first decade, 45% in the second

Table 8.1 Primary Glomerulonephritis: Histological Presentation over 3 decades

	Histology	1st Decade (D1)	2nd Decade (D2)	3rd Decade (D3)	p (χ^2) D1 vs D2 vs D3	p (χ^2) D2 vs D3
1	Minimal Change	97 (9%)	87 (13%)	151 (19%)	<0.000001	<0.002
2	Focal Global Sclerosis	72 (6%)	83 (12%)	31 (4%)	<0.000001	<0.000001
3	Mesangial Proliferative Glomerulonephritis	357 (32%)	112 (17%)	55 (7%)	<0.000001	<0.000001
4	IgA Nephritis	473 (42%)	300 (45%)	316 (40%)	0.17	0.07
5	Focal & Segmental Glomerulosclerosis	57 (5%)	41 (6%)	115 (15%)	<0.000001	<0.000001
6	Membranous Glomerulonephritis	38 (3%)	42 (6%)	90 (11%)	<0.000001	<0.001
7	Crescenteric Glomerulonephritis	5 (1%)	1 (1%)	8 (1%)	0.07	0.08
8	Others	28 (2%)	0	20 (3%)	<0.0002	<0.0001
	Total	1127 (100%)	666 (100%)	786 (100%)		

decade and 40% in the third decade. Mesangial Proliferative GN (Non IgA) was the second commonest cause of Primary GN in the first decade (32%) but has steadily declined to 17% in the second decade and only 7% in the third decade ($p < 0.000001$). This decrease in the 3rd decade of Mesangial Proliferative GN was accompanied by a significant increase in Minimal Change ($p < 0.000001$), Focal Segmental Glomerulosclerosis (FSGS) ($p < 0.000001$) and Membranous GN ($p < 0.001$) compared to the 1st and 2nd decade. In both FSGS and Membranous GN in the 3rd decade there was a 2 folds increase compared to the 2nd decade: FSGS (6% versus 15%) and Membranous GN (6% versus 11%) in the 2nd and 3rd decade ($p < 0.000001$ and <0.001 respectively). Cresenteric GN was uncommon, accounting for less than 1% in each decade. There was no documentation for ANCA related Crescenteric GN in the 1st decade. In the 2nd decade, 1 patient was negative for ANCA and in the 3rd decade, among the 8 patients with Crescenteric GN, 4 were positive for c-ANCA and another 2 for p-ANCA. Secondary causes for GN were excluded in all patients.

RENAL BIOPSY DATA FROM OTHER COUNTRIES

Table 2 presents renal biopsy data from 28 countries worldwide and in 21 countries there are available data to enable readers to study the pattern of renal biopsies between 2 periods, at the beginning and about 30 years later to allow a comparison of the data in the individual country as well as comparison with other countries. It provides an analysis of evolving trends among the various countries and the surrounding regions. The data also show the common features in histological profile among Asian countries in contrast to others in the East as well as the West. We have presented a comprehensive table and have incorporated as much data as we can from the original publications in Nephrology Journals during the past 30 years. Based on data in the various papers from different countries we have focused on

Table 8.2 An Overview of the Prevalence (%) of Primary Glomerulonephritis in 28 Countries

COUNTRY	Ref No.	Author	Period (year)	Number of Biopsies	MCD (%)	MesPN (%)	IgAN (%)	MN (%)	FSGS (%)	MesCN (%)	Others (%)	Total (%)
AUSTRALIA	19	Clarkson AR	1976–1978	623	6	18	23	8	7	5	33	100
	20	Painter D	1986–1993	634	3	16	37	13	15	3	14	100
	21	Briganti EM	1995–1997	1147	6		49	15	21	3	6	100
AUSTRIA	49	Kronenberg F	1980–1990	449	13	14	12	6	6	3	47	100
BRAZIL	30	Bahiense	1979–1999	943			12	15	30	12	33	100
	31	Mazzarolo	1990–1993	206	5		10	20	43	14	7	100
	33	Malafronte P	1999–2005	1131	9	4	18	21	30		19	100
CHINA	7	Li LS	1980–1985	8852	5	20	15	7	11	7	34	100
	40	Chen H	1979–2000	7101	1	30	40	10	6	7	7	100
	24	Li LS	1979–2002	9278	1	26	45	10	6		12	100
CZECH	50	Rychlik I	1994–2000	2217	13	11	35	9	11		22	100
DENMARK	51	Heaf J	1985–1997	2380	18	26		12	14	5	26	100
FRANCE	14	Simon P	1976–1985	663	10		27	12	12	6	45	100
	38	Simon P	1976–1980	179	13	5	29	12	12		28	100
			1981–1985	170	10	6	36	18	12		19	100
			1986–1990	131	11	7	37	25	6		15	100
HONG KONG	8	Ng WL	1974–1978	215	21	10	8	11	15	9	26	100
	37	Chan KW	1993–1997	871	14	11	39	13	10	4	8	100

(Continued)

Table 8.2   (Continued)

COUNTRY	Ref No.	Author	Period (year)	Number of Biopsies	MCD (%)	MesPN (%)	IgAN (%)	MN (%)	FSGS (%)	MesCN (%)	Others (%)	Total (%)
HUNGARY	52	Sipiczki T	1990–2002	798	8		15	14	7		56	100
INDIA	53	Chugh KS	1964–1973	369	23	14		20	1	20	23	100
	34	Narasimhan B	1986–2002	3845	16		12	14	24		34	100
	42	N Balakrishnan	1990–2001	2673	18	12	14	16	28		12	100
INDONESIA	54	Sidabutar RP	1976–1980	94	10	33		6	6	7	37	100
	9	Sidabutar RP	1985–1986	459	16	35		4	7		38	100
IRAN	55	Antonovych TT	1981–1994	623	13	2	12	18	8		47	100
	15	A. Emami Naini	1998–2001	364	11	3	15	26	12		34	100
ITALY	16	Schena FP	1987–1993	8287	8		35	21	12		25	100
	22	Stratta P	1970–1979	449	5		15	14	11		55	100
			1980–1989	840	5		27	22	8		38	100
			1990–1994	637	8		32	23	9		29	100
JAPAN	10	No author	1980–1985	1850	16	15	27	11	6	4	21	100
	25	Honma M	1976–1985	622	6	34	44	7	4	2	3	100
			1986–1995	397	6	32	46	8	5	2	1	100
			1996–2000	290	8	16	51	8	9		8	100
KOREA	11	Choi IJ	1973–1988	1412	40	10	29	13	4		5	100
	27	Choi IJ	1973–1995	1732	32	6	27	14	6		15	100
			1988–1995	1561	34	1	29	16	9		12	100
KUWAIT	41	Chang JH	1987–2006	1346	21		38	17	8	5	11	100
	35	El-Reshaid W	1995–2001	584	13		8	5	18		56	100

(Continued)

Table 8.2 (*Continued*)

COUNTRY	Ref No.	Author	Period (year)	Number of Biopsies	MCD (%)	MesPN (%)	IgAN (%)	MN (%)	FSGS (%)	MesCN (%)	Others (%)	Total (%)
MACEDONIA	56	Polenakovic MH	1975–2001	716	7	4	12	14	10		53	100
MALAYSIA	12	Prathap K/Looi M	1970–1981	1000	26	25		6	5		39	100
	28	Looi LM	1982–1991	1000	21	16	19	6	3		36	100
	29	Khoo JJ	1994–2000	281	41	15	14	6	7		16	100
PERU	36	Hurtado A	1985–1995	731	6	15	2	20	24	4	30	100
PORTUGAL	57	Carvalho E	1977–2003	1030	14	17	31	11	7	5	15	100
RUSSIA	58	Varshavskii VA	1978–1983	852	7	56		9	11	10	8	100
	43	Varshavskii VA	1970–1999	2746	6	49		13	8	18	6	100
SAUDI ARAB	32	Mitwalli AH	1989–1994	147	1	21	13	13	41	11		100
	44	Mitwalli AH	1994–1999	127	9	25	10	4	35	16	2	100
SINGAPORE	3	Woo KT	1976–1986	1127	9	32	42	3	5		9	100
	4	Woo KT	1987–1997	666	13	17	45	6	6		13	100
	Unpublished data	Woo KT	1998–2008	786	19	7	40	11	15		8	100
SPAIN	59	Rivera F	1994–1999	4824	10		24	14	15		37	100
	39	Rivera F	1994–2001	4157	10	5	14	13	11		49	100
THAILAND	13	Boonpuck V	1972–1974	572		40		5	10	1	45	100
	26	Parichatica P	1982–2005	2154		46	18	16		5	15	100
	60	Kanjanabuch T	2001–2004	506			31	13	25		31	100

(*Continued*)

Table 8.2   (*Continued*)

COUNTRY	Ref No.	Author	Period (year)	Number of Biopsies	MCD (%)	MesPN (%)	IgAN (%)	MN (%)	FSGS (%)	MesCN (%)	Others (%)	Total (%)
UNITED ARAB	18	Yahya TM	1978–1996	490	18		6	20	18		37	100
UNITED KINGDOM	61	Cameron JS	1972–1973	746	32	15		9	6	14	23	100
	62	Davison AM	1978–1984	2806	18	19	14	11	6	5	28	100
	17	Hanko JB	1976–2005	903	10		39	29	6	10	7	100
UNITED STATES OF AMERICA	45	Braden GL	1975–1979	73	4		11	38	14	4	29	100
			1980–1984	96	7		25	23	9	8	27	100
			1985–1989	143	11		13	20	10	5	41	100
			1990–1994	304	11		11	15	25	9	30	100
	5	Dragovic D	1986–2002	208	9		27	17	38		9	100
	23	Swaminathan S	1994–2003	195	5	12	25	10	20	8	20	100

Abbreviation:

Ref No:	Reference Number in the reference list	IgAN:	IgA Nephritis
Period:	Period (year) in which renal biopsies were performed	MN:	Membranous Glomerulonephritis
MCD:	Minimal Change Disease	FSGS:	Focal Segemental Glomerulosclerosis
MesPN:	Mesangial Proliferative Glomerulonephritis	MesCN:	Mesangial Capillary Glomerulonephritis

the various Primary GN, removing Secondary GN (like lupus nephritis and diabetic nephropathy) from the total numbers biopsied in order to obtain comparable data for various types of Primary GN. Most countries had included IgA Nephritis as a separate group of Primary GN. All the other Mesangial Proliferative GN that were non IgA Nephritis were classified as Mesangial Proliferative GN. A few countries however, grouped IgA Nephritis under Mesangial Proliferative GN in the initial years but subsequently in later years also had separate categories for IgA Nephritis and Mesangial Proliferative GN. These countries also have a high prevalence of IgA Nephritis and are mainly in the Asian region.

Some countries have a separate group classified under Mesangiocapillary GN (MCGN) as it is still prevalent in their population, whilst other countries have very few patients with MCGN, like Singapore (<1%) and have included them under "Others". Where MCGN is separately classified as MCGN we have included this as a separate heading named MCGN. Those countries with high prevalence of MCGN usually have low prevalence of Mesangial Proliferative GN. Both MCGN and Mesangial Proliferative GN are related to infections. Post Infectious GN or Diffuse Endocapillary GN is very uncommon in many countries and their biopsy registries do not classify such biopsies as a separate group and in the few that do so we have included these under "Others" as well. As far as possible we have strived towards the presentation of data which would enable us to make appropriate comparisons for the distribution of Primary GN among the various countries.

Figures 1–4 show the various countries from among the 17 countries where there were significant changing trends in the prevalence for Mesangial Proliferative GN [decreasing prevalence], IgA Nephritis [increasing prevalence], Membranous GN [increasing prevalence] and Focal and Segmental Glomerulosclerosis [increasing prevalence].

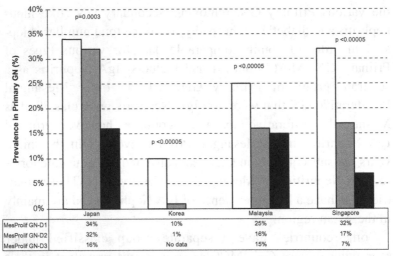

MesProlif GN: Mesangial Proliferative Glomerulonephritis (non-IgAN)

p<0.05 as significance for comparison of prevalence (%) of decade 1(D1) vs decade 2(D2) vs decade 3(D3) for each country.

Fig. 8.1   Countries with significant changing trends of Mesangial proliferative GN (Non-IgAN) over the past 3 decades

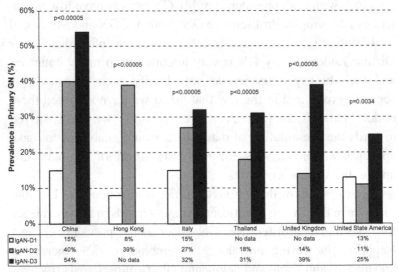

IgAN: IgA Nephritis

p<0.05 as significance for comparison of prevalence (%) of decade1(D1) vs decade2(D2) vs decade3(D3) for each country.

Fig. 8.2   Countries with significant changing trends of IgA Nephritis over the past 3 decades

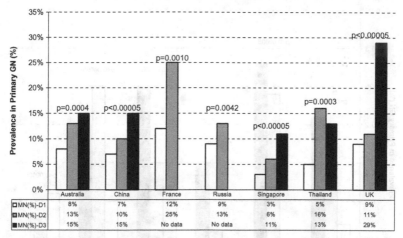

MN: Membranous Nephropathy

$p<0.05$ as significance for comparison of prevalence (%) among decade1(D1) vs decade2(D2) vs decade3(D3) for each country.

Fig. 8.3 Countries with significant changing trends of Membranous Nephropathy over the past 3 decades

THE FIRST DECADE

In Singapore we have documented 3 decades of renal biopsy data, the 1st decade shows IgA Nephritis as the most common GN (42%) with Mesangial Proliferative GN as the 2nd most common (32%). Comparing these data with that of the surrounding Asian Countries, the preponderance of IgA Nephritis and Mesangial Proliferative GN is consistent with countries like China,[7] Hong Kong,[8] Indonesia,[9] Japan,[10] Korea,[11] Malaysia,[12] Singapore[3–4] and Thailand[13] (Table 2). However, in Singapore, Mesangial Proliferative GN has been steadily decreasing as mentioned earlier ($p < 0.000001$) but IgA nephritis has always been the most common GN. In general, countries in the Asian region with a high prevalence of Mesangial Proliferative GN also have a high prevalence of IgA Nephritis.

In contrast, when compared to the Western countries like France,[14] Iran,[15] Italy,[16] UK[17] and United Arab Emirates,[18] Membranous GN seems more prevalent in these countries

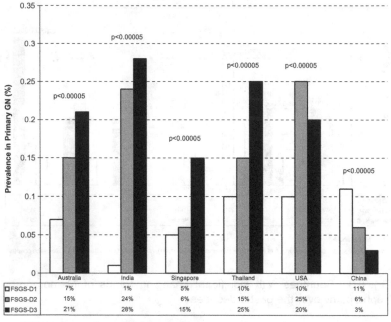

	Australia	India	Singapore	Thailand	USA	China
☐ FSGS-D1	7%	1%	5%	10%	10%	11%
◪ FSGS-D2	15%	24%	6%	15%	25%	6%
■ FSGS-D3	21%	28%	15%	25%	20%	3%

FSGS: Focal Segmental Glomerulosclerosis

p<0.05 as significance for comparison of prevalence (%) of decade1(D1) vs decade2(D2) vs decade3(D3) for each country.

Fig. 8.4. Countries with significant changing trends of Focal Segmental Glomerulosclerosis over the past 3 decades

(Table 2). A country like Australia[19-21] has a very high prevalence of IgA Nephritis and relatively less patients with Membranous GN compared to other Western countries like UK[17] and Italy[22] even though it is a Western country. This could reflect the Asian immigrants in the population. This trend is also seen in the USA[23] where recent data show the decrease in those with Membranous GN and an increase in IgA Nephritis (Table 2). The high prevalence of IgA Nephritis in some countries, just as the low prevalence in others could also reflect their policy of biopsying more patients with Asymptomatic Haematuria and Proteinuria in contrast to those which biopsy relatively less patients with Asymptomatic Haematuria and Proteinuria.

THE SECOND DECADE

In the 2nd decade, in Singapore, there is a relative decrease in patients with Mesangial Proliferative GN associated with an increase in those with Membranous GN. Mesangial Proliferative GN is still prevalent in Asian countries like China,[24] Japan[25] and Thailand[26] coexisting with low prevalence of Membranous GN and FSGS (Table 2). But in Japan,[25] Korea[27] and Malaysia[12,28-29] the prevalence of Mesangial Proliferative GN is also decreasing like in Singapore. However, in Singapore[3-4] the prevalence of Mesangial Proliferative GN has decreased and there is an observed increase in prevalence of FSGS which is not seen in Japan[25] Korea[27] and Malaysia[12,28-29] (Table 2). In some countries like Brazil,[30-31] Saudi Arabia[32] and USA[23] during this period the increased prevalence of FSGS is already well documented (Table 2).

THE THIRD DECADE

By the 3rd decade (Table 2), there appears to be a wide spread increased prevalence of FSGS in Australia,[21] Brazil,[30-31] India,[34] Kuwait,[35] Peru,[36] Saudi Arabia,[32] United Arab[18] and the USA.[5,23] But in the surrounding Asian countries like China,[24] Hong Kong,[37] Japan,[10] Korea[11] and Malaysia[28] the prevalence of FSGS is still relatively low. In Singapore, the prevalence has risen dramatically. However in countries like France,[38] Spain[39] and UK[17] the prevalence of FSGS is also relatively low (Table 2). Probably, multiple factors influence the varying trends of occurrence of FSGS in different countries.

Factors Influencing the Prevalence of Glomerulonephritis

The prevalence of primary glomerulonephritis in various countries throughout the world varies depending on the genetic profile of the population as well as their environmental exposure, hence the different patterns of glomerulonephritis amongst the various countries. As the countries evolve, the social environment and other factors in these countries may also change in keeping with improvement in living and other conditions and these changes may explain why the patterns of glomerulonephritis change over a period of time, some of this may be in response to environmental antigens though in reality there are many and varying factors in each country which influence the pattern of glomerulonephritis. Among these many factors, one of the factors which may influence the pattern of glomerulonephritis in various countries could be the Hygiene Hypothesis.[1-2] Overcrowding and poor hygiene in early life according to this hypothesis may protect from atopic diseases because exposure to microbes favours the development of a T helper 1 (Th1) dominant response. On the other hand, dominance of a T helper 2 (Th2) subset would be responsible for increasing incidence of allergies. The allergens involved could be from the diet, other putative antigens as well as those from industrialized environment in the more developed countries. The Hygiene Hypothesis proposes that early and frequent exposure to bacterial and other antigen occurring in less developed or developing countries leads to a Th1 phenotype response but better public hygiene and less infections lead to a Th2 phenotype response with increased risk for developing allergies.[1,2] These same authors[1,2] have reviewed the prevalence of glomerulonephritis in relation to the Hygiene Hypothesis and explained why certain types of glomerulonephritis like Membranoproliferative GN and Mesangial Proliferative GN are associated with poorer or developing countries (Th1 dominance) whereas Membranous GN, Minimal Change Disease and IgA nephritis are more common in industrialized countries (Th2 dominance).

As shown from the data on the 3 decades of Renal Biopsy in Singapore, one of the factors which may play a role in the evolutionary pattern of Glomerulonephritis in the population could be the socio-economic change affecting the country. This is a trend reflecting the degree of development of the nation with a population living in less developed housing facilities in the early years with exposure to parasitic, bacterial and other infective agents predisposing to Mesangial Prolififerative GN consistent with the Hygiene Hypothesis.[1,2] This would be true in Asian countries like China,[40] Japan,[10] Indonesia,[9] Malaysia,[28] Thailand[26] and Singapore[3] which have a high prevalence of Mesangial Proliferative GN (Tables 2). In some countries like Japan[10], Korea,[41] Malaysia[28] and Singapore[3] the prevalence of Mesangial Proliferative GN is already decreasing in keeping with urbanization and better housing and other amenities in these countries.

With subsequent resettlement of the people into improved living facilities with GN resulting from infections by parasites and bacteria slowly declining, but with a rise in the exposure to various types of dietary and other industrial allergens, we now witness a rising prevalence of Membranous GN (which has a T Helper 2 dominance) in these countries.

In countries like France,[38] India,[42] Italy,[22] Russia[43] and Saudi Arabia[44] there is still a relatively high prevalence of Mesangiocapillary GN (MCGN) possibly due to infections (T Helper 1 response) as in the case of countries with high prevalence of Mesangial Proliferative GN mentioned in Asian countries above. In India,[42] Post Infectious GN due to streptococcal infections used to be prevalent and this could account for the high incidence of MCGN in India as MCGN could also result from Post Infectious GN. With urbanization in these countries the incidence of MGCN is declining thro' the years.

In the 3rd decade, data from Singapore and other countries show that the prevalence of Mesangial Proliferative GN has decreased (Table 2) and in its place Membranous GN and FSGS have become prevalent. The increased prevalence of FSGS has been documented in many countries like Brazil[31], India[42], Kuwait[35], Peru[36], Saudi Arabia[32], United Arab[18] and USA[45] (Table 2). This is related to the increasing number of patients with obesity, diabetes mellitus and smoking, a pattern representing the rising affluence in these countries where FSGS represents the changing lifestyle of fast food and unhealthy diets predisposing to diseases like obesity and diabetes mellitus.

Apart from geographical and socioeconomic changes, ancestral or genetic influences also play a significant role in predisposing people to certain types of GN. FSGS has been found to have a racial predilection; African-Americans are more prone to development of FSGS compared to Whites.[46] They have a 4 fold increased risk for sporadic FSGS compared to Whites. Individuals of African ancestry also have an increased risk for FSGS in other geographic regions suggesting that genetic factors contribute to this predilection.[47] McKenzie's paper has suggested that genetic variation or mutation of the NPHS2 gene may play a role in sporadic FSGS in adults.[48]

CONCLUSION

With urbanisation and socio-economic changes and less exposure to parasitic and other infestations, the prevalence of primary glomerulonephritis in Asia and other less developed countries is changing. Antigenic exposure due to lifestyle, geographical location as well as dietary antigen are significant contributory factors which predispose to the various glomerulonephritis. The rise in prevalence of FSGS may reflect aging and obesity. Therefore apart from the geographical and genetic influence, other socio-economic factors also exert an influence on the evolution and hence the prevalence of various types of glomerular diseases in many countries. The conclusion is that the prevalence of Primary Glomerulonephritis is different all over the world because of various factors like genetics and race, environmental antigen and allergens including those of dietary and industrial origin which can all influence the pattern of glomerulonephritis.

REFERENCES

1. Abdias Hurtado, Richard J Johnson. Hygiene hypothesis and prevalence of glomerulonephritis. *Kidney International*, 2005; **68**: S62–S67.
2. Richard J Johnson, Abdias Hurtado, Justin Merszel, *et al.* Hypothesis: Dysregulation of Immunologic Balance Resulting From Hygiene and Socioeconomic Factors May Influence the Epidemiology and Cause of Glomerulonephritis Worldwide. *Am J Kidney Dis* 2003, **42**(3):575–581.
3. Woo KT, Chiang GCS, Edmonson RPS, *et al.* Glomerulonephritis in Singapore. *Ann Acad Med Singapore*, 1986, **15**:20–31.
4. Woo KT, Chiang GSC, Pall A, *et al.* The changing pattern of glomerulonephritis in Singapore over the past two decades. *Clin Nephrol* 1999, **52**:96–102.
5. Dragovic D, Rosenstock JL, Wahl SJ, *et al.* Increasing incidence of focal segmental glomerulosclerosis and an examination of demographic patterns. *Clin Nephrol* 2005, **63**:1–7.
6. Churg J. Renal Disease: Classification and Atlas of glomerular diseases. prepared by the World Health Organisation, Collaborating Centre for the Histological Classification of Renal Diseases. 1987, New York, Igaku-Shoin.
7. Li LS. Renal Disease in China: An Overview. KT Woo, AYT Wu, CH Lim (Eds.), Proc 3rd Asian Pacific Congress of Nephrology, Singapore, 1986, Pg 292–296.
8. Ng WL, Chan WC. Primary Glomerular Disease in Adult Chinese in Hong Kong. K Oshima, T Takeuchi (Eds.), Sasaki Printing and Publishing Co Ltd, Sendai, Japan. Proc 3rd Colloquium in Nephrology, Tokyo, 1979. pp 65–68.
9. Sidabutar RP. Glomerulonephritis in Indonesia. Proc 3rd Asian Pacific Congress on Nephrology, Singapore, 1986, Pg 282–291.
10. No author, Nationwide and long term survey of primary glomerulonephritis in Japan as observed in 1,850 biopsied cases. Research Group on Progressive Chronic Renal Disease. *Nephron*, 1999, **82**(3):205–213.
11. Choi IJ, Jeong HJ, Han DS, *et al.* An Analysis of 2361 Cases of Renal Biopsy in Korea. *Yonsei Medical Journal*, 1991, **32**(1):9–15.
12. Prathap K, Looi LM. Morphological patterns of glomerular disease in renal biopsies from 1000 Malaysian patients. *Ann Acad Med Singapore*, 1982, **11**:52–56.

13. Boonpucknavig V, Boonpucknavig S. Glomerular diseases in Thailand: Incidence, histology, immunopathology of renal biopsies in 500 cases. Proc of the Asian Colloquium in Nephrology, Singapore, 1974. *Ann Acad Med Singapore*, 1975, **4**(2):45.

14. Simon P, Ramee MP, Ang KS, Cam G. Course of the annual incidence of primary glomerulopathies in a population of 400,000 inhabitants over a 10-year period (1976–1985). *Nephrologie*, 1986, **7**(5):185–189.

15. Emami A, Amini Hatandi A, Ossareh S, *et al*. The relative frequency, Clinical and laboratory findings of Adult Glomerulonephritidies in Tehran. *Journal of Research in Medical Sciences*, 2006, **11**(2):87–92.

16. Schena FP and the Italian Group of Renal Immunopathology. Survey of the Italian Registry of Renal Biopsies. Frequency of the renal diseases for 7 consecutive years. *Nephrol Dial Transpl*, 1997, **12**(3):418–426.

17. Hanko JB, Mullan RN, O'Rourke DM, *et al*. Changing pattern of adult primary glomerular disease. *Nephrol Dial Transplant*, 2009, **24**(10):3050–3054.

18. Yahya TM, Pingle A, Boobes Y, *et al*. Analysis of 409 kidney biopsies: Data from the United Arab Emirates renal diseases Registry. *J Nephrol* 1998, **11**:148–150.

19. Clarkson AR, Mathew TH, Seymour AE, *et al*. Frequency and Morbidity of Renal Disease in an Australian Community. Proc 1st Asian Pacific Cong Nephrol 1979; pp 152–157. Tokyo, Japan.

20. Painter D, Clouston D, Ahn E, *et al*. The pattern of glomerular disease in New Caledonia: Preliminary findings. *Pathology*, 1996, **28**:32–35.

21. Briganti EM, Dowling J, Finlay M, *et al*. The incidence of biopsy proven glomerulonephritis in Australia. *Nephrol Dial Transplant*, 2001, **16**:1364–1367.

22. Stratta P, Giuseppe P, Caterina C, *et al*. Incidence of Biopsy-proven Primary Glomerulonephritis in an Italian Province. *Am J Kidney Dis* 1996, **27**(5):631–639.

23. Sundararaman S, Nelson Leung, Donna J, *et al*. Changing incidence of Glomerular disease in Olmsted County, Minnesota: A 30-year Renal Biopsy Study. *Clin J Am Soc Nephrol* 2006, **1**:483–487.

24. Li LS, Liu ZH. Epidemiologic data of renal diseases from a single unit in China: Analysis based on 13,519 renal biopsies. *Kidney Int* 2004, **66**(3):920–930.

25. Honma M, Toyoda M, Umezono T, *et al*. An investigation of 2093 renal biopsies performed at Tokai University Hospital between 1976 and 2000. *Clinical Nephrology*, 2008, **69**(1):18–23.

26. Parichatikanond P, Chawanasuntorapoj R, Shayakul C, *et al.* An analysis of 3,555 cases of renal biopsy in Thailand. *J Med Assoc Thai*, 2006 **89**(suppl 2): S106–S111.

27. Choi IJ, Jeong HJ, Han DS, *et al.* An analysis of 4,514 cases of renal biopsy in Korea. *Yonsei Med J* 2001, **42**(2): 247–54.

28. Looi LM. The pattern of renal disease in Malaysia. *Malays J Pathol* 1994, **16**(1):19–21.

29. Khoo JJ. Renal Biopsies in Johor: A 7-years study. *Malays J Pathol* 2001, **23**:101–104.

30. Bahiense-Oliveira M, Saldanha LB, Mota EL, *et al.* Primary glomerular diseases in Brazil (1979–1999): Is the frequency of focal and segmental glomerulosclerosis increasing? *Clin Nephrol* 2004, **61**:90–97.

31. Mazzarolo Cruz HM, Cruz J, Silva Al Jr, *et al.* Prevalence of adult primary glomerular diseases: retrospective analysis of 206 kidney biopsies (1990–1993). *Rev HospClin Fac sao Paulo* 1996, **51**:3–6.

32. Mitwalli AH, Al Wakeel JS, Al Mohaya SS, *et al.* Pattern of glomerular disease in Saudi Arabia. *Am J Kidney Dis* 1996, **27**(6):797–802.

33. Malafronte P, Gianna M-K, Gustavo N, *et al.* Paulista registry of glomerulonephritis:5-year data report. *Nephrol Dial Transplant*, 2006, **21**:3098–3105.

34. Narasimhan B, Chacko B, John GT, *et al.* Characterization of kidney lesions in Indian adults: towards a renal biopsy registry. *J Nephrol* 2006 Mar-Apr; **19**(2):205–210.

35. EI-Reshaid W, EI-Reshaid K, Kapoor MM, *et al.* Glomerulopathy in Kuwait: The spectrum over the past 7 years. *Renal Failure*, 2003 Jul; **25**(4):619–630.

36. Hurtado A, Escudero E, Stromquist CS, *et al.* Distinct patterns of glomerular disease in Peru. *Clin Nephrol* 2000, **53**(5):325–332.

37. Chan KW, Chan TM, Cheng IKP. Clinical and pathological characteristics of patients with glomerular diseases at a university teaching hospital: 5-years prospective review. *Hong Kong Med J* 1999 Sep; **5**(3):240–244.

38. Simon P, Ramee MP, Autuly V, *et al.* Epidemiology of primary glomerular diseases in a French region. Variations according to period and age. *Kidney Int* 1994, **46**:1192–1198.

39. Rivera Francisco, Lopez-Gomez, Rafaei Perez-Garcia, on behalf of the Spain registry of glomerulonephritis. Clinicopathologic correlations of renal pathology in Spain. *Kidney International*, 2004, **66**:898–904.

40. Chen H, Tang Z, Zeng C, *et al.* Pathological demography of native patients in a nephrology center in China. *Chinese Med J (Engl)* 2003, **116**(9):1377–1381.

41. Chang JH, Dong KK, Hyun WK, *et al.* Changing prevalence of glomerular diseases in Korean adults: a review of 20 years of experience. *Nephrol Dial Transplant*, 2009, **24**(8):2406–2410.

42. Balakrishnan N, John GT, Korula A, *et al.* Spectrum of biopsy proven renal disease and changing trends at a tropical tertiary care centre 1990–2001. *Indian J Nephrol* 2003, **13**:29–35.

43. Dzhanaliev BR, Varshaskii VA, Laurinavichus AA. Primary glomerulopathies: incidence, dynamics and clinical manifestations of morphological variants. *Arkh patol* 2002, **64**(2):532–549.

44. Ahmed Hassan Mitwalli. Glomerulonephritis in Saudi Arabia: a Review. *Saudi J Kidney Dis Transplant*, 2000, **11**(4):567–576.

45. Braden GL, Mulhern JG, O'Shea MH, *et al.* Changing incidence of glomerular diseases in adults. *Am J Kidney Diseases*, 2000, **35**(5):878–883.

46. Stephen M Korbet, Rosangela M, Genchi, *et al.* The Racial Prevalence of Glomerular Lesions in Nephrotic Adults. *Am J Kidney Dis* 1996, **27**(5):647–651.

47. Kitiyakara C, Kopp JB, Eggers P. Trends in the epidemiology of focal segmental glomerulosclerosis. Semin Nephrol 2003 Mar; **23**(2):172–182.

48. Louise M McKenzie, Sher L Hendrickson, William A Briggs *et al.* NPHS2 variation in sporadic focal segmental glomerulosclerosis. *J Am Soc Nephrol 2007*, **18**:2987–2995.

49. Kronenberg F, Lhotta K, Konig P. Retrospective review of 449 renal biopsies taken from 1980–1990. *Abstract 28th congress, European Dialysis and Transplant Association* Italy 1991; p 41.

50. Rychlik I, Jancova E, Tesar V, *et al.* The Czech registry of renal biopsies: Occurrence of renal diseases in the years 1994–2000. *Nephrol Dial Transplant*, 2004, **19**:3040–3049.

51. Heaf J, Lokkegaard H, Larsen S. The epidemiology and prognosis of glomerulonephritidies in Denmark 1985–1997. *Nephro Dial Transplant*, 1999, **14**:889–1897.

52. Sipiczki T, Ondrik Z, Abraham G, *et al.* The incidence of renal diseases as diagnosed by biopsy in Hungary. *Orv Hetil* 2004 Jun 27; **145**(26):1373–1379.

53. Chugh KS, Aikat BK, Sharma BK, *et al.* Pattern of Renal Disease in North India. *Ann Acad Med Singapore*, 1975, **2**:41–43.

54. Sidabutar RP, Lumenta NA. The pattern of Glomerulonephritis in "Tjikini" Hospital Jakarta. *Ann Acad Med Singapore*, 1982, **11**(1):42–45.

55. Antonovych TT, Sabins SG, Broumand BB. A study of membranoproliferative glomerulonephritis in Iran. *An Saudi Med* 1999, **19**(6):505–510.

56. Polenakovic MH, Grcevska L, Dzikova S. The incidence of biopsy proven primary glomerulonephritidies in the Republic of Macedonia- long term follow up. *Nephrol Dial Transplant*, 2003, **18**(suppl 5):25–27.

57. Carvalho E, Faria MDS, Nunes JPL, *et al*. Renal diseases: a 27-years renal biopsy study. *J Nephrol* 2006, **19**:500–507.

58. Serov VV, Varshavsky VA, Schill H, *et al*. Incidence of glomerular diseases in kidney biopsy materials using WHO classification. *Zentralbl Allg Pathol*, 1986, **132**:471–475.

59. Rivera Francisco , Lopez-Gomez JM. Frequency of renal pathology in Spain 1994–1999. *Nephrol Dial Transplant*, 2002, **17**:1594–1602.

60. Kanjanabuch T, Kittikovit W. Etiologies of glomerular diseases in Thailand: a renal biopsy study of 506 cases. *J Med Assoc Thai*, 2005 Sep; **88**(suppl 4):S305–S311.

61. Cameron JS. Clinicopathological Correlation in Glomerulonephritis: Problems and Limitations. Proc 1st Colloquium in Nephrology, Singapore 1974. *Ann Acad Med Singapore*, 1975, **4**(2):45–51.

62. Davison AM. The United Kingdom Medical Research Council's glomerulonephritis registry. *Contrib Nephrol* 1985, **48**:24–35.

CHAPTER 9

Clinical Trials and Management of Chronic Kidney Disease (CKD)

Chronic Kidney Disease (CKD) is a highly prevalent and costly disease. It is an important cause of public health concern. Thro' the years there has been the quest to treat patients with CKD using various strategies to retard progression to end stage renal failure (ESRF). This article offers a long term perspective with examples of clinical trials which have contributed to the management of CKD.

In a recent review by Wiggins *et al.*,[1] diabetic nephropathy, hypertensive renal disease and IgA nephropathy accounted for 54% of patients commencing renal replacement therapy in Australia in 2006. In Singapore,[2] data from the 5th Report of the Singapore Renal Registry (2004) showed that Diabetic Nephropathy accounted for 58.7% of new patients with ESRF initiated into the dialysis programme. Chronic Glomerulonephritis (GN) accounted for 19% and Hypertensive Nephrosclerosis 8.3%. This 3 groups form 86% of the 625 new patients requiring dialysis for 2004. Each year there are about 750 new patients with ESRF in Singapore. Retarding progression to ESRF in these 3 groups of patients with these diseases will address the needs of more than 80% of patients destined for ESRF.[2]

The 1960s

In the 1960s, dietary restriction of protein and phosphate was the key component to delay progression of renal failure. The Giovanetti[3] Diet consisted of only 18 grams of high biologic

155

value protein. Hypertension was said to well controlled as long as BP of 140/90 and below was achieved. Any pressure above this was considered hypertension and necessitated therapy. Essential Hypertension was considered benign and only malignant and renal hypertension were believed to cause progression to end stage renal failure (ESRF). A low protein diet and good control of hypertension were key factors in delaying the progression to ESRF.

1970s

In the 1970s protein restriction to 30 gm a day (0.6 gm/kg BW) became popular with the description of renal injury related to Glomerular Hyperfiltration.[5] Keto acid analogues and essential amino acid diets were often prescribed. This period also saw the use of Cyclophosphamide, Prednisolone and Imuran in the treatment of Nephrotic Syndrome and other forms of Glomerulonephritis. Documentation of platelet and endothelial cell injury in the glomeruli led to the introduction of antiplatelet agent (dipyridamole) and anticoagulants (heparin, warfarin).[5] These agents helped to retard progression to ESRF.

1980s

In the 1980s controlled trials of dietary protein and phosphate restriction were performed and the belief that high parathormone levels was one of the main causes of renal deterioration was held. However none of the trials were vigorous enough to demonstrate that protein restriction was beneficial in renal retardation.[6] There was the concern that a 0.6 gm/kg BW protein diet could lead to malnutrition and a 0.8 gm/kg BW protein diet was recommended. Control of Hypertension was recognised as the single most important factor in retarding progression to ESRF.

ACE inhibitor was introduced as a therapy which could cause efferent arteriolar vasodilatation and thereby decrease intraglomerular hypertension in glomerular hyperfiltration.[7] This could retard progression of chronic renal failure.

Hypercholesterolemia was recognised as a factor which could contribute to renal injury as it was toxic to the mesangial cells. Control of lipids and cholesterol was advocated.[9] Steroids and cytotoxic drugs were prescribed for nephrotic proteinuria as an immunological basis was implicated in heavy proteinuria.[8] In a controlled trial involving 52 pairs of patients with IgA nephritis using cyclophosphamide, anti-platelet and antithrombotic agent (low dose warfarin) Woo[9] demonstrated that the treatment group had slower deterioration of renal failure, 8 years later compared to those on no treatment.

The Early 1990s

In the early 1990s hyperfiltration injury in kidney disease was now considered as the main cause of renal deterioration and the role of Enalapril was recognised in retarding progression to ESRF in Diabetic Nephropathy[10] and IgA nephritics.[11] Proteinuria was also documented as directly nephrotoxic contributing to proximal tubular cell injury leading to glomerulosclerosis. Angiotensin II Receptor Antagonists (ATRA) introduced in the mid 1990s was an alternative for those patients who cannot tolerate ACEI because of cough.[12] Cyclosporine A was introduced in therapy of glomerulonephritis with Nephrotic Syndrome. Steroids (low dose) were introduced to reduce tubulointerstilial fibrosis in glomerulonephritis. Hypertensive nephrosclerosis resulting from Essential Hypertension[13] was documented as an important cause of ESRF, second only to Diabetes Mellitus which had become the leading cause of ESRF in USA and developed countries.

The Late 1990s

In Singapore,[14] Diabetic Nephropathy accounted for 52% of patients with ESRF with Chronic Glomerulonephritis (GN) accounting for 29% and Hypertensive Nephrosclerosis 9%. Each year there were about 750 new patients with ESRF. Retarding progression to ESRF in the 3 main causes of ESRF will address 80% of patients destined for ESRF.[15]

For patients with Diabetic Nephropathy (Diab Nx) strict control of blood sugar and use of ACEI could help retard progression of Diab Nx. ACEI was important to prevent development of Diab Nx in those patients found to have micro albuminuria.[10] Patients with persistent micro albuminuria not responding to ACEI would form the group which would progress to established Diab Nx with progressive renal failure. The importance of good blood pressure control was emphasized as one of the key features to retard progression of renal failure. In addition, control of hyper cholesterolemia was important to prevent renal damage and decrease cardiac morbidity and mortality. Anti platelet and antithrombotic therapy were used as well. In 1996 with the introduction of Angiotensin II Receptor Antagonists (ATRA), Losartan in Singapore, it was found that this could help reduce proteinuria in addition to controlling Hypertension as well.[16]

Woo's study[16] suggested that ACEI/ATRA therapy may be beneficial in patients with IgA Nx with renal impairment and non selective proteinuria as such patients may respond to therapy with improvement in protein selectivity, decrease in proteinuria and improvement in renal function. It is important to note that in this study patients with renal impairment can normalise renal function as a result of the therapy. ACEI/ATRA therapy probably modifies pore size distribution by reducing the radius of large nonselective pores, causing the shunt pathway to become less pronounced resulting in less leakage of protein into the urine.

EARLY CLINICAL TRIALS OF ACEI AND ARB

For patients with Diabetic Nephropathy (Diab Nx) strict control of blood sugar and use of ACEI could help retard progression of Diab Nx. ACEI was important to prevent development of Diab

Nx in those patients found to have micro albuminuria.[10] Patients with persistent micro albuminuria not responding to ACEI would form the group which would progress to established Diab Nx with progressive renal failure. The importance of good blood pressure control was emphasized as one of the key features to retard progression of renal failure. In addition, control of hypercholesterolemia was important to prevent renal damage and decrease cardiac morbidity and mortality.

It has been postulated that ACEI/ARB (ACE inhibitor/ Angiotensin receptor blockers) may decrease proteinuria in patients with glomerulonephritis by its action on the Glomerular Basement Membrane (GBM). In a previous study, Morelli *et al.*[11] reported that ACEI reduced proteinuria in patients with diabetic nephropathy by reducing the size of large unselective pores in the GBM. Woo *et al.*[16] performed a study to examine the relationship between the response of patients with IgA Nephritis (IgA Nx) to ACEI (Enalapril)/ARB (Losartan) therapy by decreasing proteinuria and its effect on the Selectivity Index (SI) in these patients. Selectivity Index is the ratio of IgG clearance over transferrin clearance. A ratio of <0.2 indicates highly selective proteinuria while one of >0.2 indicates non selective proteinuria. Patients with non selective proteinuria have a poorer renal prognosis. Forty one patients with biopsy proven IgA Nx entered a control trial with 21 in the treatment group and 20 in the control group. The entry criteria included proteinuria of 1 gm or more and or renal impairment. Patients in the treatment group received ACEI (5 mg)/ARB (50 mg) or both with 3 monthly increase in dosage. In the control group, hypertension was treated with atenolol, hydrallazine or methyldopa. After a mean duration of therapy of 13 ± 5 months, in the treatment group there was no significant change in serum creatinine, proteinuria or SI but in the control group, serum creatinine deteriorated from 1.8 ± 0.8 to 2.3 ± 1.1 mg/dl ($p < 0.05$). Among the 21 patients in the treatment group, 10 responded to ACEI/ARB therapy determined as decrease in proteinuria by 30% (responders) and the other 11 did not (non responders). Among the responders, SI improved from a mean of

0.26 ± 0.07 to 0.18 ± 0.07 (p<0.001) indicating a tendency towards selective proteinuria. This was associated with improvement in serum creatinine from mean 1.7 ± 0.6 to 1.5 ± 0.6 mg/dl (p < 0.02) and decrease in proteinuria from mean of 2.3 ± 1.1 g/day to 0.7 ± 0.5 g/day (p < 0.001).

After treatment, proteinuria in the treatment group (1.8 ± 1.6 g/day) was significantly less than in the control group (2.9 ± 1.8 g/day) (p < 0.05). The post treatment SI in the responder group (0.18 ± 0.07) was better than that of the non responder group (0.33 ± 0.11) (p < 0.002). Eight out of 21 patients in the treatment group who had documented renal impairment had improvement in their renal function compared to 2 in the control group (x^2 = 4.4, p < 0.05). Of the 8 patients in the treatment group who improved their renal function, 3 normalized their renal function.

Woo's study[16] suggested that ACEI/ARB therapy may be beneficial in patients with IgA Nx with renal impairment and non selective proteinuria as such patients may respond to therapy with improvement in protein selectivity, decrease in proteinuria and improvement in renal function. It is important to note that in this study patients with renal impairment can normalise renal function as a result of the therapy. ACEI/ARB therapy probably modifies pore size distribution by reducing the radius of large nonselective pores, causing the shunt pathway to become less pronounced resulting in less leakage of protein into the urine.

RECENT CLINICAL TRIALS USING VARIOUS THERAPIES

Combination therapy with ACEI and ARB was advocated for patients with proteinuria associated with Diab Nx, Glomerulonephritis and Hypertension. The objective was to reduce proteinuria to less than 1 gm a day.[18]

In 2000, the USA National Kidney Foundation recommended a target BP of 130/80 in the treatment of Hypertension.[19] Lowering systolic BP to 120 mmHg was associated with improved patient and kidney survival (Pohl).[20] Lewington[21] Reported that of 1 million subjects with no Cardiovascular (CVS) Disease, by decreasing SBP to 115 mmHg and DBP 75 mmHg, there was a linear association between decreasing SBP and DBP and reduced risk of CVS mortality. But Pohl[19] reported that SBP reduction to less than 120 mmHg did not provide added renoprotection. He found that SBP < 120 mmHg was associated with accelerated loss of renal function because of co-morbidities in these patients. In 2003, the 7th Joint National Committee[22] on detection, evaluation and treatment of high BP in the USA stated that BP above 115/75 mmHg was associated with higher incidents of adverse CVS outcome. Adequate control of high BP is both cardio as well as renoprotective. It helps to retard progression of CKD to ESRF.

Sarnak *et al.*[23] reported on the effect of a lower BP on the progression of kidney disease using data culled from the long term follow up of the Modification of Diet in Renal Disease study. This study had the longest follow up and highest degree of statistical power demonstrated. The MDRD (Modification of Diet in Renal Disease) study achieved BP separation of 8/3 mmHg, 126/77 versus 134/80 over 2 years during an average of 6 years follow up. ESRF and all cause death was reduced by 23% in the group with lower BP.

The effects of microalbuminuria is another important area relating to renal and CVS mortality. Microalbuminuria is defined as 20–200 mg albumin excretion in the urine a day. Less than 20 mg has been said to be 'normal'. There is ample data to suggest that albuminuria in the 'normal' range carries a significant risk of vascular events.[24] The degree of albuminuria reduction in response to treatment is a primary determinant of both renal and CVS outcomes. More than 2 mg/gm creatinine of albumin excretion is significantly associated with CVS death, myocardial infarct, strokes and high BP. This is applicable to both Diabetics and non Diabetics.

It has been shown that reduction of microalbuminuria slowed progression of renal disease.[25] Every halving of albumin excretion was associated with 18% lower risk of CVS Death. A 20% to 50%

reduction in albumin excretion at 6 months was associated with 50% lower risk of ESRF. If albumin excretion rate is reduced by more than 50% there is a decrease in relative risk of ESRF by 75%.[26] CVS risk follows a continuous positive relationship with albumin excretion and lowering albuminuria independently lowers risk of Renal and CVS events. The so called 'Normal' is not normal. We should identify level of BP and albumin excretion below which treatment is no longer beneficial. However, at this moment there is no clear consensus on whether we should routinely offer renoprotective therapy using ACEI/ARB for patients with raised urinary microalbumin in the absence of any overt renal disease.

Apart from control of hypertension and reduction of proteinuria, another area of great interest is the role of high levels of cholesterol in renal damage. This role has been documented in the 1980s[15] but it is only recently that this role has been better documented with evidence to demonstrate that control of hypercholesteronemia can help in retarding progression to ESRF. High LDL Cholesterol causes proliferation of mesangial cells with subsequent increased contractility of these cells eventually leading to glomerulosclerosis.[15]

Tonolo in a recent publication "Simvastatin maintains steady patterns of GFR and improves Albumin Excretion Rate (AER) and expression of slit diaphragm (SD) proteins in type II diabetes"[27] has provided new evidence. In a 4 year study of 86 microalbuminuric, hypertensive, type II diabetics, comparing the effects of 40 mg/day of Simvastatin (Group I) versus patients treated with 30 gm cholestyramine/day (Group II), it was found that those patients in Group II had a GFR decay per year of 3 ml/min/1.73 metre square compared to those in Group I whose GFR was stable. Both groups showed a significant decrease of LDL-cholesterol after simvastatin and cholestyramine therapy but only the statin was beneficial for CKD progression. The Albumin Excretion rate (AER) decreased in Group I but not in Group II (p < 0.01). The percentage of patients who had steady "normoalbuminuria", during the fourth year of follow-up instead of "microalbuminuria", was three-fold higher during simvastatin than during cholestyramine treatment (29% versus 8%, p < 0.01). Overt proteinuria developed in 15% of cholestyramine treated patients and in 4% of simvastatin treated patients (p < 0.01). Finally, the simvastatin treated group also had markedly improved mRNA expression of SD proteins. It was postulated that the improvement attributed to the simvastatin treated group could be due to the decreased overproduction of reactive oxygen species. But whatever the mechanism, the authors believe that the study supports the reno-protective role of simvastatin against the development of ESRF.[27]

Dual Therapy with Losartan and Aliskiren in Type 2 Diabetic Nephropathy may be promising. Aliskiren is a new renoprotective agent that inhibits renin, the rate limiting step in the renin angiotensin aldosterone system (RAAS). In both healthy volunteers and disease states, aliskiren reduces angiotensin II levels and plasma renin activity (PRA), without stimulating compensatory increases in PRA, Angiotensin I and Angiotensin II as seen with ACE inhibitors and ARBs (REF). In the recently published AVOID (Aliskiren in the Evaluation of Proteinuria in Diabetes) Trial by Parving *et al.*,[28] 301 patients with Type 2 Diabetes were on Losartan 100 mg daily plus Aliskiren 150 mg daily for 3 months, then 300 mg daily for another 3 months (a total trial duration of 6 months), versus those on Losartan plus placebo. A reduction of mean urinary albumin: creatinine ratio of 50% or more was found in 24.7% of those given Aliskiren, versus 12.5% of those on placebo (p < 0.001). Aliskiren allows for total blockade of the renin angiotensin system and its beneficial effect is independent of BP control. Dual inhibition with Losartan and Aliskiren may be promising.

In a recently published open label randomized controlled trial over 6 years by Woo *et al.*,[29] 226 patients with IgANx were enrolled with 112 patients treated with an ARB (Losartan 100 to 200 mg) and 114 treated with ACEI (Enalapril 10 to 20 mg). Entry criteria included proteinuria >1 gm/day and or serum creatinine >1.6 mg/dl and Chronic Kidney Disease (CKD) Stage 3 (eGFR

30 to 59 mls/min). The 226 patients were randomized to Control arm of ACEI 10 mg, ACEI 20 mg, ARB 100 mg and ARB 200 mg in the ratio of 2:3:2:3.

Patients on ARB 200 mg were designated High Dose ARB group, those on ARB 100 mg were designated Normal Dose ARB, those on ACEI 20 mg designated Normal Dose ACEI and those on ACEI 10 mg designated Control group. Two hundred and seven patients completed the trial, 40, 61, 43 and 63 were in the ACEI 10 mg, ACEI 20 mg, ARB 100 mg and ARB 200 mg groups respectively.

Determination of the ACE Insertion/Deletion genotypes was done using the method of Vleming *et al.*,[30] DNA was extracted from 0.2 ml EDTA-blood using the QIAmp DNA blood extraction kit (QIAGEN, Germany). Amplification of the I allele produced 1 band at 490 base pair (bp) for homozygote II. Amplification of the D allele produced 1 band at 190 bp for homozygote DD. Both bands at 490 bp and 190 bp were produced by heterozygote.

Patients on high dose ARB had significantly lower proteinuria, 1.0 +/− 0.8 gm/day compared to 1.7 +/− 1.0 gm/day in the other groups (p = 0.006). The loss in eGFR was 0.7 ml/min/year for high dose ARB compared to 3.2 to 3.5 ml/min/year for the other 3 groups (p = 0.006). There were more patients on high dose ARB with improvement in eGFR compared to the other 3 groups (p < 0.001) at end of the trial. Comparing patients with the 3 ACE genotypes DD, ID and II, all 3 groups responded well to therapy with decrease in proteinuria (p < 0.002) and no difference in renal survival. Only in the group on low dose ACEI (10 mg/day) was there a trend towards patients with increasing numbers of those with the I allele having increasing ESRF (p = 0.037). Data from this study suggest that adequate dosage of ACEI/ARB will override the genomic influence of ACE gene polymorphism on renal survival. ACE gene polymorphism of a patient is not a cause for concern as patients with the various genotypes DD, ID and II will respond to therapy as long as the drug dosage is adequate. High dose ARB is more efficacious in reducing proteinuria and preserving renal function when compared with normal dose ARB and ACEI and also obviates the genomic influence of ACE gene polymorphism on renal survival. At year five, 38% of patients on high dose ARB had a gain in eGFR suggesting recovery of renal function in these patients on high dose ARB. The study of high dose Losartan[29,31] over a period of 6 years shows that the loss of eGFR is significantly less when compared to normal dose Losartan (ARB) and Enalapril (ACEI). It also demonstrates that irrespective of whether it is ARB or ACEI usage, as long as the trial duration is sufficiently long (at least 5 years or more), the eGFR in a significant proportion of treated patients will improve.[29] Hitherto, the concept of renal retardation was one of delaying the onset of the time when the patients would require renal replacement therapy. But today we are employing renal retardation drugs to help improve renal function and induce regression of glomerular sclerosis and perhaps in the long term prevent renal failure.[31]

One question often raised is whether a combination therapy of both ACEI and ARB together will be just as effective as using High Dose ARB alone. One of the answers to this question may be found in the recent trial[32] regarding renal outcome in the Ongoing Telmisartan Alone and in Combination with Ramipril Global End point Trial (ONTARGET Trial) which compares the effect of Telmisartan 80 mg daily alone (n = 8542), Ramipril 10 mg daily alone (n = 8576) and on both together (n = 8542) over a duration of 56 months (almost 5 years). Doubling of serum creatinine was 13.4% in the Telmisartan group, 13.5% in the Ramipril group but 14.5% in the Combined Therapy group (p = 0.037). Initiation of dialysis was also increased among the Combination Group, 212 patients or 2.49% versus 189 patients or 2.21% for the Telmisartan and 174 patients or 2.03% for the ramipril group (p < 0.01). eGFR decline was more in the Combination group, −6.1 ml/min/year versus −2.82 ml/min/year in the Ramipril group and −4.12 ml/min/year in the Telmisartan group (p < 0.0001). However, the geometric mean increase in proteinuria (urinary albumin/creatinine ratio) was more compared with baseline in the Ramipril group +31% and the Telmisartan group +24% compared to the Combination group +21% (p < 0.0028). This should sound a note of caution to those practising Combination ACEI and ARB therapy. One should however state that the patients in this study were Diabetics with Diabetic nephropathy and established cardiovascular disease and were more than 55 years old with baseline proteinuria <1 gm/day. Ironically, one of the long term side effects of ACEI therapy is progressive renal fibrosis with worsening of eGFR while short term use of ACEI may show improvement.[33] The reverse to this answer could be from our recent paper on the beneficial effects of long term high dose ARB therapy in patients with IgA nephritis over a period of 6 years,[33] which showed that high dose ARB is more efficacious in reducing proteinuria and preserving renal function in terms of earlier and more effective improvement in eGFR in those treated with high dose ARB compared to those on normal dose ARB and ACEI. We believe that high dose ARB does so by causing regression of glomerular sclerosis.[20] Another alternative strategy which may prove to be even more effective is to employ a combination of losartan and aliskiren as shown in the AVOID Trial by Parving.[28]

RENAL FIBROSIS AND FUTURE THERAPEUTIC OPTION

Renal fibrosis is the consequence of all forms of CKD. However the very drugs that we use like ACEI and ARBs could indirectly cause renal fibrosis as they promote the increase of aldosterone which in turn causes renal fibrosis. The pathogenesis of renal fibrosis is a process characterised by excessive accumulation and deposition of extracellular matrix (ECM) components. The underlying cellular events are complexed consisting of mesangial and fibroblast activation, tubular epithelial to mesenchymal transition (EMT), monocyte and macrophage and T cell infiltration and cell apoptosis. TGFβ can stimulate mesangial cells, interstitial fibroblasts and tubular epithelial cells to undergo myofibroblastic activation to transition to become matrix producing fibrogenic cells. Inhibition of TGFβ can suppress renal fibrotic lesions and prevent loss of kidney function.

TGFβ and its downstream Smad signalling has now been shown to play a crucial role in renal fibrosis. Smad signalling in the kidney is constrained by a family of proteins known as Smad transcriptional corepressors which include SnoN, Ski and TGIF. These Smad antagonists effectively confine Smad mediated gene transcription, thereby safeguarding the tissue from unwanted TGFβ response. It has been demonstrated by Liu[34] that SnoN and Ski is diminished in the fibrotic kidney, suggesting loss of Smad antagonists as a mechanism that amplifies the TGFβ signal.

HGF or Hepatic Growth Factor is an endogenous antifibrotic factor present in our body. BMP-7 is a member of the TGFβ superfamily that also counteracts the fibrogenic action of TGFβ.

The therapy for the future will be to develop antifibrotic renal drugs which can counter the effects of TGFβ as well as the aldosterone effects induced by ACEI and ARBs. Already Eplerenome is one drug which is anti-aldosterone, apart from spironolactone. We need to add other TGFβ and Smad antagonists to prevent renal fibrosis and preserve renal function in patients with CKD[34].

CONCLUSION

It would be apparent from this review article that several important strategies are necessary to prevent progression to ESRF. These are control of hypertension, treatment of proteinuria and treatment of hypercholesterolaemia. In addition, it is necessary to stress to patients the need for a low salt diet as this will help BP control and optimize ACEI and ARB therapy. A reduced protein diet is also advisable as it will help to further reduce glomerular hyperfiltration. For diabetics with normal renal function, good glycemic control must be emphasized. We should offer therapeutic intervention earlier to patients with CKD. In the past, therapy was started only when patients developed renal failure. In recent years, therapy is offered much earlier and more aggressively whether it is in terms of reduction of BP, proteinuria or high cholesterol. Early therapeutic intervention must continue to be the corner stone if we are to solve the problem of increasing number of patients who fall prey to ESRF year after year. The use of high dose ARB and the novel renin inhibitor Aliskiren may prove to be yet another bonus in this regard. There is a need for more clinical trials involving Aliskiren. However, there are concerns that ACEI and ARBs could in the long term induce renal fibrosis. There is a great need for novel therapies which could ameliorate or prevent renal fibrosis.

REFERENCES

1. Wiggins KJ, Kelly DJ. Aliskiren: a novel renoprotective agent or simply an alternative to ACE inhibitors? *Kidney Int* 2009, **76**: 23–31.
2. Fifth Report of the Singapore Renal Registry (2004), Health Promotion Board, Singapore, 2008, p. 24.
3. Giovanetti S, Maggiore Q. A low-nitrogen diet with protein of high biologic value for serve chronic uremia. *Lancet*, 1964, **1**:1000.
4. Hostetter TH, Olson JL, Rennke HG. Hyperfiltration in remnant nephrons: A potentially adverse response to renal ablation. *Am J Physiol* 1981, **241**:F85.
5. Kincaid-Smith P. The treatment of chronic mesangiocapillary glomerulo-nephritis with impaired renal function. *Med J Aust* 1972, **2**:587–592.
6. Adler SG. A critical review of clinical trials on retarding progression of renal failure–focus on dietary protein and phosphorus restriction. Proc. 11th Asian Colloquim in Nephrology, Singapore, 1996. Yap HK, Tan CC, Woo KT (eds.), pp. 36–44.
7. Diamond JR, Karnovsky MJ. Focal and segmental glomerulosclerosis: Analogies to atherosclerosis. *Kidney Int* 1988, **33**: 917–924.
8. Hayslett JP. Prevention of glomerular damage with pharmocologic agents. In Avram MM (ed.), Prevention of kidney disease and long term survival. New York and London, Plenum Medical Book Co. 1982, pp. 93–99.
9. Woo KT, Edmondson RPS, Yap HK, Wu AYT, Chiang GSC, Lee EJC, Pwee HS, Lim CH. Effects of triple therapy on the

progression of Mesangial Proliferative Glomerulonephritis. *Clin Nephrol* 1987, **27**:56–64.

10. Lewis EJ, Hunsicker LG, Bain RP, Rohde RD. The effect of angiotensin-converting-enzyme inhibition on diabetic nephropathy. *N Engl J Med* 1993, **329**:1456–1462.

11. Rekola S, Bergstrand A, Bucht H. Deterioration rate in hypertensive IgA nephropathy: Comparison of a converting enzyme inhibitor and β-blocking agents. *Nephron* 1991, **59**:57–60.

12. Nakamura T, Obata J, Kimura H, Ohno S, Yoshida Y, Kawaihi H, Shimizu F. Blocking angiotensin II ameliorates proteinuria and glomerular lesions in progressive mesangioproliferative glomerulonephritis. *Kidney Int* 1999, **55**:877–889.

13. Luke RG. Essential hypertension: A renal disease? A review and update of the evidence. *Hypertension,* 1993, **21**(3):380–390.

14. Woo KT. Proceedings: Preventing Renal Failure, Singapore General Hospital, 2001, Pp. 6–13.

15. Woo KT, Lau YK, Wong KS, Chiang GSC. ACEI/ATRA Therapy Decreases Proteinuria by Improving Glomerular Permselectivity in IgA Nephritis. *Kidney International*, 2000, **58**:2485–2491.

16. Morelli E, Loon N, Meyer TW, Peters W, Myers BD. Effects of converting enzyme inhibition on barrier function in diabetic glomerulopathy. *Diabetes* 1990, **39**:76–82.

17. Woo KT, Lau YK, Wong KS, Chiang GSC. ACEI/ATRA Therapy Decreases Proteinuria by Improving Glomerular Permselectivity in IgA Nephritis. *Kidney Int* 2000, **58**:2485–2491.

18. Parving HH, Lehnert H, Brochner-Mortensen J, Gomis R, Anderswn S, Arner P. The effect of irbesartan on the development of diabetic nephropathy in patients with type 2 diabetes, *N Engl J Med* 2001, **345**:870–878.

19. Bakris GL. Preserving renal function in adults with hypertension and diabetes: A consensus approach. *Am J Kidney Dis* 2000, **36**:646–661.

20. Pohl MA. Independent and additive impact of blood pressure control and angiotensin II receptor blockade on renal outcomes in the Irbesartan Diabetic Nephropathy Trial: clinical implications and limitations. *J Am Soc Nephrol* 2005, **16**:3027–3037.

21. Lewington S: Age-specific relevance of usual blood pressure to vascular mortality: a meta-analysis of individual data for one million adults in 61 prospective studies. *Lancet,* 2002, **360**:1903–1913.

22. Chobanian AV, Bakris GL, Black HR. The Seventh Report of the Joint National Committee on prevention, detection, evaluation and

treatment of high blood pressure: The JNC 7 report. *JAMA*, 2003, 289:2560–2572.

23. Sarnak MJ, Greene T, Wang X. The effect of a lower target blood pressure on the progression of kidney disease: long-term follow-up of the modification of diet in renal disease study. *Ann Intern Med* 2005, **142**:342–351.

24. Forman JP, Brenner BM. 'Hypertension' and 'microalbuminuria': The bell tolls for thee. *Kidney Int* 2006, **69**:22–28.

25. Lea J, Greene T, Hebert L. The relationship between magnitude of proteinuria reduction and risk of end-stage renal disease. Results of African American study of kidney disease and hypertension. *Arch Int Med* 2005, **165**:947–953.

26. Diamond JR, Karnovsky MJ. Focal and segmental glomerulosclerosis : Analogies to atherosclerosis. *Kidney Int* 1988, **33**:917–924.

27. Tonolo G, Velussi M, Brocco E. Simvastatin maintains steady patterns of GFR and improves AER and expression of slit diaphragm proteins in type II diabetes. *Kidney Int* 2006, **70**:177–186.

28. Parving HH. Aliskiren combined with losartan in type 2 diabetes and nephropathy. *N Engl J Med* 2008, **358**:2433–2446.

29. Woo KT, Chan CM, Wong KS *et al*. High Dose Losartan and ACE gene polymorphism in IgA nephritis. *Genomic Medicine*, 2009, **2**(3): 77–81.

30. Vleming LJ, Van Kooten C, Van Es LA *et al*. The D- allele of the ACE gene polymorphism predicts a stronger antiproteinuric response to ACE inhibitors. *Nephrology,* 1998, **4**:143–149.

31. Woo KT, Chan CM, Wong KS *et al*. Beneficial effects of high dose losartan in IgA nephritis. *Clinical Nephrol* 2009, **71**(6):617–624.

32. ONTARGET Investigators. Telmisartan, ramipril, or both in patients at high risk for vascular events. *N Engl J Med* 2008, **358**: 1547–1559.

33. Hamming I, Van Goor H, Navis GJ. ACE inhibitor use and the increased long term risk of renal failure in diabetes. *Kidney Int* 2006, **70**:1377–1378.

34. Liu YH, Renal Fibrosis. New insights into the pathogenesis and therapeutics. *Kidney Int* 2006, **69**:213–217.

CHAPTER 10

Lupus Nephritis

RENAL INVOLVEMENT IN SYSTEMIC LUPUS ERYTHEMATOSUS (SLE)

Fifty to ninety percent of patients with SLE have nephritis. It affects the glomeruli, tubules and blood vessels of the kidneys. The onset can be insidious to precipitous. This is a chronic disease with remissions and exacerbations. Women are more likely to be affected by SLE.

ASSESSMENT OF THE PATIENT AT PRESENTATION

1. In the clinical assessment of the patient, one has to determine whether the patient has asymptomatic lupus nephritis (urinary abnormalities) or features of the nephrotic syndrome.
2. The younger age group and male patients do worse.
3. Determine whether the patient has hypertension.
4. If there is renal failure, determine whether it is acute, chronic or acute on chronic renal failure. Acute renal failure is potentially reversible. Acute renal deterioration in a patient with lupus nephritis could be due to sepsis, transformation of the lupus nephritis to one with a more severe histology, a crescenteric change (rapidly progressive glomerulonephritis), pre-renal failure due to the nephrotic syndrome, uncontrolled hypertension, renal vein thrombosis, drugs like non-steroidal anti-inflammatory agents (NSAIDS) or nephrotoxic antibiotics.

INVESTIGATIONS

1. Urine examination: A telescoped specimen (presence of RBC, WBC, casts and protein) points to the likelihood of diffuse lupus nephritis. Culture the urine if infection is suspected.
2. Full blood counts, platelets. If there is anaemia, proceed to a reticulocyte count, Coomb's test, peripheral blood film.
3. Serum creatinine, creatinine clearance.
4. Total urinary protein in 24 hours' urine collection.
5. Total serum protein, serum albumin.
6. Anti-nuclear factor, anti-DNA, serum complement.
7. Chest X-ray if chest infection suspected.
8. Ultrasound of the kidneys and renal biopsy.

RENAL BIOPSY

Some advocate a renal biopsy for all patients because of "silent nephritis", i.e. no urinary abnormalities but a renal biopsy shows lupus nephritis.

Others perform a biopsy only if urinary abnormalities are present. A renal biopsy is useful as it will help to determine the type and extent of the renal pathology. It helps in the planning of the management as well as the rendering of a prognosis. A biopsy also helps in the interpretation of the renal failure as to whether the renal failure is reversible (acute renal failure) or chronic.

MODIFIED WHO CLASSIFICATION
OF LUPUS NEPHRITIS [1982]

Class I.   Normal glomeruli
           — Nil change
           — Normal LM, deposits by IMF or EM

Class II. Pure mesangial alterations

Class III.   Focal segmental glomerulonephritis
— Associated with mild or moderate mesangial alterations. May be proliferative, necrotising or sclerosing (<50% glomeruli involved). Necrosis and leukocytic infiltration indicate a higher degree of activity. More aggressive clinical course than Class II. Class Ill and IV are continuation of the same lesion.

Class IV.   Diffuse glomerulonephritis
— Associated with severe mesangial, endocapillary or mesangio-capillary proliferation and/or extensive subendothelial deposits.
— Majority of glomeruli involved with hypercellularity. There are focal areas of necrosis, crescents, nuclear debris and wire loops.
— IMF may show full house immunoglobulins and EM will show subendothelial deposits.
— Patients usually have a severe clinical picture with nephrotic range proteinuria and active urinary sediment, and renal impairment occurs more frequently.

Class V.   Diffuse membranous glomerulonephritis
This lesion has a better prognosis than Class III and IV.

Class VI.   Advanced sclerosing glomerulonephritis
The prognosis is not good as many will develop renal failure.

INDICES OF ACTIVITY AND CHRONICITY

These indices or lesions (see below) represent active (potentially reversible) lesions → Activity Index, or chronic, sclerosing, fibrosing (presumably irreversible) lesions → Chronicity Index. A graded scale consists of 0, 1, 2, and 3+. The total score forms an INDEX; Activity or Chronicity Index as the case may be.

ACTIVE LESIONS (POTENTIALLY REVERSIBLE)

1. Disruption of capillary walls
2. Polymorphs and karyorrhexis
3. Haematoxyphil bodies
4. Crescents
5. Wire loops
6. Hyaline thrombi
7. Fibrin thrombi
8. Segmental fibrin deposition

Activity index is a relatively weak predictor of renal failure outcome. Mild to moderate elevations of the index represent reversible disease (with treatment). A marked elevation of index may represent disruption of glomerular capillaries which tend to heal by scarring rather than regression. Cellular crescents and severe fibrinoid necrosis are the most ominous. The presence of subendothelial deposit is evidence of activity and is an indicator for treatment.

CHRONIC LESIONS (IRREVERSIBLE)

1. Segmental sclerosis
2. Mesangial sclerosis
3. Global sclerosis
4. Fibrous crescents
5. Interstitial fibrosis
6. Tubular atrophy

Chronicity index has a graded relationship to risk of ESRF as a high index appears to increase the risk of renal functional deterioration.

ISN/RPS (2003) CLASSIFICATION
OF LUPUS NEPHRITIS

(ISN = International Society of Nephrology, RPS = Renal Pathology Society)

Class I   Minimal Mesangial Lupus Nephritis (LN)

Class II   Mesangial Proliferative LN

Class III Focal LN (<50% of glomeruli)
          III (A): active lesions
          III (A/C): active and chronic lesions
          III): chronic lesions

Class IV   Diffuse LN (≥50% of glomeruli)
          Diffuse segmental (IV-S) or global (IV-G) LN
          IV (A): active lesions
          IV (A/C): active and chronic lesions
          IV (C): chronic lesions

A single glomerular lesion with any feature of activity is enough to assign "A" for active. Similarly, a single segmentally or globally sclerotic glomerulus judged to be sclerotic as a consequence of scarred glomerulonephritis merits a designation of "C" for chronic.

Class V   Membranous LN

Class VI   Advanced Sclerosing LN
          (≥ 90% globally sclerosed glomeruli without residual activity)

LN CLASS IV-SEGMENTAL VERSUS IV-GLOBAL:

Introduction of subclassification with Class IV, i.e. IV S and IV G, Segmental and Global.

1. On biopsy, LN Class IV – S had more segmental endocapillary proliferation and fibrinoid necrosis. In contrast, LN IV-G was more commonly associated with large subendothelial "wire loop" deposits and intracapillary deposits (hyaline thrombi) suggesting higher immune complex load.
2. Patients with LN IV – S had lower activity and higher chronicity indices although differences did not reach statistical

significance. The 2 groups received similar treatment including prednisolone, cyclophosphamide and some plasmapheresis. The 5 years cumulative remission rate was 73% for patients with LN IV -G versus 48% for LN IV – S (p < 0.05).

3. Renal survival at 10 years was 75% for LN IV – G versus 52% for LN IV – S (p < 0.05). Authors concluded that patients with segmental endocapillary proliferation involving > 50% of glomeruli (now termed LN IV – S) should have more aggressive therapy.

5. However, 3 other retrospective studies (Refer to these studies in paper by Markovitz GS and D'Agati VD, The ISN/RPS 2003 Classification of lupus nephritis: an assessment at 3 years, Kid International, 2007, 49: 491–495) to differentiate between LN IV – S and IV – G have failed to show that those patients with LN IV – S have a worse outcome than those with IV – G although there have been some clinical and morphological differences between these 2 groups.

6. In the largest study comparing LN IV – S with LN IV – G by Hill GS *et al.*, Class IV–S LN versus Class IV G: clinical and morphological differences. Kid International 2005, 68: 2288–2297, involving 15 LN IV – S and 31 LN IV – G French patients, those with IV – G at baseline had more proteinuria, renal insufficiency, anemia and hypocomplementemia. They also had more membranoproliferative features, wire loop deposits and hyaline thrombi, greater immunofluorescence positivity in peripheral capillary walls and less fibrinoid necrosis. After initial biopsy, patients received steroids with or without cyclophosphamide and underwent a protocol biopsy 6 months later. Clinical outcome at 10 years follow up were similar for patients with LN IV – S and LN IV – G diagnosed at the first biopsy. What is interesting is that over the initial 6 months interval, 30 of the 46 patients converted to mesangial proliferative LN (class II). Among the 16 patients, the second biopsy showed transformation to IV – S in seven patients (all originally IV – G) and nine cases of IV – G (3 of which were transformations from IV – S).

7. The authors concluded, based on their findings as well as findings from other studies that while there were some clinical and pathological differences between LN IV – S and IV – G, outcomes were similar.
8. One of the findings regarding the use of the ISN/ RPS classification compared with the old WHO classification is that the percentage of cases of Class IV has increased from 23% based on the WHO classification to an increase to 46% with the ISN/RPS classification.

RENAL HISTOPATHOLOGY AND SURVIVAL (BALDWIN 1977)

1. Focal glomerulonephritis
   — 92% normal renal function
   — 2/3 of patients are nephrotic
   — 70% five-year survival
2. Membranous glomerulonephritis
   — proteinuria present in nearly all patients — 70% of patients are nephrotic
   — 79% five-year survival
3. Diffuse proliferative glomerulonephritis
   — 90% of patients have nephrotic syndrome
   — 82% have renal impairment
   — 30% five-year survival

SEROLOGIC PARAMETERS (BALOW)

1. Serum complement (CH50, C3, C4) usually correlates with degree of activity of glomerular disease.
2. Falling levels of complement predict lupus flare.
3. Immunosuppressive drugs usually improve C3 levels and this would correlate with reduction of disease activity.

4. Others: anti-DNA antibodies, circulating immune complexes, and C reactive protein are useful but none of the tests "alone" are specific or sensitive enough as strict guides to therapy, activity or prognosis.

CORRELATION BETWEEN SEROLOGIC MARKERS AND DISEASE ACTIVITY (HAYSLETT)

1. High titres of anti-DNA and haemolytic complement (CH50) is associated with active disease and their absence indicates inactivity.
2. An increase in anti-DNA or fall in CH50 heralds relapse by several weeks.
3. The solid phase C1q binding assay for circulating immune complexes also correlates with activity.
4. Normalisation of anti-DNA and CH50 with treatment is associated with a better outcome.

ASSESSMENT OF A PATIENT FOR THERAPY

When assessing a patient for therapy one has to consider:
1. Whether the patient has nephrotic syndrome, hypertension or renal impairment.
2. Determine if active disease is present.
3. A renal biopsy will help to determine the type of lesion, the activity index and the chronicity index.

ASSESSMENT FOR PREGNANCY

1. Does patient have active disease? Check urinary sediment and lupus markers.
2. What is the renal function like?

3. Does she have hypertension?
4. Is there proteinuria and if so, is it heavy?
5. Are complement levels and anti-DNA titres low or normal?
6. A renal biopsy will enable one to assess the activity and chronicity indices.

PREGNANCY IN WOMEN WITH SLE

1. Pregnancy increases exacerbations of SLE. These exacerbations are higher during pregnancy and in the post-partum period.
2. Patients with complete remission a few months prior to conception have lower incidence of relapses (25% to 35%).
3. Those with active disease in pregnancy have 50% to 60% incidence of exacerbations.
4. There is a 90% foetal survival for those with inactive SLE and 50% to 75% for those with active SLE.
5. The presence of lupus anticoagulant causes thrombosis in the placenta resulting in intrauterine deaths and abortions.

TREATMENT OF LUPUS NEPHRITIS

1. High dose prednisolone (45 mg or 60 mg) for 3 months, then reduce to 20 mg over 3 months for those with nephrotic syndrome and those who have mild to moderate Class IV nephritis maintain with 10 mg a day.
2. Prednisolone and oral cyclophosphamide (2 mg/kg body weight) for 6 months, then prednisolone alone for non-steroid responsive nephrotic syndrome and those with moderate Class IV lupus nephritis. Those who fail Cyclophosphamide can be offerred Cyclosporine A [CyA] at 5 mg/kg BW for 3 months with dose reduction over the next 3 months.

As an alternative to CyA, some physicians are using Mycophenolate Mofetil [MMF] at a dose of 0.5 gm to 1.5 gm twice daily for 6 months. Patients can be maintained with MMF at a lower dose (0.25 to 0.5 gm twice daily) for another 6 months. Always monitor the patients for sepsis when on MMF. There may be a potential role for Tacrolimus [FK 506] at a dose of 0.1 to 0.2 mg/kg BW a day for those who fail to respond to CyA and MMF.

3. Prednisolone and oral cyclophosphamide for 12 months, then prednisolone alone for moderate to severe Class IV (those who have crescents, fibrin thrombi and sclerosis on renal biopsy). Patients with diffuse sclerosing lesions or renal impairment should also be offered the same treatment. If fail, try Cyclosporine A and maintain up to 1 year.

4. Pulse methyprednisolone (0.5 gm I.V. daily for 6 days) with oral cyclophosphamide and prednisolone for a year for those with acute renal deterioration where biopsies show active Class IV with crescents and fibrin thrombi (High activity index).

5. Oral cyclophosphamide with maintenance prednisolone or Azathioprine with prednisolone for those with biopsies showing sclerosis and fibrous crescents with mild renal impairment (High chronicity index).

6. Plasmapheresis for those with rapidly progressive glomerulonephritis or pulmonary haemorrhage.

7. Patients with Class II (Mesangial Proliferative LN) or Class V (Membranous LN) should have only low dose steroid therapy unless they are nephrotic, in which case remission could be induced with high dose prednisolone. Cyclophosphamide or Azathioprine for 6 months could be used if there is no response to prednisolone.

8. Patients with Class VI (Advanced Sclerosing LN) with serum creatinine above 400 micro Mol/L or 4.5 mg/dl should not be treated aggressively. They require protein restriction, control of hypertension and treatment for sepsis, as well as plans for long-term renal replacement therapy.

CLINICAL TRIALS IN LUPUS NEPHRITIS

[A]. The Aspreva Lupus Management Study [ALMS] Group [Appel GB *et al.*, Mycophenolate mofetil [MMF] versus cyclophosphamide for induction treatment of lupus nephritis. J Am. Soc. Nephrol. 2009, 20:1103–1112].

1. This is a randomised controlled trial of 6 months of steroids in a tapering dose with open label MMF (up to a dose of 3 gm/day) versus monthly IV Cyclophosphamide (CYC) pulses of 0.5 to 1.0 gm/m^2 in a 24 week induction study. Both groups received Prednisolone at 60 mg with tapering doses. The primary end point was a prescribed decrease in protein/ creatinine ratio and stabilization or improvement in serum creatinine. Secondary end points included complete renal remission, lupus activity and damage as well as safety.

2. The study enrolled 370 patients with Class III, IV and V Lupus Nephritis. Overall, there was no difference in the response rate between the 2 groups: 104 (56.2%) of 185 patients responded to MMF compared with 98 (53.0%) of 185 to IV CYC. Secondary end points were also similar between the 2 groups.

3. MMF was not superior to Cyclophosphamide. MMF group had more SLE relapses, Prolonged proteinuria > 1gm/day, more with elevated serum creatinine > 177 microMol/l compared to the Cyclophosphamide group, meaning that these patients were more likely to deteriorate with time [Rovin BD, Lupus Nephritis: are we beyond cyclophosphamide? Nature Reviews, Nephrology, 2009 5: 492–494].

4. The study showed that the incidence of adverse effects and serious infections and deaths were similar in both groups. Although most patients in both groups experienced clinical improvement, the study did not meet its primary objective of showing that MMF was superior to IV CYC as induction treatment for LN.

5. In another trial, the ALMS trial, Blacks or mixed-race patients on IV cyclophosphamide did worse than on MMF.

However, Robin *et al.*, in his Institution, found that severe lupus nephritis treated with oral cyclophosphamide for 3 months (a cumulative dose similar to 6 months of IV cyclophosphamide) followed by long term MMF or azathioprine, the response rate among African Americans and European Americans were the same.

6. Among Asians, daily oral cyclophosphamide showed a tendency towards more rapid improvement in proteinuria and better preservation of renal function compared with IV cyclophosphamide [Mok CC *et al.*, Treatment of diffuse proliferative lupus nephritis: a comparison of two cyclophosphamide- containing regimens. Am J Kidney Dis. 2001, 38: 256–264.

   [B]. 1. In the Euro Lupus Trial by Houssiau (Houssiau FA *et al.*, Immunosuppressive therapy in lupus nephritis: the Euro-Lupus Nephritis Trial, a randomised trial of low-dose high–dose IV cyclophosphamide (CYC). Arthritis Rheum 2002, 46: 2121–2131) where 90 patients, 85% with Class IV LN were randomised to either standard doses of CYC consisting of 6 doses of monthly IV pulses followed by 2 quarterly pulses or Low Dose CYC of fixed pulses of 500 mg biweekly X 6, followed by maintenance with Azathioprine (AZA). There was no significant difference in renal remission with High Dose (54%) versus Low Dose (71%) and renal flares occurred in 29% and 27% respectively. High Dose group had trend towards more infections. Low Dose therapy regimen equally effective with less infections.

2. Chan TM (Chan TM *et al.*, Efficacy of mycophenolate mofetil in patients with diffuse proliferative lupus nephritis, Hong Kong-Guangzhou Nephrology Study Group. N Engl J Med 2000, 343:1156–1162) randomised 42 patients with Class IV LN to either MMF (induction with 2 gm/day for 6 months followed by 1gm/day for 6 months or Oral CYC (2.5 mg/Kg BW/day) for 6 months followed by AZA for 6 months. MMF and CYC were found to have equivalent efficacy with no differences in complete or partial remissions

or relapses. A 5-year follow up with addition of another 22 patients showed long term benefits of MMF with similar rates of relapse and relapse- free survival in both groups. Leukopenia, amenorrhoea and infections were more frequent in the CYC group with 2 deaths occurring in this group.

[C]. The LUNAR Trial using Rituximab, a chimeric monoclonal antibody which selectively targets CD20 expressing B cells in 144 patients in US, Canada, Mexico, Argentina and Brazil with Class III and IV LN where patients received 2 infusions of either Rituximab or placebo every 6 months, in addition to steroids and MMF did not achieve its target of improvement in renal function, urinary sediment and proteinuria at 52 weeks (Chloe Harman, Lupus Nephritis Trials end in disappointment, Nature Reviews, 2009, 5 [6]: 303).

[D]. The ASPEN Trial using Abetimus which comprises 4 double-stranded oligodeoxyribonucleotides attached to polyethylene glycol, and is designed to induce tolerance to pathogenic anti double- stranded-DNA autoantibodies both in the circulation and the surface of autoreactive B cells. The study involved 943 patients with LN from 203 centres in North and South America, Europe, Asia and Australia. Patients were given a dose of 300 mg or 900 mg per week of Abetimus or a placebo for 52 weeks. However the trial was stopped after an interim analysis showed the results to be of no benefit (Chloe Harman, Lupus Nephritis Trials end in disappointment, Nature Reviews, 2009, 5 [6]: 303).

INCREASED RISK OF MORTALITY

The following are features associated with an increased risk of ESRF:

1. Severe proteinuria during early clinical course
2. Renal impairment
3. Diffuse Lupus Nephritis (Class IV)

4. High chronicity index (sclerosis, crescents, interstitial fibrosis and tubular atrophy)
5. Younger age at disease onset
6. Male gender

PREDICTORS OF MORTALITY

The following are predictors of mortality in any patient with SLE:

1. Severe proteinuria during early clinical course
2. Renal impairment
3. Anaemia from any cause
4. Central nervous system disease (any form)
5. Younger age at disease onset
6. Disease duration prior to SLE diagnosis

PROGNOSIS

1. The overall 10-year survival rate is 70%.
2. The risk of ESRF within 10 years is 30% for those with diffuse proliferative lupus nephritis.
3. Young age and male gender increase the risk of renal failure.
4. Patients with insidious progression of azotaemia are likely to develop chronic irreversible disease.
5. A swift decline in renal function means active, treatable and potentially reversible lupus nephritis.

REFERENCES

1. Markowitz GS. The ISN/RPS 2003 Classification of lupus nephritis: an assessment at 3 years, Kid International, 2007, **49**:491–495.
2. Harman C. Lupus nephritis trials end in disappointment. Editorial. *Nature Reviews Nephrology*, 2009, **5**:303.

3. Walsh M, Jayne D. Rituximab in the treatment of anti-neutrophil cytoplasm antibody associated vasculitis and systemic lupus erythematosus: past, present and future. *Kidney Int* 2007, **72**:676–682.
4. Rovin BD, Lupus Nephritis: are we beyond cyclophosphamide? *Nature Reviews Nephrology*, 2009, **5**:492–494.
5. Chan TM *et al.*, Efficacy of mycophenolate mofetil in patients with diffuse proliferative lupus nephritis, Hong Kong-Guangzhou Nephrology Study Group. *N Engl J Med* 2000, **343**:1156–1162.
6. Houssiau FA *et al.*, Immunosuppressive therapy in lupus nephritis: the Euro-Lupus Nephritis Trial, a randomised trial of low-dose high–dose IV cyclophosphamide (CYC). *Arthritis Rheum* 2002, **46**:2121–2131.

CHAPTER 11

Urinary Tract Infection

The diagnosis of urinary tract infection is based on the demonstration of bacteria in the urine. Urine specimens can be obtained in one of 3 ways.

1. Mid Stream Urine

The patient should start with a full bladder, preferably the morning specimen. In the case of a female patient, a tampon should be used to prevent vaginal secretions from contaminating the urine specimen. The labia should be separated. In the uncircumcised male, the foreskin should be retracted. The exposed surface should then be cleansed with normal saline. After this the patient voids the first 200 ml of urine. Without stopping the micturition stream, the container is passed under the stream and the urine collected. The mid stream specimen of urine is then sent for urine microscopy as well as for culture and sensitivity. If colony counts exceed 10^5 it denotes an infection.

2. Suprapubic Aspiration

This is the best method for determining significant bacteriuria. Any bacterial growth regardless of the numbers is significant.

3. Catheterised Specimen

If for any reason the mid stream urine cannot be obtained or a suprapubic aspiration is contraindicated, then one may have to resort to a catheterised urine specimen. This method of obtaining urine should be the last resort as it carries the danger of introducing urinary tract infection. Remember to instill 100 ml of 0.2% neomycin in the bladder before removing the catheter.

EVIDENCE OF URINARY TRACT INFECTION

Direct evidence of urinary infection is provided by demonstration of bacterial growth in the urine.

Indirect evidence is provided by the demonstration of pyuria exceeding 3 WBC per high power field. For the modified Addis count where the cell count in 1 ml of urine is determined, the following are abnormal: WBC > 2000/ml, RBC > 800/ml and casts >1000/ml.

The mid stream urine should be cultured within 30 minutes. If at night, the urine specimen should be refrigerated if it cannot be sent off to the laboratory. Sometimes one can have a colony count of less than 10^5 which could still represent an infection, eg. if the patient has symptoms in the afternoon and he drinks a lot of fluid, the counts may be low. A mixed growth in general means a contaminated specimen. If 3 organisms are isolated together there is only a 5% incidence of this being due to an infection.

STERILE PYURIA

In a patient with sterile pyuria one has to exclude anaerobes, bacteriophage and mycoplasma. For the isolation of such organisms one requires special culture medium. Fungal infection is another cause of sterile pyuria. Yet another cause of sterile pyuria is Chlamydia trachomatis or C trachomatis. A patient who has earlier received antibiotics from his general practitioner before coming to see you may also not grow any organisms from his urine as the antibiotic is still present in his urine. Sometimes bacteriuria may be intermittent. Tuberculosis is of course a well-known cause of sterile pyuria and one should always remember to send urine for AFB cultures. In a woman, cancer of the cervix is something to remember and a vaginal examination may be indicated. Reflux nephropathy, analgesic nephropathy and renal stones are other causes of sterile pyuria.

SYMPTOMS

The symptoms of urinary infection in an adult are frequency of micturition, dysuria, bladder discomfort, loin pain, and fever with rigors. The presence of gross haematuria usually means involvement of the bladder indicating the presence of cystitis. This in a woman may be due to sexually related bladder infection or honeymoon cystitis.

In a patient with acute symptomatic urinary tract infection, about 25% of cultures will be sterile or there will be no significant counts. Of the other 75%, colony counts will exceed 10^5, half of whom would have cystitis and the other half an upper tract infection (pyelonephritis).

RADIOLOGY

An intravenous pyelogram is traditionally indicated in a male even if it is a first infection. In the case of a female the IVP is indicated only on the second infection. This is because females with a shorter urethra are more easily prone to develop cystitis during the sexual act as the urethra is very close to the anus and organisms are often accidentally introduced during sexual intercourse.

The IVP may show chronic atrophic pyelonephritis through the presence of unilateral or bilateral asymmetrical scars associated with distortion of the pelvicalyceal system. The scars are most often present in the upper poles of the kidneys, then the lower poles, followed by the mid zone. Sometimes an IVP may show renal stones, papillary necrosis or polycystic kidneys.

A Woman with Recurrent Infection

In a woman of child bearing age or for that matter, any female capable of the sexual act, if she has lower tract symptoms (cystitis) and the IVP is normal, the infection is often related to sexual intercourse. In such a case the patient should be given advice on sexual hygiene. Within 15 minutes of sexual intercourse she should empty her bladder. The couple may have to prolong the period of foreplay to ensure that there is adequate lubrication, otherwise they may have to resort to the use of lubricant in the form of KY jelly or other lubricant gel.

If the patient returns with a history of recurrent cystitis in spite of the above measures, then one would have to prescribe a tablet of nitrofurantoin postcoitally. If she returns again with infection the next step is to prescribe a tablet of nitrofurantoin every night. If the infection recurs, then she would require a tablet in the morning and another in the night. Nalidixic acid can also be used as a prophylactic agent though nitrofurantoin is preferable as there is less likelihood of the organism developing resistance. However, nitrofurantoin sometimes gives rise to the unpleasant side effects of nausea and vomiting in individuals who are susceptible.

Other side effects of NTF include chronic interstitial pneumonitis, acute pulmonary hypersensitivity reactions, liver damage, blood dyscrasias, skin reactions and neuropathy. Like Nalidixic Acid it should not be given when there is renal impairment. Half a tablet of Bactrium can also be used for prophylaxis. Another useful antibiotic for prophylaxis is Cefuroxime (Zinnat) given in a nightly dose of 250mg. Cephalexin is another oral cephalosporin which is popular for prophylaxis. This may be more appropriate than NTF if one is worried about side effects of NTF.

A Man with Recurrent Infection

In a man with recurrent urinary infection in the presence of a normal IVP, one has to suspect prostatitis and proceed to do a prostatic massage. In the choice of antibiotics remember to choose those that cross into the prostatic bed, namely, ciprofloxacin, erythromycin, trimethoprim and oleandomycin. In the treatment of prostatic infection one has to continue for a period of 6 weeks to even 3 months.

TREATMENT

For the acute infection most reports state that there is no difference whether one treats the patient for 6 weeks, 2 weeks or even 1 week. If the patient responds to the antibiotic, the urine should be sterile within a few hours. Symptoms may persist for another 24 to 48 hours. Pyuria however takes about a week to disappear. In general, for lower tract infections like cystitis 1 week therapy is sufficient. But for severe infections like pyelonephritis after the initial per-enteral injections of 5 days to a week, patients should have another week of oral antibiotics. In severe complicated infections treatment with oral antibiotics may have to continue for up to a month or 6 weeks depending on the underlying complication.

One should start off with the simple antibiotics like zinnat (cefuroxime), nalidixic acid or ampicillin. If symptoms are severe one may want to start with bactrium or ciprofloxacin. A mid stream urine is taken before the commencement of antibiotics and if there is no response, the subsequent choice of antibiotics is dictated by the results of culture and sensitivity. It may be that one may have to prescribe more potent antibiotics like an aminogly-coside such as gentamicin or amikacin or use a cephalosporin. When using an aminoglycoside one should always check the serum creatinine as the dose may have to be reduced in the presence of renal impairment. It is imperative that the levels of gentamicin or amikacin be monitored in the presence of renal impairment so as to prevent nephrotoxicity.

If culture and sensitivity results are not known and the patient is very ill or septicaemic, one should proceed to a combination of an aminoglycoside and ampicillin intravenously or a cephalosporin. Oral antibiotics like ciprofloxacin (quinolone) 500 mg BD or Zinnat (cefuroxime axetil) 250 mg BD may also be used in a severe infection, provided the patient is not septicaemic. Cedax or Ceftibufen dihydrate 400mg daily for 1 week for severe UTI caused by strains of susceptible organisms often resistant to other usual antibiotics. It is contraindicated in those who are hypersensitive to cephalosporins. For more resistant strains of organisms one would have to use antibiotics based on sensitivity. For gram negative bacilli, adequate cover is provided by quinolones, gentamycin or amikacin. Other antibiotics include broad spectrum cephalosporins like ceftrixone, astreonam, the β-lactum-β-lactamase inhibitor combinations (ampicillin-sulbactum, ticarcillin-clavulanate, and piperacillin-tazobactum); and imipenem-cilastin. The last few antibiotics should be kept for more complicated and severe infections.

Single Dose Therapy

Another mode of treatment is Single Dose Therapy. This treatment should be confined to patients who present with symptoms of cystitis. The treatment consists of a single intramuscular injection of 0.5 gm of kanamycin. A single oral dose of Ciprofloxacin 500 mg, Amoxycillin 3 gm or bactrium (4 tablets) may also be used. In Asian women however, a large dose of bactrium may cause headaches with nausea and vomiting.

If there is no response to Single Dose Therapy when the patient returns after a week the patient should have an IVP to exclude any anatomical abnormality. By this time results of cultures and sensitivity would also be ready if it had been sent off earlier.

There are now 2 forms of short course therapy, a single dose and a 3 day course. Evidence suggest that a 3 day course is superior with either TMP-SMX [bactrium or septrin] or quinolone. Those on Single dose therapy tend to recur more often. However, there are now more resistance to TMP-SMX compared to the past.

CONDITIONS ASSOCIATED WITH PYELONEPHRITIS

Conditions associated with pyelonephritis are obstruction to the urinary system, developmental causes like congenital valves, cystic disease and vesicoureteric reflux. Other causes are pregnancy, diabetes mellitus, stones, gout and analgesic abuse. The above list should be thought of in patients with recurrent infections.

Vesicoureteric Reflux

In man, the vesicoureteric valve is extremely competent due to the long intramural segment. Under certain conditions, reflux is demonstrated, e.g. during cystitis when the inflamed mucosal valve flap and the intramural ureter is rendered a rigid plastic tube. The refluxing valve is often due to a congenital weakness and the natural history of vesicoureteric reflux is one of spontaneous cure as the valve matures with the growth of the patient.

There are other causes of vesicoureteric reflux apart from a congenital defect. These could be acquired ureteric, bladder or urethral defects, bladder neck obstruction, diverticulum, ureterocele, ectopic ureter, duplex kidneys and renal stones.

In the West, vesicoureteric reflux accounts for 30% of renal failure in children and 15 to 20% in adults (about 10% in Singapore). The radiological term of chronic pyelonephritis which refers to the presence of asymmetrical scars in the kidneys associated with distortion of the pelvicalyceal system should in practice refer to chronic atrophic pyelonephritis which is due to vesicoureteric reflux. In other words acute pyelonephritis should not give rise to renal scars. It is only chronic atrophic pyelonephritis caused by vesicoureteric reflux which causes renal scarring.

Reflux nephropathy or chronic atrophic pyelonephritis affects 1 in 300 of the White female population. Of the number affected, about 10% have a bad prognosis. We do not have any local figures but it is suspected that the incidence is much lower here. However, there is a possibility that the condition may be under diagnosed as micturating cystourethrograms are not performed as frequently. In the West, apart from being an important cause of renal failure it is also a cause of renal hypertension. It has also been found to cause glomerulonephritis where the patients have proteinuria, sometimes in the nephrotic range, and the glomerular lesions are those of focal and segmental glomerulosclerosis. The cause of these glomerular lesions could be due to hyperfiltration, atypical bacterial forms, Tamm Horsfall proteins or an autoimmune basis.

The most important aspect of reflux nephropathy is that it is an important cause of persistent and recurrent urinary infection which can sometimes be very debilitating to the patient plus the fact that it is a cause of chronic renal failure.

The Scarring Process in Man

It has now been shown that in order to form renal scars, 3 conditions must be present. The patient must have composite (compound) renal papillae which allow intrarenal reflux. On this background there must be reflux of infected urine before renal scars can be formed.

Once scars are formed they will progress inexorably and lead to eventual contraction or fibrosis. A 3 cm scar may with time become only a 2 mm fibrous tissue. The patterns of the scars could be confined to the upper poles, bipolar, bilateral focal but unequal, or generalised.

Fresh scars are uncommon after the age of 5 years. The prognosis is poorer if there is no compensatory hypertrophy and the kidneys are progressively getting smaller. In other words, if the patient's infection is suppressed or prevented with prophylactic antibiotics and the reflux has disappeared as the vesicoureteric valves mature, the kidney may grow.

The standard tests for assessing VUR has been the voiding cystourethrogram or the radionucleoclide cystourethrography, both with significant radiation exposure. Recently, contrast enhanced voiding ultrasonography and magnetic resonance cystography have been developed and they provide equally useful information [Teh HS *et al*. Magnetic resonance cystography. Novel imaging technique for evaluation of vesicoureteric reflux. Urology 2005, 65:793].[31] Magnetic resonance imaging as a new approach is good for children because of lack of radiation exposure.

Jean Smellie *et al* have shown only 2 fresh scars in 75 compliant children on low dose prophylactic antibiotics followed up for 15 years. Children who have UTI but unscarred kidneys after age 3 years have only an estimated risk of developing new scars of 2% to 3%, so very low incidence as long as they continue prophylactic antibiotics.

Treatment

As part of the management, a micturating cystourethrogram should be performed and the reflux graded. Grade I is when there is reflux up to the pelvic brim. Grade II is reflux up to the renal pelvis but without causing distension of the pelvis. Grade III is when there is distension of the renal pelvis. Grade IV is when there is intrarenal reflux. However, there can be variability of grading from time to time as bacterial toxins during an infection may cause ureteric dilatation and increase the grading severity.

Children should be on prophylactic antibiotics till after the age of 5 years. After that if they still get infection they should be on prophylactic antibiotics until they are free of infection for 3 years in a stretch. The same applies to adults, especially in the presence of Grade III or IV reflux.

There is no place for routine ureteric reimplantation. The only indication is when the patient has Grade IV reflux in the presence of severe uncontrolled infection and progressive scarring. Another indication is the adult who has pain in the kidney during micturition due to distension of the renal pelvis resulting from urine refluxing during micturition.

Controlled trials have shown that the results of surgery for reimplantation of the ureters are no better than in patients treated medically with prophylactic antibiotics. Besides, the natural history of vesicoureteric reflux is one of spontaneous cure as the vesicoureteric valves mature.

Patients with vesicoureteric reflux with reflux nephropathy, especially if they already have renal impairment may do poorly during pregnancy and may deteriorate to end stage renal failure as a result of pregnancy. It may be safer to advise termination of pregnancy therefore in the presence of renal impairment especially if the patient is also hypertensive.

MANAGEMENT OF RECURRENT URINARY TRACT INFECTION

In the management of a patient with urinary tract infection (UTI), the clinician should take note of two salient features. The first is that clinical improvement does not equate with bacteriologic eradication and the second, follow-up urine cultures are necessary to ensure a cure. The first will determine the choice of antibiotics and the duration of treatment, and the second will help the clinician decide when to do follow-up urine cultures and sensitivity.

Relapsing Recurrences due to Urologic Abnormalities

One should always consider three common causes: renal stone disease, vesicoureteric reflux and prostatitis. A relapse often occurs about two weeks after an infection. In a female, she should receive another 6-week course of treatment and in a male, another 12 weeks. These 6 weeks would ensure proper eradication of UTI due to vesicoureteric reflux and 12 weeks for chronic prostatitis.[1] Relapse occurs because the bacteria are deep-seated within the stone, the prostate or within the kidney tissue in the case of reflux nephropathy. A short course of antibiotic will kill the organism but those within the stone or organ will still survive and cause a relapse if not properly eradicated.

Reinfections

Patients with frequent reinfections will have altered bacteria flora, reflecting faecal bacterial reservoir and impact of antibiotics. Sulphonamides, penicillin and cephalosporins will eradicate gram negative organisms in the gastrointestinal tract (GIT) but they are replaced by enterobacteraceae or pseudomonas species. The next "infection" usually occurs within 2 to 4 weeks and would be resistant to the above antibiotics. The choice of antibiotics would depend on the results of culture and sensitivity. Nitrofurantoin, trimethoprim and quinolones (nalidixic acid, ciprofloxacin) less commonly select resistant organisms in the GIT.[2]

Prophylaxis

Prophylaxis of symptomatic lower tract infection in women is effective. Women with 2 or more symptomatic upper tract infections in a year should have prophylaxis. Nitrofurantoin 50 mg, cotrimoxazole 240 mg or ½ tablet, Zinnat (cefuroxime axetil) 250mg, nalidixic acid 500 mg following sexual intercourse is effective. If the patient continues to have recurrent infection the antibiotic can be prescribed thrice weekly or even nightly if necessary. In males, there are no definitive studies regarding the value of preventing asymptomatic infection to reduce occurrence of acute pyelonephritis. For patients with vesicoureteric reflux, prophylaxis prevents infection of kidneys, protects or preserves renal function and in a growing child, allows resumption of normal renal growth.[3]

Continuous Suppression

Permanent suppression is recommended in patients with frequent relapses (3 or more episodes a year) or for those where the source of infection cannot be removed, like stones, vesicoureteric reflux, prostatitis or obstructive uropathy.

The suppressive regimen consists of nightly, twice daily or full dose suppressive therapy with nitrofurantoin, cotrimoxazole or nalidixic acid, ciprofloxacin or cefuroxime axetil (Zinnat). For example, a patient with chronic prostatitis, after treatment of the infection for 6 to 12 weeks with antibiotics can be put on cotrimoxazole one tablet (480 mg) nightly for years with no infection. It is important to review the patient every 3 to 4 months with urine culture and sensitivity. In the event of a breakthrough infection occurring, a new antibiotic is prescribed to treat the infection. After that, the patient is put on suppressive antibiotics again. Cotrimoxazole can still be used as the suppressive agent once the infection is eradicated. After 2 years on suppressive therapy, in the absence of infection, the antibiotic can be stopped to see if infection recurs. If it does, the patient will require treatment followed by further suppressive therapy.

Patient with Renal Impairment

Aminoglycosides like gentamicin and amikacin should be avoided if possible. If they have to be used, the dose should be reduced and serum creatinine and antibiotic levels monitored. Nitrofurantoin is contraindicated because it is of no use since it is poorly concentrated in the failing kidney. But more importantly, it causes very severe and painful peripheral neuropathy in patients with renal impairment.[4]

Penicillins can be used. The newer ones with a broader spectrum of activity like piperacillin, mezlocillin and azlocillin are also active against most strains or pseudomonas and strep faecalis.[5] They are preferred over the third generation cephalosporins like ceftriazone and ceftazidime if either of these are infecting pathogens. The first generation cephalosporins are nephrotoxic but the second generation is less so and the third generation are safe but dosage has to be reduced in renal failure. Cotrimoxazole consists of trimethoprim which is not nephrotoxic but sulphamethoxazole is. In mild renal impairment only half the usual dose of cotrimoxazole (480 mg) twice daily should be used. Quinolones are safe drugs to use in renal failure.

Causes of Recurrent UTI

Recurrent UTI could be due to or associated with the following: obstruction of the urinary tract, vesicoureteric reflux, renal calculi, diabetes mellitus, analgesic nephropathy, polycystic kidneys, cystitis, prostatitis, pregnancy, neurogenic bladder, urinary catheterisation, benign prostatic hypertrophy and uterovaginal prolapse among the elderly.

Obstruction of the Urinary Tract

Obstruction at all levels, from renal tubules to urethral meatus, is the most important factor predisposing to infection. Stasis compromises bladder and renal defence to Sepsis. In patients with renal cortical scars as in reflux nephropathy, there is no increased susceptibility to infection. However in those with renal papillary scars (analgesic nephropathy, diabetic papillary necrosis) there is an increased susceptibility to infection because of intratubular obstruction.

Causes of obstruction could be due to congenital lesions (valves, bands, stenosis, bladder neck obstruction), extrinsic compression of the ureters (tumours, retroperitoneal fibrosis), localised intrarenal obstruction to urinary flow (nephrocalcinosis, uric acid nephropathy, polycystic kidney and analgesic nephropathy).

Vesicoureteric Reflux (VUR)

This is a common cause of UTI. In patients with VUR, bladder infection may induce reflux because the inflamed intramural portion of the ureter is rendered a rigid plastic tube by the inflammation thus allowing reflux when the bladder contracts during micturition. Reflux disappears once infection is controlled. This is therefore a vicious cycle. Infection produces reflux or aggravates it, which in turn maintains the infection by producing residual urine which predisposes to infection because of urinary stasis.

If urinary infection is controlled, reflux tends to diminish as a result of the ureteral and bladder wall growing thicker with age. Prophylactic antibiotics are useful in preventing infection. About 20% of children not on prophylaxis develop new scars compared to those on prophylaxis.[6-8]

Infection and Nephrolithiasis

Damage to renal papillae produced by infection can cause calcified foci which with time become renal stones. The renal stones then cause UTI, incidence varying from 2% to as high as 47%.[9] About 50% of infections are due to proteus mirabilis. UTI with urea splitting organism causes triple phosphate (struvite) stones. There is a 25% mortality over 5 years in patients with stones induced by bilateral renal infection. The risk of stone recurrence after surgery is 40% to 60%. The rate of persistent UTI is 40% because bacteria survive deep inside the stone.[10] In the management of such patients it is important to continue suppressive antibiotic therapy to prevent infected stones.

Xanthogranulomatous Pyelonephritis

This is a rare condition which occurs when infection affects a kidney which is partially obstructed by calculi. Most common in adults in the 5th to 7th decade. About 70% of patients have history of renal stones, diabetes or obstructive uropathy.

Patients with this condition have fever with chronic urinary tract infection and a mass in the loin which is seen on the IVP as a tumour mass. Angiography however does not suggest a tumour.

Urine cultures grow *Proteus* in 60% of the cases and *E. coli* in the rest. Methicillin resistant Staph aureus can also cause this condition.

The gross pathology reveals large kidneys with adhesions and abscesses. Histology reveals foam cells, foreign body giant cells with necrotic debris and polymorphs. Some glomeruli will have masses of clear cells like in a carcinoma but with no mitosis. However there have been rare reports of renal cell cancer or transitional cell cancer of the renal pelvis associated with this condition. Nephrectomy may be needed if the kidney is non-functioning. Recurrence is rare. It can occur in transplanted kidneys.

Malakoplakia

A condition often confined to urinary bladder mucosa appearing as a soft yellow slightly raised often confluent plaques of 3 to 4 cm in diameter. Cause usually due to enteric bacteria.It occurs commonly in middle aged women with a history of chronic UTI. The plaques are composed of closely packed large macrophages with occasional lymphocytes and multi nucleate giant cells. The macrophages have abundant foamy PAS reactive -positive cytoplasm. Michaelis –Gutmann bodies result from deposition of calcium phosphate and other minerals on the phagosomes.

Identical lesions have been found in the kidneys, prostate, bones, lungs, intestines, testes and skin. E coli is the most common organism found in the urine. In rare occasions bilateral involvement have caused a presentation with acute renal failure.

This is a disease of uncertain etiology and has been associated with autoimmune disease, immunodeficiency, malignancy, HIV infection and rheumatoid arthritis.

Treatment consists of treating or removing the underlying condition and the use of appropriate antibiotics based on urine culture and sensitivity.

Renal Tuberculosis

The genitourinary tract is the most common extra pulmonay site for tuberculosis and accounts for about 10% of all new cases reported every year. It is often present for many years in the patient before a diagnosis is made by which time there already exists significant destruction of the urinary tract.

It often presents as sterile pyuria and the symptoms include dysuria, haematuria and loin pain. In about 20% of renal TB, there are no associated symptoms. About 50% present with urinary abnormalities and 90% yield positive cultures for mycobacteria tuberculosis. Abnormal intravenous pyelogram is present in about 95% of patients.

The pathology consists of granulomatous inflammation and caseous necrosis which begin in the medulla and papillary occasionally resulting in papillary necrosis. From here it extends to the cortex. When the lesions coalesce, large caseous cavities are the result. Radiological diagnosis is based on intravenous pyelogram and the CT Scan.

Treatment consists of an initial 2 months course of rifampicin, isoniazid and pyrazinamide followed by another 4 months of daily rifampicin and isoniazid. This regimen is suitable for women. In men, because of involvement of the prostate gland it is advisable to continue treatment for another 3 to 6 months. In patients with caseating destruction of the kidneys a total of 18 months therapy is advisable.

Patients with drug resisitant TB should have initial therapy with isoniazid, rifampicin and pyrazinamide to ensure use of at least 2 bactericidal agents plus one of the following: ethambutol, ofloxacin or streptomycin. If two bactericidal agents are used, treatment should be for 12 months. If only one bactericidal agent is used, treatment should be for 24 months.

Tuberculosis heals by fibrosis and subsequently, if obstructive uropathy should arise, the patient will require surgery to relieve obstruction and preserve renal function.

Diabetes Mellitus

Diabetes mellitus is said to be associated with an increased frequency of UTI. However, this is based on evidence from uncontrolled or poorly controlled studies. A diabetic with no neurological complication affecting the bladder and has not undergone instrumentation is not at greater risk of developing UTI. However, following urinary catheterisation or in the presence of an autonomic bladder the incidence of ascending infection is frequent and severe. Underlying nephrosclerosis in a diabetic kidney also increases the possibility of papillary necrosis which predisposes to infection.

Analgesic Nephropathy

This condition is associated with recurrent or asymptomatic UTI. UTI occurs in 15% to 60% of patients with analgeic nephropathy[11]. In a patient with analgesic nephropathy associated with UTI and deteriorating renal function, one has to exclude urinary tract obstruction and septicemia. The cause of urinary obstruction in a patient with analgesic nephropathy could be the result of a sloughed papilla, a calcified papilla or renal stones, transitional cell carcinoma in the renal pelvis or ureter and lastly, pyonephrosis. Analgesic nephropathy is one of the causes of sterile pyuria.

Cystitis

Acute cystitis or urethritis is common in women. An infection is termed a relapse if it occurs within 3 weeks of cessation of treatment. Reinfection accounts for about 80% of recurrent UTI. The organism is often from the perineal flora. Other foci of infection are the kidneys, prostate or the presence of any urologic abnormality. Nuns have an annual incidence of 0.4% cystitis compared to 1.6% in women aged 13 to 54 years.[12] This is because during sexual intercourse, bacteria is massaged into the urinary bladder through the anterior urethra.

E coli causes 79% of cystitis, Staph saprophyticus 11%, Klebsiella 3%, mixed organisms 3%, Proteus mirabilis 2%, enterococcus 2% and other bacteria 2%. Uropathogenetic E coli has virulent features like increased adherence to cells, resistance to bactericidal human serum and K capsular antigen which is anti-phagocytic and causes persistent infection in a certain proportion of women with recurrent cystitis.[13]

In men, prostatic fluid itself inhibits bacterial growth and the mucus in the bladder has anti-mannose activity which discourages bacterial growth. Some females are prone to UTI because of a defect in local defence which makes them vulnerable to periurethral colonisation. This defect may be due to a lack in a particular antibody. Another reason may be the virulence of the particular strain of bacteria. Once infected, the bacteria persist.[14]

Bacterial Virulence of Escherichia Coli

1. Virulent or uropathogenic clones of E coli possess a variety of special features that enable them to wreak havoc in the host. The virulent clones are of a limited number of serotypes belonging to the O serotypes and account for about 80% of cases of pyelonephritis, compared to 28% of fecal strains, 60% of cystitis isolates and 30% of asymptomatic bacteriuria.

2. Also a limited number of K or capsular antigens are found on these uropathogenic clones for more than 70% of pyelonephritis isolates. A variety of other factors contribute to their virulence such as surface adhesins that mediate attachment to specific receptors in the uroepithelium, molecules

that preferentially capture metabolites and growth factors that enhance growth and proliferation and toxins that injure the tissue of the urinary tract by inducing an inflammatory response.

3. The most clearly defined virulence factors of uropathogenic E coli are surface adhesins that mediate attachment to receptors on uroepithelial cells and gut mucosa, thus accounting for colonization of the bowels, vagina and periurethral tissue. These sites of colonization are the reservoirs where the invading organisms arise.

4. The ligand- receptor interactions allow the bacteria to resist the flushing action of the urine flow and bladder emptying. The majority of these adhesins are found at the tip of the fimbria extending from the bacterial surface.

5. Another binding site for the E coli is fibronectin which provides another mechanism for attachment of the bacteria to the extracellular matrix.

6. Other mechanisms include the production of hemolysin, the presence of iron binding protein aerobactin and iron –regulating gene products which can resist the bactericidal effect of normal human serum.

7. Another critical determinant of the effects of UTI on the host is the inflammatory response to the presence of replicating bacteria resulting in the release of noxious cytokines like interlukins IL 6 and IL 8, tumour necrosis factor (TNF).

8. P fimbria and endotoxin play a role in initiating the inflammatory response to the replicating bacteria.

9. Men with prostatitis, women with pyelonephritis and those with spinal cord injuries with UTI all share the same virulence factors of E coli.[28,29,30]

Treatment of Cystitis

The principle is to use the least toxic and least expensive antibiotic like ampicillin, cefuroxime axetil (zinnat) and ciprofloxacin.

The patient should be encouraged to drink plenty of water to promote a good flow of urine to prevent urinary stasis which encourages bacterial growth. In recent years, ampicillin has been found to be less effective because of resistant strains of E coli.[13] Fifty percent of Staph saprophyticus and all Klebsiella species are now ampicillin resistant. However, augmentin which is a combination of amoxycillin and clavulinic acid is effective. The clavulinic acid destroys penicillinase produced by the bacteria and allows the ampicillin component to act on the cell wall of the bacteria.

Nitrofurantoin is highly effective but 40% of patients experience nausea.[15] Cotrimoxazole has a propensity to cause gastrointestinal upset and rash. It is also effective against Chlamydia trachomatis. The quinolones (pefloxacin, ciprofloxacin)) are related to nalidixic acid and cinoxin. They are also highly effective against C trachomatis.

If a patient has symptoms of acute dysuria, suggestive of cystitis, she should be treated for UTI though the urine culture shows $<10^5$ colony counts of bacteria growth as one-third of patients with UTI has negative urine cultures.[16]

Cystitis and Urethritis

Females are 50 times more likely to have UTI than males. About 20% of females aged 24 to 60 years have at least one episode of UTI per year. After the age of 60 years the frequency is equal in both sexes.

One-third of patients with cystitis have gross haematuria. Some of these progress to upper UTI. About 40% of those with symptoms of UTI would have less than 10^5 colony counts of bacteria in the urine culture. They should still be treated as for cystitis. Fifty percent of patients with the "acute urethral syndrome" with negative cultures subsequently develop significant bacteriuria on follow-up.[16] There are 2 groups of patients with acute urethral syndrome. About 70% of them have pyuria with positive cultures.

Many of these 70% may have infection with C trachomatis or with infection due to E. coli or Staph saprophyticus but with less than significant bacteria counts (10^2 to 10^4/ml). The remaining 30% of patients with acute urethral syndrome have no known etiologic agent for their symptoms.

If urine cultures are negative for bacteria and the patient has symptoms of dysuria suggesting the urethral syndrome, one should apart from C. trachomatis, also consider N. gonorrhoea, Herpes simplex, Mycoplasma and Ureaplasma. These organisms can also cause the acute urethral syndrome. Sometimes a complaint of "dysuria" is actually due to pain caused by urine flowing over the inflamed vagina as in Candida vaginitis.

Relapsing Lower Tract Infection

In a woman with relapsing lower tract infection one should suspect an upper tract infection (pyelonephritis) and in the case of a man one should suspect prostatitis. In both sexes, a structural abnormality, stones, diverticulae should also be considered.

A patient who relapses after a week of treatment should be treated for another 2 weeks, cotrimoxazole or ciprofloxacin are the better choices. If there is another relapse the patient should receive a 6-week course of treatment and an intravenous pyelogram (IVP) should be performed. Thereafter the patient should be followed up with repeat urine cultures at 2 weeks, 4 weeks, 12 weeks and 6 months to ensure eradication of the infection.

In the case of patients with chronic prostatitis they should be treated with antibiotics like cotrimoxazole, erythromycin, oleandomycin and ciprofloxacin (17). Instead of the standard erythromycin one could use azithromycin, 4 courses of 3 day therapy with a break of 1 week in between. With these antibiotics, adequate therapeutic levels can be achieved within the prostate. Treatment should be for at least 4 weeks for acute prostatitis and

12 weeks for chronic prostatitis to ensure eradication of the infection.

Recurrent Urinary Tract Infection in the Females

Two groups of women should be considered. Those with structural or functional abnormality of the urinary tract and those with normal IVP who have lower tract infection. In some, there may be a relationship to sex or use of diaphragm but in the majority there is often no apparent cause. Infection tends to cluster in time, that is, it tends to occur more and more frequently with shorter intervals in between and then it will go off for long periods without a recurrence.

Patients should be given advice regarding sexual hygiene like voiding of the urine within 15 minutes of sexual intercourse, prolonging the period of foreplay to ensure adequate lubrication, drinking enough fluids to pass more urine to reduce urinary stasis at night and wiping from front to back to avoid introduction of perianal flora into the urethral opening.

Women with frequent lower UTI should have prophylactic antibiotics post coitally if infections are related to sex. Nitrofurantoin one tablet post coitally is a useful prophylactic agent. Others are trimethoprim or cotrimoxazole (½ tablet or 240 mg) and nalidixic acid 500 mg. Women who suffer 2 or more infections a year could be taught the use of self administered single dose therapy, 4 x 480 mg of cotrimoxazole orally or 3 gm of amoxycillin or 500 mg of Ciprofloxacin orally as a single dose therapy.[18] For those who still continue to suffer recurrent UTI with prophylactic nightly antibiotics, we would prescribe suppressive therapy cefuroxime axetil 250mg or 500mg bd, cotrimoxazole 480 mg bd or ciprofloxacin 250mg or 500mg bd. This should continue for 1 year to 2 years and thereafter antibiotics stopped and reinfections monitored. If reinfection occurs, it should be treated with a course of antibiotics and the suppressive regimen continued for another 1 to 2 years and then reviewed again.

E coli is the commonest organism responsible for pros
Others are Proteus, Klebsiella, Enterobacter, Pseudomon
Serratia. The route of infection is

  (i) by ascending urethral infection
 (ii) reflux of infected urine into the prostatic duct and i
      prostate
(iii) invasion by rectal bacteria, and
 (iv) hematogenous route

During sexual intercourse a man can be infected by gono
urethritis through sexual contact with an infected female
harbouring the gonococci in the cervix. Reflux of infected u
another route. The presence of an indwelling catheter would
bacteria to directly infect prostatic ducts by peri-urethral ext
along the catheter. In acute prostatitis, a rectal examinatic
reveal a tender prostate. Prostatic massage or instrumentati
cystoscopy should not be performed during acute prostatitis

In a patient with prostatitis one should exclude prostat
culi, cancer of the prostate, prostatomegaly due to benign
plasia and chronic prostatitis. If epididymitis is present the
is likely to have chronic prostatitis.[17] Urethral discharge in
could be due to urethritis, urethro-prostatitis, or prostato
(very often the result of infrequent ejaculation). Chronic ba
prostatitis is a common cause of relapsing UTI in a male wi
mal IVP. If a patient has a large residual urine volun
enlarged prostate is often the cause. In a male with positive
cultures from mid-stream urine with no symptom of UTI,
nosis of prostatitis is very likely. Under these circumsta
prostatic massage should be performed. Four specimens
be obtained: void bladder urine (VBI) when urine is passed
the mid-stream urine (MSU), the mid-stream urine (
expressed prostatic secretion (EPS) resulting from the m
and the fourth specimen which is the urine passed followi
massage (VB3).[19,20]

Relapsing Urinary Tract Infection due to Prostatitis

Infection should be by the same pathogen with symptoms of dysuria, urgency, frequency of micturition, nocturia, suprapubic, perianal, scrotal, penile pain or hemospermia. Once treatment is stopped, symptoms recur soon after in a patient with a relapse.

Acute prostatitis should be treated for 4 to 6 weeks to prevent chronicity. Cotrimoxazole 2 tablets twice daily is a useful agent. Alternatively, one could start off with injection gentamicin plus intravenous amoxycillin for a week followed by oral cotrimoxazole once cultures confirm the sensitivity of the bacteria to the antibiotic. Other agents like erythromycin or azithromycin, doxycycline, cephalosporin and quinolones could be used in acute prostatitis. In acute prostatitis most antibiotics can penetrate the inflamed prostate gland because of the acute inflammation of the gland.

For chronic prostatitis treatment should be with trimethoprim, erythromycin, oleadomycin or ciprofloxacin for 12 weeks.[17] Azithromycin, the new form of Erythromycin could be used at a dose of 500 mg daily for 3 days with a break of one week. A total of 9 courses would cover 3 months. If there is no cure after 12 weeks and relapse still occurs, the infection should be treated and thereafter the patient should receive suppressive therapy with trimethoprim one tablet daily or twice daily on a long term basis for 2 years, and thereafter stopped to see if there is a relapse. If so, the patient should continue to receive therapy for another 2 years.

Non Bacterial Prostatitis

This is caused by the same organisms causing non gonococcal urethritis (NGU); apart from fungus and anaerobes. Organisms causing NGU are C. trachomatis, Ureaplasma, Mycoplasma, Trichomonads, H. simplex and Cytomegalovirus (CMV). C trachomatis causes 40% to 50% of NGU and Ureaplasma causes

Urine cultures should be performed to exclude gonococc
special cultures performed for C. trachomatis and Ureaplas

Treatment for NGU consists of either erythromycin or te
cline for 2 weeks. But in the case of non bacterial pro
resulting from organisms causing NGU, treatment should
12 weeks. Trimethoprim and ciprofloxacin could also be
During therapy the patient should abstain from sex and al
The sexual partner should also be treated. Relapse could be
the organism becoming resistant to the antibiotic, poor
compliance, H. simplex infection which would require th
with iodoxyuridine or it could mean that the sexual partn
not been or has been inadequately treated.

Pregnancy

Asymptomatic bacteriuria occurs in 4% to 7% of pr
women. About one-third of these women run the risk of de
ing acute pyelonephritis in the later stages of pregnancy.[22]

Screening is important as this will reduce the inciden
pyelonephritis to less than 5% in 75% of patients.[22] This wi
vent the foetal morbidity due to prematurity.

An increased rate of spontaneous abortion in pregnancies
plicated by bacteriuria has been reported. There is also a
frequency of low birth weight babies born to such mother
is also associated with increased fetal; mortality rate.

In pregnancy, estrogen and progesterone induce dilatat
ureters and the renal pelvis. This will increase progres
towards term. The bladder capacity also doubles and the b
becomes distorted due to compression by the gravid uterus

The following antibiotics are safe in pregnancy; short
sulphonamides, amoxycillin, nitrofurantoin and cephalexin
those with overt pyelonephritis they should have parenteral
tion with β-lactum drugs, aminoglycosides or both.

Upper Urinary Tract Infection and Neurogenic Bladder

Patients with spinal cord injury require either continuous or intermittent urethral catheterisation. Renal infection is secondary to chronic upper tract infection and many patients form stones.[24]

In the past decade the use of non-sterile intermittent self catheterisation has been introduced.[25] The patients were not treated with routine prophylactic antibiotics so as to reduce incidence of emergence of resistant strains of organisms. However, others employ low dose prophylactic antibiotics with cotrimoxazole to prevent infection.[26] Continuous long term suppression with antibiotics has been used to prevent recurrent symptoms. Antibiotics used include cotrimoxazole, amoxycillin and cephalosporins.

Infection by proteus must always be suppressed as such infections predispose to stone formation which are difficult to eradicate as the bacteria lie within the stone. Some advocate treatment only for symptomatic infection. They argue against suppressive antibiotic therapy as it selects multiresistant organisms.

Catheter Associated Urinary Tract Infection

This constitutes 35% to 40% of all hospital acquired infections. It is the most common source of gram negative bacteremia. Bacteria gain entry in the following ways:

(i) at time of catheterisation
(ii) they enter around catheter in the urethral mucus (periurethral route)
(iii) via contamination of the collecting system; bacteria ascend through the lumen of the catheter, hence the importance of using a closed drainage system

Antecedent rectal or periurethral colonisation also plays an important role as it does in female with cystitis. After a single in-out catheterisation, bacteriuria occurs in 1% of healthy persons compared to 3% to 20% among the pregnant, the elderly, debilitated and those patients with urologic abnormalities.[26]

About 50% of females and males who are catheterised for 2 weeks become bacteriuric.[26] The overall incidence increases with the duration of catheter in place and is related to the patient's condition.

Prevention of Catheter Urinary Tract Infection

The following have been advocated:

(i)   Closed drainage system. This prevents bacteriuria up to 10 days
(ii) Twice daily application of polyantimicrobial cream to urethral meatus
(iii) Systemic antibiotics in the short term not long term because this will predispose to infection with resistant strains
(iv) Lubricating gels for catheter

Treatment of Catheter Urinary Tract Infection

The infected catheter should be removed, antibiotic therapy initiated and a new catheter reintroduced together with a new closed drainage system. If the patient has fever and loin pain, parenteral antibiotics should be initiated immediately and therapy continued for a week. Resistant bacteria and fungi (Candida, Torulopsis) are frequently isolated in patients on multiple courses of antibiotics. The choice of a suitable anti-fungal agent is guided by results of sensitivity tests.

Lower tract funguria (cystitis) usually responds to amphotericin B bladder washout. First, empty the bladder of urine by means of a urinary catheter. Amphotericin B is then introduced in a dosage of 15 mg in 100 ml of distilled water through the urinary catheter. The catheter is then removed. The amphotericin will stay in the bladder and is passed out together with the urine after a few hours. Lower tract fungaria causing cystitis should respond after an amphotericin bladder wash out. After one week the urine culture should be negative for fungus. If fungus persists, it would mean that the infection is in the upper tract (pyelonephritis). If that is the case then, the patient should be treated as for an upper tract fungal infection as for systemic candidiasis (if candida is the organism grown). Intravenous amphotericin is administered following a test dose and then progressively increased until a total dosage of about 1 gm has been given, usually over a period of 6 weeks or more. Alternatively, if the organism is sensitive to 5-fluorocytosine, it could be administered intravenously for the first 2 weeks and then oral therapy given for the remaining period. This has the advantage of early discharge of the patient from hospital.

Some may not like the idea of bladder catheterisation with amphotericin washout which could induce bacteriuria. A 10 to 14 day course of fluconazole in a dose of 200 to 400 mg a day may be preferable.

Urinary Tract Infection and the Elderly

Ageing is associated with an increased prevalence of bacteriuria. It is about 10% in males and 20% in females over the age of 65 years.[27] Young female adults have 30 times greater prevalence of bacteriuria compared to young male adults. Many post-menopausal women have significant amount of residual urine volume in their bladder after voiding as a consequence of childbirth and loss of pelvic tone. The lack of estrogen also causes a marked change in the susceptibility of the uroepithelium and the vagina to pathogens. This is also due to the loss of lactobacilli which causes a rise in the vaginal pH. In young women one would consider other uropathogens and C trachomatis. But in the older women one has to consider TB, fungal infection, diverticulitis and diverticular abcess impinging on the bladder or ureter.

Estrogen replacement therapy, either as local cream or systemic with oral therapy would restore the atrophic genitourinary tract mucosa of the post menopausal woman and is associated with reappearance of lactobacilli in the vaginal flora with a fall in vagina pH with decreased colonization to E coli. Thus estrogen therapy can counter recurrent UTI in the elderly woman. Cranberry juice has been shown to reduce the frequency of both bacteruria and pyuria in the elderly woman. In addition to acidification effect, it also helps to inhibit the attachment of bacterial adhesins to the female uroepithelium [Avorn J *et al.* Reduction of bacteruria and pyuria after ingestion of cranberry juice. J.A.M.A. 1994, 271:571].[32]

The following causes account for an increased prevalence of UTI in the elderly:

 (i) Obstructive uropathy
 (ii) Loss of bactericidal activity of prostatic secretion
(iii) Poor bladder emptying due to utero-vaginal prolapse, cystocele and prostatomegaly
(iv) Soiling of perineum from faeces
 (v) Increased bladder catheterisation

CONCLUSION

Every episode of a UTI has the potential to become a recurrent or chronic disease. Patient education is a very important aspect of the management as in many diseases which have the propensity to become chronic. Patients should be taught to anticipate subsequent episodes by teaching them to look out for early symptoms. They must understand the reasons for recurrence in order to avoid infection.

It is equally important too that the attending physician should be aware of certain aspects of the management to minimise the possibility of relapse, recurrence and chronicity. Clinical improvement does not equate bacteriologic eradication. Follow-up urine cultures are necessary to ensure cure. Depending on the circumstances of the case, whether it is a lower tract infection due to cystitis (1 week treatment), upper tract infection (2 weeks) or prostatitis (6 to 12 weeks), the physician would have to prescribe an antibiotic for varying duration. The choice of the antibiotic will depend on whether one is treating a simple recurrent cystitis in a female with normal IVP, or a patient with acute or chronic prostatitis. The choice of an antibiotic will also depend on whether it is prescribed for the current infection or for prophylactic or suppressive therapy because the emergence of multiresistant organism has to be considered. Therapy has to be accompanied by follow-up cultures and sensitivity performed at the right time and the correct periodic interval; 1 week, 2 weeks, 4 weeks, 12 weeks and 6 months to detect asymptomatic bacteriuria and at any time when the patient has a breakthrough infection.

Managed properly, the patient is likely to have a marked reduction in the incidence of relapses and recurrences, apart from the possibility of preventing a relapse or recurrence in a patient with a first or new infection. Even so, for many patients who have had a UTI, they would be prone to relapses and recurrences, often requiring long term prophylactic or suppressive antibiotics.

REFERENCES

1. White NJ, Stamm WE. eds. Cystitis and urethritis. In: Diseases of the kidney. Boston: *Little Brown and Co* 1988, 1109–1133.
2. Lacey RW, Lord VL, Howson GL, Luxton DEA, Trotter JC. Double blind study to compare the selection of antibiotic resistance by amoxylline or cephradine in the commensal flora. *Lancet*, 1983, **2**: 529–532.
3. Winberg J, Bollgren I, Kallenius G, Molby R, Svenson SB. Clinical pyelonephritis and focal renal scarring. *Paed Clin North Am* 1982, **29**:801–814.
4. Woo KT. ed. Drugs and the kidney. In: Handbook of clinical nephrology, Singapore: PG Lim Publishing, 1991, 182–187.
5. Sattler FR, Moyer JE, Schramm M, Lombard JS, Appelbaum PC. Aztreonam compared with gentamicin for treatment of serious urinary tract infections. *Lancet*, 1984, **1**: 1315–1318.

6. Smellie JM, Ransley PG, Normand ICS, Prescod N, Edwards D. Development of new renal scars: A collaborative study. *Br Med J* 1985, **290**:1957–1960.
7. Naimaldin A, Burge DM, Atwell JD. Reflux nephropathy secondary to intrauterine vesicoureteric reflux. *J Paed Surg* 1990, **25**:287–290.
8. Bailey RR, Lynn KL, Smith AH. Long term follow-up of infants with gross vesicoureteric reflux. In: Bailey RR. ed. Second CJ Hodson Symposium on Reflux Nephropathy. Christchurch, New Zealand: Typeshop, 1990, 33–36.
9. Blandy JP, Singh M. The case for a more aggressive approach to staghorn calculus. *J Urol* 1976, **115**:505–506.
10. Rous SN, Turner WR. Retrospective study of 95 patients with staghorn calculus disease. *J Urol* 1977, **118**:902–907.
11. Murray TG, Goldberg M. Analgesic associated nephropathy in the USA: Epidemiologic, clinical and pathogenetic features. *Kidney Int* 1978, **13**:64–71.
12. Kunin CM, McCormack RC. An epidemiological study of bacteriuria and blood pressure among nuns and working women. *N Engl J Med* 1968, **278**:635–642.
13. Latham RH, Running K, Stamm WE. Urinary tract infections in young women caused by Staphyloccus saprophyticus. *JAMA* 1983, **250**:3063–3066.
14. Stamey TA, Fair WR, Timothy MM. Antibacterial nature of prostatic fluid. *Nature*, 1968, **218**:444–449.
15. Aronoff GR. Antimicrobial therapy for patients with renal disease. *Hosp Pract* 1983, **18**:145–150.
16. Stamm WE, Running K, McKevitt M, Counts GW, Turk M, Holmes KK. Treatment of acute urethral syndrome. *N Engl J Med* 1981, **304**:956–958.
17. Meares EM Jr, Prostatitis: new perspectives about old woes. *J Urol* 1980, **113**:141–147.
18. Bailey RR. Single dose therapy of urinary tract infection. In: Recent advances in Paediatrics. London: Churchill Livingstone, 1986, 75–83.
19. Meares EM Jr, Stamey TA. Bacteriologic localization patterns in bacterial prostatitis and urethritis. *Invest Urol* 1968, **5**:492–518.
20. Meares EM Jr, Barbalias GA. Prostatitis: Bacterial, nonbacterial and prostatodynia. *Semin Urol* 1983, **1**:146–151.
21. Berger RE, Urethritis and epididymitis. *Semin Urol* 1983, **1**:138–145.
22. Stamm WE. Prevention of urinary tract infections. *Am J Med* 1984, **76**: 148–154.

23. Zinner SH. Bacteriuria and babies revisited. *N Engl J Med* 1979, **300**:853–855.
24. Barkin M, Dolfin D, Herschron S, Bharatwal N, Comisarow R. The urologic care of the spinal cord injury patient. *J Urol* 1983, **129**:335–339.
25. Maynard FM, Diokno AC. Urinary infection and complications during clean intermittent catheterization following spinal cord injury. *J Urol* 1984, **132**:943–946.
26. Krieger JN, Kaiser DL, Wenzel RP. Nosocomial urinary tract infection, secular trends, treatment and economics in a university hospital, *J Urol* 1983, **130**:102–106.
27. Romano JM, Kaye D. Urinary tract infection in the elderly: Common yet atypical. *Geriatrics* 1981, **36**:113–115.
28. Andreu A, Stapleton AE, Fennel C *et al.* Urovirulence determinants of Escherichia coli strains causing prostatiitis. *J Infect Dis* 1997, **176**:464.
29. Terrai A, Yamamoto S, Mitsumori K *et al*, Escherichia coil virulence factorsand serotypes in acute bacterial prostatitis. *Int J Urol* 1997, **4**:289.
30. Hull RA, Rudy DC, Wieser IE *et al.* Virulence factors of Escherichia coli isolates from patients with symptomatic and asymptomatic bacteriuria and neuropathic bladders due to spinal cord and brain injuries. *J Clin Microbiol* 1998, **36**:115.
31. Teh HS *et al.* Magnetic resonance cystography. Novel imaging technique for evaluation of vesicoureteric reflux. *Urology* 2005, **65**:793.
32. Avorn J *et al.* Reduction of bacteruria and pyuria after ingestion of cranberry juice. *JAMA* 1994, **271**:571

CHAPTER 12

Sex and the Kidney

RELATIONSHIP BETWEEN SEXUAL INTERCOURSE AND RENAL DISEASE

The relationship between sex and the kidney has existed since the oldest profession in the world came into existence. Men who frequent brothels run the risk of infection of the urethra (urethritis) and the prostate gland (prostatitis). The infection is due to the gonococci which cause gonorrhoea. Males are infected when they have sexual intercourse with a female who harbours the infection in the cervix of her uterus without any symptoms.

One of the most feared infections is AIDS for which there is still no cure. AIDS is a disease caused by a virus called HIV, or human immuno-deficiency virus. The disease destroys part of the body's immune system, leaving victims incapable of defending themselves against infections and certain cancers. HIV is found in seminal and vaginal secretions and can be transmitted in a heterosexual or homosexual relationship.

However, a more common infection is due to Chlamydia trachomatis. In females it can give rise to vaginitis with white or yellowish vaginal discharge with itch simulating fungal or candidial vaginitis with UTI. The female can transmit C trachomatis infection to the male during sexual intercourse. In the unsuspecting male it may persist in a carrier state with him infecting other women he has sex with and the man may have no symptoms or the infection can present as cytitis or prostatitis. Treatment should be prescribed for both the man and the woman at the same time in order to prevent further reinfection between the partners. The following drugs are useful: bactrium, ciprofloxacin, erythromycin, azithromycin, amoxicillin and doxycycline should be given in a course of 1 to 2 weeks depending on the severity of the infection.

HONEYMOON CYSTITIS

This refers to a condition in a woman who has urinary infection in the bladder following sexual intercourse. On awakening the next morning she has pain or discomfort in the bladder as well as pain each time she passes urine. There may be blood in the urine and the frequency of urination is also increased. The term "Honeymoon" refers to young brides who are at greater risk from the infection, presumably because of inexperience.

In clinical practice, however, this condition can occur in any female who has sexual intercourse. This is because in a woman the urethral opening has a very intimate relationship to the anterior wall of the vagina and both are very close to the anus. During intercourse bacteria may be introduced into the urethra thereby causing infection of the bladder. The bacteria are *Escherichia coli* which normally live in the part of the large bowel called the colon. Some are always found around the anus where they are passed out with the faeces. When the penis touches the area around the anus it picks up the bacteria which subsequently get introduced into the vagina during intercourse. When the penis contaminated with *E. coli* comes into contact with the female urethra the bacteria could then enter the urethra to cause urethritis or ascend into the bladder to cause cystitis.

What can be done for women prone to recurrent Urinary Infections?

If there is no abnormality on the IVP and if she has been engaged in sexual intercourse, then the infections are likely to be related to sexual activity.

In the case of some women, the spouse may prefer to have anal intercourse first before vaginal intercourse, thereby introducing bacteria into the urethra.

Advice on sexual hygiene is usually given to the women to prevent recurrent attacks of cystitis:

1. Empty the bladder within 15 minutes of coitus. Drink water to promote a good flow of urine to flush the organisms from the bladder.
2. Prolong the period of sexual foreplay before the actual sexual intercourse. This is especially important if either one or the other partner tends to be dry and lacking in genital lubricant. The foreplay will ensure adequate lubrication and will reduce friction and make penetration by the penis easier so that it is less likely to linger around the urethral opening to provide bacteria the opportunity of entering the urethra.
3. If adequate lubrication is not forthcoming, especially in slightly older women, then KY Jelly or other similar lubricating jelly can be applied on the genitalia. It is important not to apply too much of the jelly, otherwise the genitalia becomes too slippery and much sexual pleasure will be lost.
4. After each bowel movement wipe the anus from front to back. Similarly after passing urine wipe the area from front to back.
5. Wash with soap the area around the urethra, vagina and anus (perineum) after each bowel movement.
6. Do not use vaginal deodorants, dettol, strong soap, or antiseptic lotions for washing as they may cause irritation and inflammation of the urethra.

The doctor may prescribe an antibiotic tablet (nitrofurantoin usually) to be taken immediately after coitus. This will kill any bacteria introduced into the urethra and bladder. Half a tablet of bactrium will do just as well.

In the case of a married woman who gets repeated infection many years after marriage it may be that the spouse has acquired a new preference for having anal intercourse before vaginal intercourse. The couple should be told that after anal penetration the penis should not be introduced into the vagina. Ensure that the penis is washed thoroughly with soap and water before subsequent vaginal penetration.

Anal Intercourse and Urinary Infection in a Male

A male who practises anal intercourse with a woman may himself sometimes get urinary tract infection because bacteria from her anus could find their way into his urethra and from there into the bladder. Usually, however, this is uncommon as bacteria in the male urethra is also flushed out with the emission of semen. Moreover the long male urethra also makes ascending infection less likely.

Oral Intercourse and Urinary Infection

Usually this is uncommon as saliva from the woman's mouth itself inhibits bacterial activity. However vigorous oral activity by the female may cause a soreness at the urethral opening. Occasionally, there may be minor trauma at the urethral opening which could be infected giving rise to pain on passing urine. Oral sex may also cause the transmission of HIV infection from a woman harbouring HIV to the man as a small abrasion on the penis may be a portal of entry for the HIV into the bloodstream of the man.

Urinary Tract Infection in Sexy Young Males

Until recently, UTI in young men was believed to be confined to those with an underlying abnormality of the urinary tract. It is now recognised that uncomplicated cystitis can occur in young men and "can even mimic urethritis." Risk factors include anal intercourse, HIV infection, lack of circumcision, having a sexual partner with colonization of the vagina with uropathogens. Seven day treatment regimen are usually adequate and imaging is only necessary in those who fail to respond to therapy. Prostatitis have to be considered in those who fail to respond to therapy or have recurrent infection. [Smyth EG and O'Connell N. Complicated urinary tract infection. Current Opinion in Infectious Diseases, 1998, **11**(1):63–66.]

In a woman who has repeated bruising to the urethral opening following Sexual Intercourse what could be done?

Varying the position of sexual intercourse may avoid bruising. One way is to have intercourse with the male penetrating the female from a posterior position. This way, the urethral opening is spared from friction but the female may suffer discomfort from pressure on the bladder. Emptying the bladder before coitus will help.

Significance of Blood Stained Semen

When a male ejaculates, sometimes the seminal fluid may be blood stained. The commonest cause is an infection of the urinary bladder (cystitis or prostatitis). Sometimes a rupture of a small blood vessel, usually a vein may also cause some blood to be present in the ejaculate. He should seek medical treatment as he may require investigations if he does not respond to a course of antibiotics.

Impotency

Impotency is the term used when a male is incapable of perform-ing the sexual act. Impotency occurs with increasing frequency over the age of 40, affecting 50% of males in their late sixties. In most cases no organic explanation can be found. The younger man may require psychiatric evaluation. Systemic disease like diabetes, causing diabetic autonomic neuropathy and drugs given for hypertension and specific neurological problems should be excluded. Measurement of hormone levels and hormonal treatment are usually not very useful. A healthy male can often have a normal sexual life up to the age of 70. For those who have associated medical conditions they may not be able to perform as well from the age of 60. For females a normal healthy sexual life span can extend to 60 to 65 years. Some men are sexually active and even productive up to the age of 80 years. As people survive longer, their sexual life span is similarly prolonged.

CAUSES OF IMPOTENCY

There are many causes of impotency:

- Psychological.
- Injury or tumours in the brain (especially temporal lobe).
- Spinal cord injury or tumours.
- Drugs which depress the brain (barbiturates, alcohol).
- Drugs which block the action of nerves, especially drugs used in the treatment of hypertension (guanethidine, bethanidine, methyldopa, clonidine, beta adrenergic blocking drugs like atenolol as well as alpha adrenergic drugs like terazoxin).
- Interference with blood supply to lower part of body: disease and narrowing of blood vessels due to arteriosclerosis (aorto-iliac arteriosclerosis, bilateral lumbar sympathectomy).
- Inappropriate hormones: lack of male hormones (androgen) or excessive female hormones (oestrogen).

CHAPTER 13
Hypertension and the Kidney

1. Hypertension was first characterized when Riva-Rocci [Gaz Med Torino, 1896, 47:981] developed the prototype of the sphygmomanometer and so allowed the measurement of blood pressure. Korotkov [Korotkov N. A contribution to the problem of methods for the determination of the blood pressure. Izv Imperatorskoi Voenno Meditsinskoy Akad 1905, 11:365] by describing the sounds heard over the brachial artery as the pressure on the cuff was reduced thus giving his name to these sounds. A systolic value of 140 mm Hg and a diastolic value of 90 mm Hg is taken as the upper value of what is considered normal BP. If BP is controlled at this level it has been shown to protect patients against the development of myocardial infarction [MI] and strokes. However, it has been ascertained that for patients with Chronic Kidney Disease the BP should be targeted at 130/80 mm Hg for renoprotection.

2. Population studies have shown that BP is a continuous variable with no absolute dividing line between what is considered normal and abnormal. So for an individual whose BP is 90/60 mm Hg, if it has recently increased to 120/90 mm Hg, this represents an increase of 30 mm Hg for the systolic and 10 mm Hg for the diastolic BP and there should be cause for concern. The individual should be investigated and treated. In the case of a pregnant patient this would indicate preeclampsia and there should be cause for alarm as untreated the patient may develop eclampsia with disastrous consequences.

3. Recent guidelines [Hypertension 2003, 21:1011–1053] from the Joint National Committee on Prevention, Detection,

Evaluation and Treatment of High Blood Pressure [JNC7] have designed a classification for BP for Adults. Normal is when systolic is <120 or diastolic is <80 mm Hg, prehypertension is when systolic is 120–139 or diastolic is 80–89 mm Hg, Stage 1 is when systolic is 140–159 or diastolic 90–99 mm Hg and Stage 2 is when systolic is ≤160 or diastolic ≥100 mm Hg.

4. As one grows older, the systolic BP will increase but BP for women tend to be lower than men. After age 60, this difference disappears. The diastolic BP would increase until age 50. After this it plateaus and decreases with advancing age. From here the systolic BP rises steadily with age year by year as we age. Interestingly, this is the time when we need to check our vision. Many will be surprised that their myopia has improved and we are at the age there is a need to decrease the power of the lenses, otherwise we shall be wearing over-corrected spectacles. From age 45 onwards the systolic BP becomes a more and more important determinant of cardiovascular risk. At this time we shall be needing our reading glasses for near vision due to presbyopia.

5. The National Health and Nutrition Examination Survey [NHANES] in a 1999 to 2000 Study [Hypertension, 1995, 25:305–314] showed that 65% of people over the age of 60 years were hypertensive and the Framingham Study showed that BP was normal for only 6.9% of people older than 80 years. As we age our arteries and arterioles harden and lose their elasticity and so our systolic BP rises progressively with age. In contrast, our diastolic BP decreases with age. Hence, as we age the pulse pressure [diffence between the systolic and diastolic BP] increases. There is a J shaped relationship, meaning an excess of mortality due to Coronary Artery Disease [CAD] at both low and high levels of diastolic BP [Kannel WB, JAMA 1996, 275:1571–1576].

6. Left Ventricular Hypertrophy [LVH] is a bad prognostic sign as it is associated with a high incidence of cardiovascular disease [CVD] and strokes causing increased mortality.

7. Plasma Renin Activity [PRA] is an indicator of the activity of the Renin Angiotensin System [RAS] and has an important

role in CVD. High PRA is associated with high CVS risk with increased incidence of myocardial infarction [MI]. Contrary to what is thought, elderly patients with hypertension also have associated high PRA. Medium levels are found in 60% of old people with hypertension, 8.4% have high and 31.5% low levels of PRA. There is therefore a role for the use of ACEI and ARBs in this group of patients.

8. Cerebral Vascular Accidents [CVA] or Strokes is the third commonest cause of death in patients with hypertension, apart from myocardial infarction and heart failure. Hypertension causes microaneurysms and fibrinoid necrosis of the penetrating arteries supplying the basal ganglia, deep cerebral white matter and pons. In Systemic Hypertension, ischemic strokes account for 80% of all strokes with 20% due to haemorrhagic strokes. Patients with severe uncontrolled hypertension are more prone to haemorrhagic strokes.

9. The Metabolic Syndrome refers to the condition where several CVS risk factors cluster together and doctors should recognize such patients as they are at great CVS and other risks. There are 6 components as designated by The National Cholesterol Program's Adult Treatment Panel III [ATP-III], namely obesity, atherogenic dyslipidemia, raised BP, insulin resistance [FBS > 110 mg/dL], proinflammatory state [raised C reactive protein or CRP level], and prothrombotic state [increased plasma activator inhibitor I or PAI–I].

10. Chronic Kidney Disease [CKD] is another common complication of hypertension. About 40% to 50% of all deaths from CKD is due to cardiovascular disease [CVD]. In a patient on dialysis, the CVS death risk is 50 to 500 times for age matched general population. Both the decline in GFR as well as the degree of albuminuria are predictors of CVS mortality in patients with CKD. The term Cardio Renal Syndrome is now applicable for patients with CKD as the degree of CVS morbidity and mortality can be predicted from the degree of GFR decline and amount of albuminuria, including microalbuminuria.

11. In patients on dialysis, whether it is hemodialysis [HD] or peritoneal dialysis [PD] the presence of hypertension will

result in higher mortality rates [MR] compared to the general population with hypertension, where the relationship between MR and degree of uncontrolled hypertension, both systolic and diastolic is linear and graded compared to HD and PD patients where the MR is exaggerated. One of the main reasons is that the patient on dialysis has accelerated rate of atherogenesis which is 10 times that of someone in the general population. The prevalence of hypertension is up to 80% in HD patients and up to 50% in the PD patients. For the transplanted patients, as many as 50% of them would have hypertension and this is the group that will face graft loss over the next 6 years or so [Opelz G. Kidney Int 1998, 53:217–222].

Microalbuminuria

1. This is defined as urinary albuminuria excretion between 30 and 299 mg. Microalbuminuria in the patient, whether it is in the patient with essential hypertension or diabetes mellitus heralds the onset of nephropathy. This means that the patient now has CKD and faces increased risks of developing CVD with the added increased risks of CVD morbidity and mortality.

2. It occurs in 6 to 40% of patients with hypertension and the prevalence rises with increasing age and duration of hypertension. Therefore microalbuminuria can be considered a marker of CVD risk in both the patient with essential hypertension and the patient with diabetes mellitus.

3. Once the patient develops microalbuminuria one has to look out for associated prevalence of CAD, LVH, MI, peripheral vascular disease, lipid abnormalities.

4. A patient with essential hypertension has microalbuminuria because he has developed Glomerular Hyperfiltration just like the diabetic who develops microalbuminuria. This is initially associated with increased eGFR even in the range of 150 to 200 ml/min. At this stage patients should be treated

with ACEI or ARB as this will help to decrease Proteinuria as well as to reduce the Glomerular Hyperfiltration. Untreated these patients will gradually have a decline in the eGFR and this is accompanied by positive dipstick for albumin meaning that the patient has now progressed to the stage of macroalbuminuria or the traditional proteinuria where total or 24 hours proteinuria now exceeds 150 mg/day.

CAUSES OF HYPERTENSION

1. Essential hypertension.
2. Renal parenchymal causes are acute and chronic glomerulonephritis (GN), chronic pyelonephritis, diabetic nephropathy, lupus nephritis, obstructive uropathy and polycystic kidneys. Other causes are systemic sclerosis, haemolytic uraemic syndrome and haemangiopericytoma.
   Renovascular causes are renal artery stenosis due to atheromatous changes, fibromuscular dysplasia, Takayasu's disease or hypoplastic kidneys.
3. Endocrine causes are Cushing's syndrome, Conn's syndrome, phaeochromocytoma, carcinoid syndrome, hyperparathyroidism.
4. Drug induced causes: Eg. oral contraceptives, liquorice, corticosteroids, prostaglandin synthetase inhibitors, monoamine oxidase inhibitors.
5. Others: Coarctation of the aorta, toxaemia of pregnancy.

RENAL EFFECTS OF HYPERTENSION

1. Hypertension decreases renal plasma flow.
2. When hypertension is uncontrolled, glomerular filtration is impaired. This will cause glomerulosclerosis. With time renal impairment occurs.
3. Deterioration of renal function is especially rapid in patients with malignant hypertension or accelerated hypertension.

4. Malignant hypertension (diastolic BP >120 mm Hg in the presence of papilloedema) can complicate hypertension due to whatever cause. This includes patients with essential hypertension. Hence it is very important to ensure that hypertension is well controlled at all times. This is especially so among patients with glomerular disease as uncontrolled hypertension accelerates the progression of glomerular lesions causing diffuse sclerosing glomerulonephritis. This type of uncontrolled hypertension can cause accelerated progression to ESRF, sometimes within a matter of weeks to months and is referred to as **Accelerated Hypertension** and behaves like **Malignant Hypertension** in the way it causes renal damage. Whether it is Accelerated or Malignant Hypertension, if the BP can be brought under control again [provided it has not gone on uncontrolled for too long] the renal function can be restored.

INVESTIGATION OF THE PATIENT WITH HYPERTENSION

History

Take a thorough history of the disease, its onset, how well the control has been and whether the patient was compliant with his medication. Very often there is no preceding history which could provide a clue to the cause of hypertension. A history of urinary abnormalities some years ago may point to glomerulonephritis as the cause. Paroxysms or symptoms related to sympathetic overactivity may alert one to the possibility of phaeochromocytoma. Flushing of the face with diarrhoea may be a clue to carcinoid syndrome.

Enquire about a family history of hypertension, diabetes mellitus or kidney disease (polycystic kidneys, hereditary nephritis). A strong family history of hypertension makes the diagnosis of essential hypertension more likely. Ask about drug history. In women, a history of oral contraceptive usage is important. Was there a history of toxaemia of pregnancy?

Physical Examination

1. In addition to routine examination, look for evidence of end organ damage due to hypertension — left ventricle hypertrophy, heart failure, changes of hypertensive retinopathy on fundoscopy (Keith and Wagner's grading I to IV; look for macular star as it is associated with renal insufficiency), cerebral vascular insufficiency and atheroselerosis of peripheral blood vessels.

2. Check for delayed femoral pulses and prominent collateral circulation as it points to coarctation of the aorta. Absent radial pulse and vascular bruits in the neck may be clues for a diagnosis of Takayasu's disease.

3. Listen for an abdominal bruit which would indicate renal artery stenosis.

4. Certain conditions like Cushing's syndrome or carcinoid syndrome will be diagnosed more easily when the physical signs are obvious. Enquire about steroid therapy in a patient with features of Cushing's.

5. Patients who have stigmata of systemic lupus erythematosus often have characteristic facies due to steroid therapy or because of the erythematosus rash on the face, or evidence of vasculitis and Raynaud's phenomenon.

6. Stigmata of chronic renal failure will not be missed if one remembers renal failure as a cause of hypertension.

Investigation

1. Urine microscopy and cultures.
2. Full blood count.
3. Blood urea and serum creatinine.
4. Serum electrolytes. Hypokalaemic alkalosis in a hypertensive, not treated with diuretics should alert one to the possibility of Conn's syndrome.
5. Fasting blood glucose to exclude diabetes mellitus because diabetics have a higher incidence of hypertension and diabetic nephropathy has to be excluded.

6. Serum calcium. Hypercalcaemia is a cause of hypertension and a cause of acute hypercalcaemia should be looked for.
7. Creatinine clearance or estimated Glomerular Filtration Rate (eGFR) to assess renal function and Total Urinary Proteinuria [TUP] or Protein/Creatinine Ratio (PCR) to exclude proteinuria indicating renal disease. Sometimes the PCR may not render an accurate result of the actual degree of Proteinuria as it is only a spot examination in which case one may have to resort to the TUP as a check on the actual Proteinuria.
8. Urinary VMA (vanillyl-mandelic acid) and catecholamines should be measured in a young hypertensive to exclude phaeochromocytoma.
9. Five HIAA (hydroxy indole acetic acid) to exclude carcinoid syndrome.
10. ECG, Chest X-ray are necessary to assess cardiac status.
11. Intravenous pyelogram may be necessary if renal disease is suspected. An alternative is an Ultrasound examination of the kidneys and urinary bladder to exclude abnormalities in the urological system.

Special Investigations

1. Plasma renin assay is essential in the investigation of a patient with hypokalaemic alkalosis associated with hypertension. A low plasma renin activity (PRA) may indicate Conn's syndrome. A high PRA may indicate ischaemic renal lesions. Computerised axial tomography is valuable in the assessment of a patient suspected to have adrenal masses.
2. If renal artery stenosis is suspected as a cause of hypertension, a rapid sequence IVP or a DTPA radio-isotope scan can be performed to demonstrate the decreased perfusion on the side with the stenotic artery. The kidney with the stenotic artery is smaller then the normal side by at least 1.5 cm. The nephrogram is faint, the pyelographic phase is delayed, but

there is increased concentration of the contrast on the delayed film. However, both techniques fail to detect 20% to 30% of proven cases of renal artery stenosis. A renal arteriogram is the most diagnostic procedure for renal artery stenosis.

3. The plasma renin activity can be used to predict the blood pressure response to surgery. PRA from the renal veins and the peripheral veins have to be sampled. A clear gradient of PRA between the renal vein and the peripheral vein as well as suppression of renin activity from the uninvolved kidney indicates that the stenotic side is the cause of the hypertension and response to surgery is good.

4. Saralasin (a competitive antagonist of angiotensin II) infusion test is another useful way of establishing that the blood pressure is angiotensin dependent. A fall of diastolic blood pressure of 10 mm Hg in response to saralasin predicts good response to surgery.

5. Captopril Test: An ACE inhibitor eliminates Angiotensin II induced glomerular arteriolar vasoconstriction. In the kidney with renal artery stenosis, a decrease in renal function (GFR) is seen after captopril administration. Captopril is given in an oral dose of 50 mg and the radiopharmaceutical used in the renogram is Technetium (Tc)-99m DTPA or Tc-99m MAG3. A routine (pre-captopril) renal scan is performed. This is followed 4 to 48 hours later with a second scan performed after administration of captopril (post-captropril scan). Some institutions perform post captopril scan first. If it is normal, the study is stopped.

TREATMENT OF RENAL ARTERY STENOSIS

1. Anti-hypertensive drugs are the first line of management.
2. If hypertension proves difficult to control, percutaneous transluminal angioplasty (PTCA) with a balloon catheter should be performed.

3. Surgery is resorted to if PTCA fails. Bypass procedures can be performed, especially in bilateral renal artery stenosis. Autotransplantation of the affected kidney has also been successful in selected cases.
4. If there is hardly any function left in the stenosed kidney, as in the case of segmental hypoplasia, nephrectomy can be performed.

Medical Management of Hypertension

There is a need to monitor the serum cholesterol, control obesity, reduce salt intake and stop smoking.

A. **Endocrine causes** of hypertension are identified and treated.
B. There are at least 9 main groups of **Hypotensive Drugs** which can be employed in the treatment of hypertension, namely:

(1) **Diuretics** (see chapter on Diuretics)
   A diuretic can be used for mild hypertension.

(2) **Beta Adrenergic Antagonists or Beta Blockers**
   Beta Blockers can be classified as follows:

o Non-specific	— propranolol
o Cardioselective	
— produce less bronchoconstriction	— metoprolol, atenolol
o Alpha Beta Blocker	
— postural hypotension is more common because of alpha blockade	— labetalol
o Intrinsic sympathomometic	
— useful for those with compromised cardiac function	— pindolol, oxyprenolol
o Renal vasodilating	
— increases renal blood flow	— nadolol, tertatolol

(3) **Alpha Adrenergic Antagonists or Alpha Blocker** (doxazosin, prazosin, terazosin, phentolamine, labetalol is both an α and a β blocker)

Terazosin is a selective long acting α_1 adrenergic antagonist usually given in a dose of 1 to 2 mg at night, increasing gradually to 5 to 10 mg for control of BP. Peak serum level is at 1 hour with a half life of 12 hours. This is a useful third line or fourth line drug to use where hypertension is difficult to control or where there are contraindications to the use of other agents. It is also useful in the dialysis population. Among elderly males with prostatic hypertrophy, it has the additional advantage of causing relaxation of the smooth muscle within the prostate allowing easier passage of urine.

(4) **Direct Acting Vasodilators** (hydrallazine, minoxidil, nitroprusside, indapamide) Vasodilators tend to cause fluid retention and is usually combined with a diuretic. Minoxidil causes hirsutism and is best avoided in females.

(5) **Calcium Antagonists** (nifedipine, amlodipine, felodipine, diltiazem, verapamil) Only long acting Nifedipine LA should be used as the short acting preparation has been reported to cause episodic rises in BP associated with significant morbidity, Some patients however cannot tolerate long acting [LA] nifedipine because of severe giddiness and flushing with headaches.

Another useful long acting calcium channel blocker or calcium ion antagonist is Amlodipine (Norvasc) which has minimal side effects like headaches and palpitations. However, both Amlodipine and nifedipine can cause swelling of legs which can be quite troublesome for some patients to the extent that the drug has to be discontinued.

6) **Angiotensin Converting Enzyme (ACE) Inhibitor** (captopril, enalapril, ramipril, perindropril)

This is a class of anti-hypertensives which inhibits conversion of angiotensin I to angiotensin II. Its side effects consist of taste disturbances, cough, skin rash and when high doses are combined with immunosuppressive agents, as in patients with lupus nephritis, leucopenia and agranulocytosis may occur. When using captopril, one should start with a small test dose (6.25 mg) at night to assess the initial response to the drug as there may be severe postural hypotension. This is more likely to happen in those patients who are volume depleted. Not many patients are on captopril nowadays with the advent of newer ACE inhibitors.

Enalapril, Ramipril or Perindropil which are long acting ACE inhibitors are easier drugs to use. ACE inhibitors may cause acute renal failure. This is due to relief of angiotensin II dependent vasoconstriction of the glomeruli's efferent arterioles, resulting in decrease in intraglomerular BP and therefore decreased GFR, hence the renal failure. The renal failure is reversible with cessation of ACE Inhibitor therapy. Caution should therefore be exercised in patients with renal impairment as the renal function may worsen further. Reversible renal failure also occurs when ACE inhibitor is used to treat patients with hypertension with a single kidney. In fact, this principle is used as a test for the presence of renal artery stenosis in a transplant patient with hypertension as such a patient will have renal impairment on being treated with ACE inhibitor. Monitor the serum creatinine and serum K^+ of patients with renal impairment who are on ACE Inhibitors. Hyperkalaemia is due to the anti-Aldosterone effect of ACE inhibitor.

(7) **Angiotensin Receptor Blockers (ARBs)** or Angiotensin II receptor antagonist (losartan, valsartan, candesartan, telmisartan). This class of anti-hypertensives binds selectively to the Angiotensin receptor, thus preventing the binding of angiotensin II at the receptor site. It blocks all physiologically relevant actions of Angiotensin II. Its renoprotective effect in conditions associated with glomerular hyperfiltration is similar to ACE inhibitors. Like ACE inhibitors its side effects include acute renal failure and hyperkalaemia. It is useful in patients who cannot agree with ACE inhibitors due to the side effect of cough.

(8) **Renin Inhibitors** (aliskiren, zankiren, remikiren)
Aliskiren is a specific inhibitor of renin. It can be used as a hypotensive and renoprotective drug, decreases proteinuria and retards progression of renal failure. It interferes with the first and rate limiting step in the renin angiotensin system and **prevents conversion of renin to angiotensin I.** This action of Aliskiren is therefore at an earlier step before the action of ACEI and ARB. A direct renin inhibitor would offer more complete RAS blockade. However it has been felt that such blockade with Aliskiren may lead to a reactive rise in renin. This is not a cause for concern as Aliskiren in a daily dose of 150 mg will afford adequate inhibition as **Aliskiren itself also catalyses renin.** This would explain the lowering of PRA with the use of Aliskiren unlike ACEI and ARBs which in fact cause a rise in renin. Renin is profibrotic to the kidney and is therefore undesirable. The half life of Aliskiren is 40 hours. Studies have shown that renin inhibition is >99% at 5 hours after the 300 mg and 600 mg Aliskiren doses and still >95% at 24 hours after these doses [Jan Danser *et al*. Hypertension, 2008, 51] [Fisher NDL. Circulation, 2007, 116:556]. The circulating Aliskiren levels during once daily therapy of 150 mg would be more than sufficient to obtain adequate renin blockade, even at trough level. The Aliskiren induced rise in renin is well below the 20–100 fold rise required to overcome the 95% or 99% of renin inhibition. Therefore a rise in Angiotensin II and or BP during prolonged Aliskiren is unlikely. Aliskiren lowers BP and prevents proteinuria by reducing TGF β by suppression of TGF β gene expression. Aliskiren can be prescribed in a dose from 150 mg to 600 mg a day, with some diarrhoea at higher doses. What is important to know is that with ACEI and ARB blockade, there is a reactive rise in renin associated angiotensin peptides together with a rise in PRA which in the long term would lead to renofibrosis accompanied by renal deterioration. This is not so with the use of Aliskiren. In fact patients who have been on ACEI or

ARB when Aliskiren is added, there is a decrease in the PRA levels previously raised when they were on ACEI or ARB alone. Hence with Aliskiren, we can achieve renoprotection without the risk of raised PRA. To go another step, if patients with CKD do not respond well when on ACEI or ARB alone, one can safely add Aliskiren for reduction of proteinuria and renoprotection. Hence Aliskiren provides renoprotection in patients with CKD comparable to ACEI and ARB. **There is therefore wisdom in initiating therapy with Aliskiren and only of proteinuria is uncontrolled or renal dysfunction not improving should we then introduce an ARB. This would lessen one's worry about long term ARB therapy inducing renal fibrosis.**

(9) **Selective Aldosterone Receptor Antagonists (Eplerenone)**
   Eplerenone is a potassium sparing diuretic which is also a Selective Aldosterone Receptor Antagonist. It can be used as a hypotensive and renoprotective drug. **Aldosterone causes renofibrosis through upregulation of Angiotensin II receptor responsiveness**. Angiotensin II is the mediator for the Renin Angiotensin Aldosterone System [RAAS] which produces Angiotensinogen II which is the most powerful vasoconstrictor in the body and causes progressive renal damage. Eplerenone, being a selective aldosterone receptor antagonist can prevent development of proteinuria and retard progression of renal failure. Hence, Elperenone can protect the kidney in addition to ACEI and ARB therapy by inhibiting the effect of Aldosterone that persist despite therapy in these drugs. Spironolactone too would have the ability to block the action of Aldosterone but Eplerenone is a more specific aldosterone blocker. Eplerenone is 24 times less potent than spironolactone in blocking mineralocorticoid receptors and has a lower incidence of gynecomastia, breast pain, impotency in males and diminished libido and menstrual irregularities [IwamotoT *et al.* Trends Cardiovasc Med. 2005, 15:273–277].

Choice of Anti Hypertensive Drugs

1. In general one can broadly divide patients into two groups, those whose hypertension is associated with high Plasma Renin Activity [PRA] and would respond well to ACEI and ARBs in contrast to those who are salt sensitive or volume related hypertension and would respond better to calcium channal blockers or calcium antagonists or vasodilators. Most would employ ACEI or ARBs as the first line and calcium Antagonists as the second line. Beta Blockers would constitute the third line and if patients do not respond well, one may then add a small dose of a diuretic like 12.5 mg of hydrochlorothiazide. I usually do not like to resort to a diuretic as patients tend to become volume depleted with renal impairment. Some may develop serious hypokalaemia which may prove disastrous, especially if the patient is elderly and already has cardiovascular disease. The hypokalemia will only compound their problems. My next choice of therapy would be an alpha adrenergic blocker like terazosin, 1 mg for an initial first dose and then increasing to 5 to 6 mg or more. It is also useful for the patient with prostatic hyperplasia as it relaxes the smooth muscles of the prostate and ease the passage of urine.

2. Nowadays, it is not good enough to bring the BP down to 140/90. The target should be 130/80 and if a patient is a diabetic the BP should be around 120/80 for added renoprotection. It is important to remember that proteinuria and eGFR have to be addressed as well using the same drugs for treatment of hypertension, though with the addition of Aliskiren the Renin inhibitor and Eplerenone the Aldosterone Antagonist we could secure even better protection for the kidneys including those already with renal impairment or Stage 3b CKD with eGFR 45 ml to 30 ml/min and below. Most patients with hypertension or CKD will require multidrug therapy in addition to those that lower LDL – Cholesterol or treat diabetes for those who are diabetic.

3. For the older patient, the problem is one of gradually increasing systolic BP as the arterial stiffening progresses with increase in peripheral vascular resistance. The elderly will have high systolic BP and lowering of diastolic BP as age progresses with widening of pulse pressure. There is also proximal aorta stiffening associated with hypertrophic cardiomyopathy resulting in impaired diastolic function, hence impairing cardiac output [Rich GM *et al.* Ann Intern Med. 1992, 116:813–820]. These patients would do well with a calcium channel blocker like Amlodipine. For the elderly male, Terozosin an alpha adrenergic blocker, may be more useful as it would also relieve prostatic symptoms. The use of Amlodipine may sometimes cause troublesome ankle edema. Both ACEI and ARBs are also useful in the elderly patient. Beta Blockers should be used with caution as they impair baroreceptors in the elderly and worsen orthostasis causing postural hypotension.

4. An Obese hypertensive patient has other problems like a hyperdynamic circulation with increased peripheral resistance with expanded plasma volume and salt sensitivity. Calcium channel blockers with ACEI or ARB would help reduce peripheral resistance. Be careful with the use of Beta Blockers as they may potentiate weight gain and also impair glucose tolerance.

5. For patients with Coronary Artery Disease [CAD], the use of Beta Blockers is ideal since coronary artery perfusion occurs during diastole and Beta Blockers would slow the heart rate and enhance perfusion during diastole. Agents like ACEI and ARBs would reduce mortality rates in patients with cardiovascular disease [CVD] and strokes who have CVD with LVH.

6. For CKD patients the target for BP control should be 130/80 and if they have diabetes it should be 120/80. Both ACEI and ARBs can be used. For patients who need additional agent to control proteinuria or retard progression of renal impairment, Aliskiren would be helpful. Eplerenone is another useful drug as discussed earlier in the chapter.

Refractory Hypertension

1. This is a term used to described hypertension in a patient which fail to respond to the usual standard treatment despite the first 4 lines of hypertensive therapy discussed above, including the introduction of 12.5 mg of hydrochlorothiazide diuretic which acts both as a vasodilator and a drug to decrease expanded plasma volume.

2. Among the conditions to exclude would be patients' non compliance which may also be related to failure or lack of understanding of the importance of taking the hypertensive medication. Apart from the educational level of the patient, sometimes their own prejudices or preconceived notions as to the actual need for medication would bias them to the need for medication. All these factors or reasons would cause the patient to be less or non compliant. In some cases, it is simply a case of poor doctor patient relationship. A change of doctor would be useful.

3. Improper measurement of BP. If the cuff is too small for a big or obese patient, the reading will be inaccurate. The cuff should encircle 80% of the arm for accurate measurement of BP.

4. Elderly patients may have their BP readings too high because their hardened sclerotic arteries are not easily compressed by the cuff and as a result the BP readings are high giving rise to Osler's Syndrome of Pseudo Hypertension [Messerli FH *et al.* N Engl J Med 1985, 312:1548–51].

5. White coat hypertension is when the patient's BP is found to be high at the Clinic but when patient checks it at home it is normal. This is often attributed by patient to their anxiety or apprehension when coming to hospital. In my opinion, this may be true for most patients but we should be cautious as the patient's BP machine may not be the same as the standard ones used in the clinic which has been verified to be accurate. Also, some patients are in denial and claim their BP at home to be normal because they choose to believe the lower readings at home. It has been found that a proportion of white

coat hypertensive patients actually have LVH and they do not have the appropriate nocturnal dip in BP [Glen SK *et al.* Lancet 1996, 348:654–657].

6. Excess salt intake in some patients may cause volume overload. In addition the ACEI and the ARBs that patients are taking may not be effective. If this is suspected, try 12.5 mg of hydrochlorothiazide to reduce blood volume and restore the efficacy of the usual hypertensive medication.

7. Obesity: The patient can be 5 to 10 Kg overweight, i.e. he is obese. In this case, simple weight reduction will lower the BP. However for the truly obese patient, there may be associated problems of obstructive sleep apnea which when treated will allow the BP to be more easily controlled.

8. Drug interaction: many drugs like appetite suppressants, anti depressants, analgesics especially NSAIDS, oral contraceptives, licorice, immunosuppressants like Cyclosporine A, erythropoietin can raise BP. Their removal will restore normal BP in the patient. NSAIDS often interfere with the anti hypertensive action of ACEI/ARBs and diuretics.

9. Secondary causes of hypertension like phaeochromocytoma, hyperaldosteronism, hyper or hypo thyroidism, hyperparathyroidism, coarctation of the aorta, renal artery stenosis have to be excluded in all patients with difficult to treat or refractory hypertension.

10. In Summary: always exclude all secondary causes of hypertension where the cause can be treated or removed, excessive intake of salt, volume expansion and drug interactions.

Urgency and Emergency

It is important to remember that in long standing hypertension, autoregulation of blood flow to major organs is impaired. If blood pressure in these patients is brought down too rapidly, the perfusion to a vital organ may drop so drastically as to result in impaired function. This will explain renal deterioration in some patients who have their hypertension suddenly too well controlled.

However, in certain situations it is absolutely important to control hypertension rapidly. One should differentiate Hypertensive Urgency from Emergency.

Hypertensive Urgency

This is a clinical situation where the BP is very high like 200/120 but there is not yet any target organ damage. These patients will need treatment with oral rapid onset drugs like captopril [onset of action <15 mins] or clonidine [onset of action <30 to 60 mins] or enalapril [onset of action <60 mins] or labetalol [onset of action <1 to 2 hours]. They can be monitiored at the specialist out patient clinic [SOC] and if the BP is not responding to out patient therapy, it would be safer to admit the patient for urgent in-patient management. But always start the patient on oral medication while waiting for transfer to the admitting ward in case of delay in medication and the patient converts to someone with Hypertensive Emergency.

Hypertensive Emergency

This is a clinical situation or syndrome with marked elevation of BP resulting in ongoing target organ damage like hypertensive encephalopathy, stroke, myocardial infarction, acute renal failure, retinal haemorrhage, papilledema. At this stage, any delay in BP control will result in irreversible target organ damage and even resulting in death. The patient has to be admitted to intensive care for emergency therapy.

These are clinical situations with Hypertensive Emergencies:

1. Dissecting aneurysm
2. Hypertensive encephalopathy

3. Eclampsia of pregnancy
4. Subarachnoid haemorrhage associated with hypertension
5. Malignant hypertension with rapidly deteriorating renal function

Drugs Used in Emergency Treatment of Hypertension

1. Hydrallazine [0.5 to 1.0 mg/min infusion or 10 mg to 50 mg intramuscularly] is a direct vasodilator and is given intravenously or intramuscularly. It has rapid onset action [1 to 5 mins] and its effect lasts from 3 to 6 hours.
2. Sodium Nitroprusside [0.25 to 10 μg/Kg/min infusion] is a most potent parenteral vasodilator. Its action is immediate and lasts 2 to 5 mins. It requires intra-arterial blood pressure monitoring.
3. Nitroglycerine [5 to 100 μg/min infusion] is a dilator of both arterial and venous blood vessels. It dilates both epicardial coronary vessels and their collaterals increasing supply to ischemic region. It has onset of action in 1 to 2 minutes and lasts from 3 to 5 minutes.
4. Enalaprilat is the active metabolite of oral ACE inhibitor enalapril. It is given as an IV dose infusion for 5 mins in an IV dose of ¼ of the oral dose [0.625 mg to 5 mg bolus over 5 mins]. Onset of action is 5 to 15 mins. Duration of action is 6 hours. In patients with renal impairment the dose should not exceed 0.625 mg.
5. Labetalol which is an α and β adrenergic antagonist is given in a dose of 2 mg /min infusion or 0.25 mg/Kg. Its onset of action is 5 mins with duration of action from 3 to 6 hours.
6. Rapid oral drugs : Labetalol, Clonidine, Diltiazem, Captopril, Enalapril, Prazosin can all be used.
7. Sublingual Nifedipine is **no longer used** because it induces strokes and myocardial infarction. The cerebral blood flow is carefully autoregulated even when blood pressure is low. A rapid reduction of BP will decrease cerebral blood flow

precipitating cerebral ischemia and infarction. Similarly, a sudden lowering of BP will interfere with coronary perfusion during diastole resulting in myocardial infarction and arrhythmias.

8. Diazoxide is a pure arterial vasodilator. It is also **seldom used** now because its rapid action causes a reduction in BP which is accompanied by increase in cardiac output and heart rate which provokes cardiac ischemia.

ROLE OF SODIUM AND POTASSIUM IN HYPERTENSION

Story of Evolution

Man over the last million years consumed only 5% of the sodium we now eat. He was a forager and ate mainly vegetable which contained large amounts of potassium. Three hundred to four hundred years ago, salt became readily available from the sea and salt mines. Salt was found to have the magical property of preserving food. Today, because of instinctive appetite and the easy availability of processed food, we are used to eating large amounts of salt in our diet.

SODIUM AND BLOOD PRESSURE

Communities with a high salt intake have an increased risk of developing hypertension. Primitive communities which eat less salt and have a higher potassium intake have a lower risk of developing hypertension. The sodium/potassium ratio in the diet is a better determinant of blood pressure than either sodium or potassium alone.

HOW DOES SALT RAISE BLOOD PRESSURE?

The abnormality causing hypertension is believed to reside in the kidney and patients with essential hypertension have difficulty in excreting sodium. Professor HE de Wardener and GA MacGregor think they have an inherited defect to get rid of sodium (*Kidney International* 1980, 18:1–9).

A high sodium intake increases the secretion of natriuretic hormone. This hormone causes the kidney to excrete sodium. But at the same time natriuretic hormone also inhibits the sodium pump (sodium potassium ATPase) in the smooth muscle cells of the arterioles. This in turn leads to an increase in intracellular calcium which causes increased contractility of the arteriole smooth muscle, giving rise to increased peripheral resistance and hence hypertension.

Does Salt Restriction Lower Blood Pressure?

There is considerable evidence that severe reduction of sodium intake lowers raised blood pressure. The Kempner rice and fruit diet which has low sodium and protein and high potassium has also been shown to lower blood pressure in hypertensive individuals. MacGregor conducted a study on 19 patients (*Lancet* 1982, 1:351–354) in a double blind trial where sodium intake was reduced by half (160 mmol/day to 80 mmol/day) for 2 weeks, and documented a fall in blood pressure of the patients with reduced sodium intake.

Role of Potassium

Potassium is also important in blood pressure regulation. In the 1930s it was used as a diuretic. Even then there was already a suggestion that increasing potassium intake might lower blood pressure. In rats, increasing the intake of potassium blunts the effects of sodium on blood pressure and this can prevent a rise of blood pressure due to high sodium intake.

MacGregor in a study of 23 patients (*Lancet* 1986, II:567–570) in a double blind crossover trial of slow K versus placebo, where patients were given 8 slow K tablets per day (64 mmols of K^+) reported that patients given slow K had a small but significant fall in blood pressure.

Presently patients with hypertension (and normal renal function) are urged to increase potassium intake by taking more fruits and vegetables. Oranges, banana and skim milk are useful sources of potassium. Experimentally, rats given a high potassium diet were protected from blood vessel lesions of hypertension in the brain, heart and kidney in spite of raised blood pressure whereas control rats not on a high potassium diet had the vascular lesions of hypertension.

Daily oral sodium bicarbonate preserves glomerular filtration rate by slowing its decline in early hypertensive nephropathy

In a 5 year double blind prospective study of hypertensive patients with mean eGFR of 75 ml/min, patients matched for age, ethnicity, albuminuria and eGFR receiving daily placebo or equimolar sodium chloride or sodium bicarbonate, 40 patients in each of the 3 groups, NaHCO3 in a dose of 3.5 gm for a 70 Kg subject, it was shown that those on NaHCO3 had slower decline of eGFR compared to the other 2 groups. All patients were also maintained on ACEI.

REFERENCE

Mahajan A *et al*. *Kidney Int* 2010, **78**:303–309.

Essential Hypertension: A Renal Perspective

There is now evidence that essential hypertension results from an inherited renal tendency towards excessive vasoconstriction or an inability to appropriately increase renal blood flow. Studies of African-Americans show that their hypertension is seen at an earlier age, increases more quickly with time, has a higher prevalence, is more severe and is associated with more adverse cardiovascular and renal effects; excluding primary atherosclerotic disease (Hypertension 1993; 21:380–90).

Recently Johnson and Schreiner (Kidney International, 1997, 52:1169–1179) — hypothesized that Essential Hypertension is a form of Acquired Tubulointerstitial Disease. The Hypothesis is that HPT is a 2 phase disease. The first phase is episodic HPT which is due to a Hyperactive Renin Angiotensin and Sympathetic Nervous System. Later on, a second phase sets in whereby there is persistent hypertension due to an inability to excrete salt. What causes people with 1st Phase Hypertension to develop 2nd Phase Hypertension or established Essential Hypertension, that is, the transition from the 1st to the 2nd Phase is the result of catecholamine induced interstitial disease. Excess catecholamine due to over- stimulation of the Sympathetic Nervous System causes increased peritubular capillary pressure and a reduction of peritubular capillary blood flow causing preferential ischaemia in the juxta-medullary region since it does not antoregulate well to changes in renal perfusion pressure. This causes local injury to the tubulo-interstitium and peritubular capillary which triggers the release of vasoconstrictors (angiotensin II, adenosine) and inhibition of vasodilators (nitric oxide, prostaglandins, dopamine) that further augment ischemia. The end result of this injury is that there is an increase in Tubulo-Glomerular (TG) Feedback with enhanced NaCl resorption and blunting of Pressure Natriuresis (PN) with decreased NaCl excretion. The combined effect of increased TG feedback and decreased of PN leads to defective NaCl excretion with persistent Hypertension. What happens is that ischemia of the tubulo-interstitium with time leads to Glomerular Hyperfiltration and proteinuria and finally chronic renal failure. The proteinuria in patients with Essential Hypertension is a sign of Acquired Tubulo-Interstitial Disease. It also explains why patients with

Essential Hypertension develop renal failure. Hence Essential Hypertension is no longer held to be a benign disease. In the past it was thought that, as long as BP was well controlled a patient with Essential Hypertension will not develop kidney failure. But this is no longer so. There are studies in patients with Hypertension which show that a significant number of patients do develop chronic renal failure. The classical example is in the African-American in the USA where there is a high incidence of ESRF due to Hypertensive Nephosclerosis. In a study in UK (QJM, 1993; 86:271–275) by Innes *et al*, among 185 renal biopsies (2.5% of 7339 biopsies) with Benign Nephrosclerosis due to Essential Hypertension, more than 1.5 gm of proteinuria occurred in 40% of patients. Seven had Nephrotic Range Proteinuria, 25% had microscopic hamaturia, 51% had renal impairment. All these 185 patients had long standing Essential Hypertension, none with co-existing renal disease.

In Singapore we estimate the incidence of Hypertensive Nephrosclerosis is at least 9%. The incidence of new ESRF patients in Singapore is about 750 a year, 9% would mean about 68 patients a year.

Revisiting Mechanisms of Essential Hypertension

Calo LA in an Editorial in Clinical Nephrology [Revisiting essential hypertension- a "mechanistic-based" approach may argue for a better definition of hypertension. Clinical Nephrology 2009, 72(2):83–86] has proposed that we adopt a more rational mechanistic based definition of Essential Hypertension. He has argued that the term 'essential' is unsatisfactory as it is a label for unknown causes. By now with a better understanding of the biochemical and physiological mechanisms involved in BP control the term essential is losing its value and its utility as it only describes a small number of hypertensive patients.

He has cited four pathways in the pathophysiology of hypertension in support of his proposal.

1. Role of NO and endothelial cell NO synthetase (eNOS).
    Deletion of eNOS gene rendered animals hypertensive and
    made them insulin resistant. This links NO to arterial pressure
    and glucose as well as lipid homeostasis, therefore represent-
    ing the link between metabolic and cardiovascular diseases.
    NO availability has been found to be reduced in hypertensive
    patients. The reverse, increase in NO and increased insulin
    sensitivity has been demonstrated in Bartter's/Gitelman's
    patients who are hypotensive.
2. The role of Adrenergic Nervous System Overactivity.
    This is a major contributing factor in hypertension induced by
    sodium retention resulting from hyperinsulinemia. Increase in
    norepinephrine in hypertensives reduced insulin sensitivity.
3. Oxidative stress with increased production of reactive oxygen
    species (ROS).
    This is an intrinsic part of the pathophysiology of hyperten-
    sion. Induced elevation of renin and angiotensin II (Ang II)
    result in a large number of ROS related changes. NAD(P)H
    oxidase, induced by Ang II. All these are upregulated in the
    kidney and cardiovascular system (CVS) and the resulting
    increased ROS production then causes CVS and renal dam-
    age. Antioxidant therapy in animals can reduce hypertension
    in animals. In Bartter's and Gitelman's syndrome, where
    antioxidant generation is blunted, normo/hypotension is pres-
    ent and there is no CVS remodelling or renal damage.
4. Role of Rho-kinase .
    Rho-kinase is a mediator involved in vascular tone and CVS
    remodelling. It increases calcium sensitisation of smooth
    muscle contraction. An imbalance between Rho-kinase and
    vasorelaxant NO favouring Rho-kinase pathway will induce
    hypertension and insulin resistance and glucose intolerance.
    Rho-kinase is associated with CVS remodelling and athero-
    genesis.

All these mechanisms contribute to development of hypertension in the context of genetic and environmental factors. He has

also observed that certain drugs like ACE inhibitors and ARBs used in the treatment of hypertension also exert other beneficial effects on insulin resistance, oxidative stress, CVS remodelling and renal damage. Personally I am in support of his viewpoint as our work on regression of renal failure and restoring the decline in eGFR as well as improvement in the permselectivity of patients with IgA nephritis treated with the ARB Losartan would lend credence to his thesis.

REFERENCES

1. Calo LA. Revisiting essential hypertension- a "mechanistic-based" approach may argue for a better definition of hypertension. *Clinical Nephrology*, 2009, **72**(2):83–86.
2. Riva Rocci. *Gaz Med Torino*, 1896, **47**:981.
3. Korotkov N. A contribution to the problem of methods for the determination of the blood pressure. *Izv Imperatorskoi Voenno-Meditsinskoy Akad*, 1905, **11**:365.
4. Recent guidelines from the Joint National Committee on Prevention, Detection, Evaluation and Treatment of High Blood Pressure [JNC7]. *Hypertension*, 2003, **21**:1011–1053.
5. Rich GM *et al. Ann Intern Med* 1992, **116**:813–820.
6. Messerli FH *et al. N Engl J Med* 1985, **312**:1548–51].
7. IwamotoT *et al. Trends Cardiovasc Med* 2005, **15**:273–277.
8. Opelz G. *Kidney Int* 1998, **53**:217–222.
9. Mahajan A *et al.* Daily oral sodium bicarbonate preserves glomerular filtration rate by slowing its decline in early hypertensive nephropathy. *Kidney Int* 2010, **78**:303–309.

CHAPTER 14

The Cardiorenal Syndromes

The term cardiorenal was used initially to describe the hemody-namic and neurohumoral connection between the heart and the kidneys. Recently, the term has been used very broadly by vari-ous people with differing interpretations. Some have proposed using the term only for patients with coexisting severe cardiac and renal dysfunction and others have proposed defining it as advanced congestive cardiac failure complicated by acute renal impairment. Yet others have suggested including a specific level of serum creatinine before the term CRS is used. In August 2004, the US National Heart, Lung and Blood Institute tasked a work group to develop recommendations for future investigations. This group focused its attention on situations in which renal responses are thought to be related to primary changes in cardiac function. As a result the term CRS describes "a state in which therapy to relief CHF symptoms is limited by further worsening renal function" [Claudio Ronco, Andrew A House and Mikko Haapio, Cardiorenal and Renocardiac Syndromes: the need for a com-prehensive classification and consensus. Nature Clinical Practice Nephrology 2008, 4(6):310–311].

Acute or chronic dysfunction of the heart or kidney can cause dysfunction in either organ resulting in the cardiorenal syndromes. Ronco *et al* [Ronco C *et al*. Cardiorenal syndrome: refining the def-inition of a complex symbiosis gone wrong. Intensive Care Med. 2008, 34:957–962] have devised a Classification of Cardiorenal Syndromes into 5 types. The classification consists of 4 subtypes reflecting probable primary and secondary pathology and their chronologies, and a fifth subtype that includes systemic conditions in which cardiac and renal involvement are considered secondary. Ronco *et al*'s definition for the CRS is: "a pathophysiologic disorder of the heart and kidneys whereby acute or chronic dysfunction in one organ may induce acute or chronic dysfunction in the other organ."

Type 1. Acute Cardiorenal Syndrome. An abrupt worsening of a cardiac condition which leads to acute kidney injury [AKI].

Type 2. Chronic Cardiorenal Syndrome. Chronic cardiac dysfunction which causes chronic and progressive renal impairment.

Type 3. Acute Renocardiac Syndrome. An abrupt worsening of kidney function causing acute cardiac dysfunction.

Type 4. Chronic Renocardiac Syndrome. Chronic kidney dysfunction which leads to cardiac dysfunction.

Type 5. Secondary Cardiorenal Syndrome. A systemic condition like diabetes or sepsis which causes both cardiac and renal dysfunction.

1. Acute Cardiorenal Syndrome [Type 1] can be caused by a sudden decrease in cardiac output like severe hypotension leading to renal hypoperfusion. Abrupt worsening of cardiac function like acute cardiogenic shock or acute decompensation of the heart like CHF can lead to AKI. Drugs prescribed for congestive heart failure including loop diuretics can precipitate intravascular volume depletion and give rise to AKI. Radiological or surgical intervention for the heart may cause renal impairment. Coronary angioplasty with the use of radiocontrast might cause renal dysfunction.
2. Chronic Cardiorenal Syndrome [Type 2] can be due to low cardiac output resulting in hypotension and renal hypoperfusion causing AKI. Chronic abnormalities in cardiac function like CHF can cause progressive and potentially permanent kidney disease.

3. Acute Renocardiac Syndrome [Type 3]. Acute Kidney Injury [AKI] has been associated with a high prevalence of Coronary Artery Disease [CAD] [Mittalhenkle A *et al*. Clin J Amer Soc Nephrol, 2008, 3:450–456]. Abrupt worsening of renal function like acute kidney ischemia or acute glomerulonephritis can cause an acute cardiac disorder like heart failure, arrhythmia or ischemia. Here AKI is the primary pathology and the heart is affected secondarily. During hemodialysis, excessive fluid removal can cause hypotension with myocardial ischemia and arrhythmias.

4. Chronic Renocardiac Syndrome. It is now established that albuminuria, including microalbuminuria and decreased GFR are independent predictors of Cardiovascular Disease [CVD] [Mann JF *et al*. Ann Intern Med, 2001, 134:629–636]. Hence many patients with CKD have increased cardiovascular morbidity and mortality and this group forms the bulk of patients with Cardiorenal Syndrome. Chronic glomerular or interstitial disease can contribute to decreased cardiac function, cardiac hypertrophy and or increased risk of CVS events. The suggested contributors include anemia, abnormal calcium-phosphate metabolism, chronic ECF overload, oxidant stress, proinflammatory cytokines, uremic toxins. Patients with renal disease, especially those on dialysis have accelerated atherogenesis predisposing them to cardiovascular disease. These patients are often in fluid overload because of fluid and dietary indiscretion leading often to salt and water overload leading to cardiac decompensation.

5. Secondary Cardiorenal Syndrome [Type 5]. Here a systemic condition causes both cardiac and renal dysfunction. Secondary implies a dysfunction of non-cardiac and non-renal origin that occurs in both the heart and the kidneys. The dysfunction can be reversible or permanent, eg, diabetes mellitus, amyloidosis, SLE and sepsis. Patients with diabetes mellitus accounts for a large proportion in this group because diabetes affects the kidneys and heart very often. Hypertension is another condition that also affects the heart and

the kidneys. Other causes include SLE and sepsis which can affect both the kidneys and the heart. In the old days, streptococcal throat infection causes Post Streptococcal Glomerulonephritis and Rheumatic Heart Disease [RHD]. RHD is seldom seen in the young in Singapore but it still occurs in less developed countries.

Cardiologists and nephrologists are frequently treating the same patients. In the acute setting cardiac or renal dysfunction is associated with increased mortality. It is important to recognise CRS in its earliest phases so that the cardiologist and the nephrologist can come and work together to tide the patient over a difficult period. The intensivist may be the person who will recognise the complex problem and the need for a coordinated management of the patient. We need to develop a better understanding of the pathophysiologic mechanisms of CRS in order to improve the treatment and prognosis for our patients.

Reference: Claudio Ronco, Andrew A House and Mikko Haapio, Cardiorenal and renocardiac syndromes: the need for a comprehensive classification and consensus. Nature Clinical Practice Nephrology 2008, 4(6):310–311.

CARDIOVASCULAR DISEASE {CVD} AND CHRONIC KIDNEY DISEASE {CKD}

1. Patients with CKD have high cardiac morbidity and mortality. Uremia itself causes cardiomyopathy due to the effects of the uremic toxin. **Uremic Cardiomypathy** presents either as an enlarged dilated left ventricle with or without systolic dysfunction or as hypertrophic ventricle with normal left ventricular volume and diastolic dysfunction [London GM *et al.* Seminar Dialysis 1999, 12:77–83]. The probability of a patient on hemodialysis having angina or myocardial infarction is high, about 10% a year [Churchill DN *et al.* Am J Kidney Disease 1992, 19(3):214–234] and

for this group of patients their 5 year mortality can be as high as 90%.

2. The blood vessels of patients with kidney failure and on dialysis are subject to the ravages of **rapid atherogenesis** with arteriosclerosis leading to narrowing of the coronary vessels with ischemia. This is associated with LVH and systolic dysfunction. The Coronary Artery Disease [CAD] predisposes to diastolic dysfunction and systolic failure. LVH is often present in patients with moderate renal failure and by the time they reach ESRF about 75% would have LVH [Foley RN *et al.* Kidney Int 1995, 47(1):1860–192]. Following LVH, with time fibrotic changes occur associated with arrhythmias. The ventricular wall thickens causing LV stiffness and there is abnormal diastolic function with eventual cardiomyopathy and LV failure [Katz AM. Ann Intern med 1994, 121:262–371].

3. Another aspect of CKD is that the **secondary hyperparathyroidism** with high serum **phosphate** and high calcium phosphate product together with raised parathyroid hormone due to hyperparathyroidism cause **calcification** of the blood vessels including those of the coronary arteries and the aorta as well as the aortic and mitral valves. Patients with poorly controlled serum phosphate are the ones most vulnerable and the use of **Vit D analogues themselves also predispose to calcification of blood vessels including that of the coronaries and aorta.** Hyperparathyroidism also has been recently shown to cause myocardial fibrosis causing arrhythmias and diastolic dysfunction [Weber KT. J Am College of Cardiol 1989, 13:1637–1644].

4. **Interstitial Fibrosis** of the myocardium is another prominent feature in the hearts of patients with CKD. The interstitium constitutes 25% of normal myocardium. When there is too much proliferation of fibroblasts in the interstitium of the heart just as interstitial fibrosis in the kidneys the next thing to happen after proliferation is that the fibroblasts undergo fibrosis. Progressive fibrosis equates with loss of functional tissue from myocardial fibrosis. Several factors contribute

especially to myocardial fibrosis in dialysis patients, namely ischemia, angiotensin II, aldosterone, catecholamines, hyperparathyroidism and TGFs. The result of myocardial fibrosis is impaired diastolic function due to delayed relaxation phase of the cardiac cycle. Prolongation of the action potential in turn causes a delay in polarisation which in turn causes tachyarrhythmias. The impairment of diastolic function is worsened by any existing LVH which also occurs commonly in dialysis patients.

5. Many patients on hemodialysis are often subject to salt and water or fluid overload. As a result their left ventricular ejection becomes less. This is partly due to diminished myocardial contractility where the myocardial fibres depends on Starling's forces to maintain a normal cardiac output. These patients subject to loss of systolic function often also have ischemic heart disease. To be fit to receive a kidney transplant the patient must have an ejection fraction of 50%. Sometimes, on initial starting of dialysis the ejection fraction may be poor, much below 50%, but with regular dialysis and dieting as well as fluid restriction and correction of anemia, after some months of dialysis, some patients do improve and their **left ventricle ejection fraction** can improve to above 50%. So do not write the patient off from the transplant register too early. Give him a chance.

6. In patients with coronary artery disease [CAD] without CKD, transient myocardial ischemia may lead to LV dysfunction that can persist after return of normal perfusion. This prolonged dysfunction is known as **myocardial stunning** [Braunwald E *et al*. The stunned myocardium: prolonged postischemic ventricular dysfunction. Circulation 1982, 66: 1146–1149]. Hemodialysis is capable of inducing subclinical myocardial ischemia, due to ultrafiltration and hemodynamic instability. Standard thrice weekly hemodialysis is a process that might lead to repetitive myocardial stunning resulting in chronic LV dysfunction with loss of ejection fraction. In a study by Burton *et al* [Hemodialysis induced recurrent cardiac

injury is associated with increased rates of ventricular arrhythmias, Renal Failure 2008, 30:1–9], 22/70 patients who
did not have HD induced myocardial stunning at 1 year had
no reduction in LV EF and 100% survival compared to 43/70
who had myocardial stunning where 28% had died by one
year. Dialysis induced myocardial stunning was associated
with lower intradialysis BP and more arrhythmias and heart
failure [McIntyre CW. Effects of hemodialysis on cardiac
function. Kidney Int 2009, 76(4):371–375].

7. **Dialysis hypotension** occurs in the setting of patients who
    have developed systolic failure, diastolic dysfunction,
    ischemic heart disease, LVH and myocardial fibrosis.
    Clinically they present with heart failure, dilated cardiomy-
    opathy, hypotension during dialysis and with time hypo-
    tension even when not on dialysis. They are also prone to
    arrhythmias due to myocardial fibrosis. These are the patients
    who have recurrent dialysis hypotension. They are not the
    same as the occasional patient who had a weekend binge and
    turned up for dialysis with fluid overload, 3 or 4 kg in excess
    of their dry weight. These patients because of the need to
    increase ultrafiltration may develop hypotension which responds
    rapidly on saline infusion.

8. **Dialysis hypertension** used to be thought of as salt and water
    related. This is true for many patients starting on dialysis. As
    the weeks go by, a patient newly initiated on dialysis will find
    his or her hypotensive medication slowly being withdrawn
    one by one and to keep taking the same dose would be to
    invite hypotension. As a result most physicians would tend to
    treat hypertension in the dialysis patient less aggressively,
    often attributing this to salt and water overload. But for the
    patient who has started on dialysis with stable dry weight,
    once hypertension occurs we should treat it as for any other
    patient as such uncontrolled hypertension is what causes the
    increased morbidity and mortality due to cardiovascular
    disease in the dialysis patient. Hypertension occurs in about
    60 to 80% of CKD patients. By the time they reach ESRF

about 80% are hypertensive. So about 80% of hemodialysis patients are hypertensive compared to 50% of those on peritoneal dialysis. This may explain why the CVS mortality for HD patients is much higher than for PD patients during the first 2 to 3 years on dialysis. Sometimes we may encounter a patient who has hypertension after hemodialysis. This is due to activation of the renin angiotension system because of excess salt and water removal during dialysis. About 50% of renal transplant patients also have hypertension. Poorly controlled hypertension is associated with delayed graft loss. [Mitsnefes M and Feig DI. Nature Reviews, Nephrology 2010, 6(1):7–8].

BP in CKD Stage 5 has been well discussed in a recent report from the Global Outcomes Controversies Conferences [Levin NW *et al*. Kidney Int 2010, 77:273–284].

REFERENCES

1. Claudio Ronco, Andrew A House and Mikko Haapio. Cardiorenal and renocardiac syndromes: the need for a comprehensive classification and consensus. *Nature Clinical Practice Nephrology*, 2008, **4**(6):310–311.
2. Mitsnefes M and Feig DI. Nature Reviews, *Nephrology*, 2010, **6**(1):7–8.
3. Ronco C *et al*. Cardiorenal syndrome: refining the definition of a complex symbiosis gone wrong. *Intensive Care Med* 2008, **34**:957–962.
4. McIntyre CW. Effects of hemodialysis on cardiac function. *Kidney Int* 2009, **76**(4):371–375.
5. Levin NW *et al*. BP in CKD Stage 5: Report from the Global Outcomes Controversies Conferences. *Kidney Int* 2010, **77**:273–284.

CHAPTER 15

Diuretics

Diuretics are useful agents and are indicated for patients with oedema due to salt and water retention from various causes. They are also popular as therapy for patients with mild hypertension or as an adjunct to other hypotensive agents. This chapter discusses the action and side effects of diuretics and their role in the treatment of hypertension.

Diuretics can cause disorder in acid-base balance as well as disturbances in fluid and electrolyte balance. Before prescribing diuretics to a patient one must always enquire about a history of diabetes mellitus or gout as diuretics can worsen these conditions. Potassium losing diuretics can also cause hypokalaemia in patients on digoxin which may precipitate arrhythmias.

A patient on diuretics should be assessed regularly with regards to his volume status and sodium stores to make sure he is not dehydrated or salt depleted. Baseline data like blood urea, electrolytes, uric acid and calcium should be obtained before commencing treatment. Similarly the lipid profile of the patient should also be ascertained. This is because diuretics can cause derangement in these parameters.

Thiazides

1. Thiazides inhibit sodium chloride (NaCl) reabsorption in the distal convoluted tubule of the kidneys. It has a second site of action in the proximal tubule when combined with a loop diuretic (see Fig. 11.1).

261

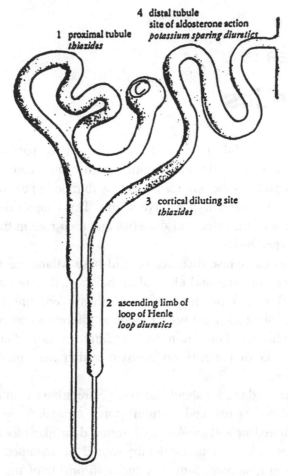

Fig. 15.1   Sites of action of diuretics

2.   There is an active reabsorptive process for calcium in the distal convoluted tubule. Thiazides augment this action and cause hyper-calcaemia. This is the result of a sodium/calcium exchange system plus an ATP-dependent calcium pump.

3.   Thiazides also have an extra-renal action causing vasodilatation of blood vessels and thereby achieving a mild blood pressure lowering effect.

Side Effects of Thiazide Diuretic

1. It causes weakness, fatigue, impotency and paresthesia.
2. Potassium depletion; metabolic alkalosis due to volume contraction and secondary aldosteronism.
3. Hypokalaemia causes ventricular ectopics.
4. Leads to decreased insulin secretion and impaired glucose tolerance test.
5. Causes elevation of total cholesterol, low density lipoprotein (LDL) cholesterol and triglycerides and predisposes the patient to atheroma formation.
6. Elevation of uric acid.
7. Causes hyponatraemia and dehydration if given in excess.
8. Causes hypomagnesaemia which can induce arrhythmia.
9. Causes hypercalcaemia.
10. Occasionally, patients may be allergic to thiazides, developing skin rash, haemolytic anaemia, thrombocytopenia, acute pancreatitis, jaundice and interstitial nephritis.

Loop Diuretic (Frusemide, Ethacrynic Acid, Bumetamide)

1. Inhibits NaCl reabsorption in thick ascending limb at the loop of Henle.
2. Side effects are hypokalaemic metabolic alkalosis, magnesium wasting, hypercalcaemia and ototoxicity.
3. Other side effects include hypersensitivity, myelosuppression, skin rash, liver dysfunction, paresthesia and interstitial nephritis.
4. Combined with thiazide, both agents increase NaCl delivery out of the proximal tubule.
5. Bumetamide is more potent on a weight to weight basis. 1 mg of bumetamide = 40 mg of frusemide. It has an additional site of action at the proximal tubule. All loop diuretics produce diuresis even in severe renal failure, but high doses have to be used.

Spironolactone (Aldactone)

1. It antagonises the action of aldosterone at the distal tubule thereby preventing the reabsorption of sodium.
2. Its main side effect is hyperkalaemia as it is a potassium sparing diuretic.
3. Should be used with caution in patients with renal impairment. These patients tend to have hyperkalaemia since potassium is retained in renal failure. Caution is needed in prescribing spironolactone to patients on potassium supplements as there is a risk of hyperkalaemia.
4. Monitor electrolytes for hyperkalaemia.

Indapamide (Natrilix)

1. This is an indoline derivative of chlorosulphonamide with both diuretic and anti-hypertensive activity.
2. it has a mild diuretic action at the distal tubule and a vasodilator action due to a direct inhibitory action on smooth muscle stimulated by noradrenaline and angiotensin II by reducing transmembrane calcium current.
3. It is more active than spironolactone and frusemide in inhibiting thromboxane A2 and stimulates prostacycline to a greater extent than frusemide.
4. Its extra-renal anti-hypertensive effect is useful in patients with renal failure and it does not have the dose-related side effects of thiazide in the treatment of hypertension.
5. Given in a small dose of 2.5 mg a day, it has only mild diuretic but significant vasodilator hypotensive effect. If the dose is doubled or if given twice a day the diuretic effect becomes more manifest. Long acting Indapamide is also available.

Diuretic Therapy and Vascular Disease

1. What is the net effect of diuretic therapy on risk factors for vascular disease?

2. Ames (1983) and the Framingham data (*Annals New York Academy of Science* 1963, 107:539–556) showed that though diuretics lower BP, they also increase serum cholesterol and impair glucose tolerance test. The probability of developing vascular disease increased from 7.8% to 8.6%. Morgan (1980) showed that patients with mild hypertension on diuretics had a mortality double that predicted and the incidence of myocardial infarction increased 3 fold.

Beta Blockers and Cardiac Protection

1. Beta blockers are associated with raised total and LDL cholesterol, triglycerides and decreased HDL cholesterol - factors promoting atheroma.
2. However, this is counterbalanced by cardio-protective effect of beta blockers.
3. Beta blockers reduce cardiovascular morbidity and mortality following myocardial infarction.

Comparison of Beta Blocker and Diuretic

1. There is no difference in the degree of control of BP.
2. In the control of mild hypertension, diuretic causes impotency, gout and glucose intolerance, whereas beta blockers cause cold extremities, breathlessness and lethargy and impotence.
3. One may therefore decide to choose the drug on the basis of side effects. It is probably safe to use diuretics for mild hypertension provided the patient has normal lipid profiles. These profiles will have to be monitored periodically while the patient is on treatment with diuretics.

Current Role of Diuretics in Hypertension

1. There is some agreement that diuretics are of value in the treatment of hypertension in spite of the potential side effects.

They should probably be used as an adjunctive therapy when the usual combination of Calcium channel blockers, ARBs and beta blockers are inadequate to bring the BP to a desired level of 130/80. I much prefer the addition of alpha terazosin rather than a small dose of thiazide diuretic simply because thiazides have more side effects.

2. Low dose diuretic has less side effect, eg. 12.5 mg hydrochlorthiazide. If this proves effective it may make thiazide more popular, though I am not a great fan myself.

3. For a young patient, some may consider vasodilator or calcium channel blocker as a first line treatment, an ARB as second line and β blocker as the next line though some may prefer low dose diuretic as third line. B blockers and diuretics may both cause impotency.

4. Angiotensin Receptor Antagonist (ATRA) are also more effective with diuretics.

6. Though diuretics may have lost the number one place to vasodilators as the choice therapy for hypertension, they still play, a somewhat important role in the treatment of the disease, especially when combined with a hypotensive drug.

7. There may a place for low dose diuretics which do not cause biochemical cardiovascular risk or impotence.

Treatment of Renal Hypertension

1. Treatment of hypertension in patients with renal insufficiency reduces morbidity and mortality and helps to arrest the progression of renal damage.

2. Use beta blockers, calcium channel blockers, or ATRA.

3. When GFR <30 ml/min, thiazides are usually ineffective.

4. Potassium sparing diuretics are dangerous and loop diuretics are preferred.

5. An alternative is indapamide.

Treatment of Essential Hypertension

1. For mild essential hypertension, thiazide can be used provided patient has normal lipid profile. Adequate control is obtained in two-thirds of patients. Nowadays, most doctors would like to start with a calcium channel blocker like amlodipine 5 to 10 mg a day as the first drug. Yet others may prefer an ARB like Losartan 50 to 100 mg a day.

2. If there is no response to the thiazide, use calcium channel blocker, ARB a β blocker. Salt and water retention may be a consequence of a calcium channel blocker or vasodilator.

3. Thiazide also has a direct effect on vascular smooth muscle causing vasodilatation.

4. Borderline hypertensives respond to salt load with rise in BP. A diuretic may be useful. Thiazide may be preferred as it has a 12 to 18 hours' duration of action.

5. There is however, the problem of renal potassium wasting due to diuretic induced potassium depletion which may give rise to ventricular ectopy. Dietary potassium supplement or oral potassium chloride is necessary. Check renal function to exclude renal impairment before prescribing potassium chloride supplements.

6. Alternatively, one could use potassium sparing diuretics like triamterene or diazide (a combination of triamterene plus thiazide). Triamterene and amiloride (also a potassium sparing diuretic) inhibit entry of sodium into the distal tubule and collecting duct by acting directly at the mucosal surface. However, triamterene has its side effects. It is associated with renal calculi (Ettinger, 1980). Among 181 renal calculi (0.4% or 56,000 calculi), 1/3 contained mainly triamterene. It also causes birefringent crystals and brownish casts which resemble granular casts in urine (Fairley 1983, Fairley and Woo, *Clinical Nephrology* 1986, 26:169–173). These casts can be differentiated from true granular casts as they show birefringence when examined under the microscope using polarised

light. Presumably, the formation of triamterene casts is a pre-disposing factor to calculi formation. In addition, Triamterene may be associated with anuric renal failure as experimentally, the site of formation of triamterene casts in the rat was mainly in the medullary and papillary collecting ducts. Its other side effects are interstitial nephritis and nephrotoxicity especially with NSAID.

7. Beta blockers are often the first step in the treatment of essential hypertension in the United Kingdom, Scandinavia and the United States. However, others may prefer to start treatment with calcium channel blocker to avoid the side effects of beta blockers altogether. Alternatively, some may choose an ACE inhibitor like enalapril, or an ARB like Losartan.

Tailor Treatment to Patient

1. Whatever the mode of therapy, one should always tailor the treatment to the patient. For the young patients with high sympathetic activity and high plasma renin activity (PRA), they may respond better to a beta blocker.

2. For the old patients with low PRA, calcium channel blockers or angiotensin receptor blockers [ARBs] may be preferable as older patients are more prone to the side effects of beta blockers like congestive heart failure and peripheral ischaemia.

3. Old patients with low PRA may respond well to calcium channel blockers or ARBs.

4. Small doses of ACE inhibitors or ARB are also useful in the elderly. Check renal function and serum potassium.

5. In general, for most patients with mild hypertension a dose of a calcium channel blocker like Amlodipine 5 to 10 mg a day should suffice. If the hypertension is mild to moderate, then an ARB like Losartan 100 mg daily could be added. Despite this, if BP is still not brought down to the ideal target of 130/80 mm Hg then one should add a β blocker like

Atenolol 50 mg to 75 mg to 100 mg a day. A β blocker may cause impotency or be contraindicated in a patient with heart block or asthma. Amlodipine may cause troublesome edema, flushing and headaches in some patients. Flushing and headaches due to calcium channel blockers occur less commonly with Amlodipine compared to Nifedipine LA but edema seems to occur more frequently with Amlodipine than Nifedipine LA. If BP is still a bit high at this stage, one could use 12.5 mg of hydrochlorthiazide, but even at such a low dose one would still have to monitor the loss of K^+. Also in elderly patients, beware of causing dehydration which could result in a loss of eGFR with a rise in serum creatinine.

6. In cases of resistant hypertension, alpha [α] terazosin in a starting dose of 1 to 2 mg at night and slowly increasing up to 4 mg to 5 mg twice daily may be useful. α Terazosin is also useful for elderly males with prostatic hyperplasia with symptoms of prostatism. However it may also cause impotency in males. One of the troublesome side effects of terazosin is nasal congestion or stuffy nose with rhinitis which may be dose related.

Diuretic Resistance

1. Diuretic resistance implies an inadequate clearance of edema despite a full dose of diuretic. The principal causes are

   (i) incorrect diagnosis [venous or lymphatic edema], inappropriate or excess NaCl intake [Na^+ intake >120 mmol/day],

   (ii) Inadequate drug reaching tubule like in noncompliance, inadequate dose or infrequent dosing, poor absorption [uncompensated congestive heart failure or CHF], decreased renal blood flow [CHF, cirrhosis of liver, elderly], reduced functional renal mass [acute renal failure, CKD, nephritic syndrome].

   (iii) Inadequate renal response like in low eGFR [Acute renal failure or AKI, CKD], decreased effective ECV [edematous states], activation of the Renin angiotensin aldosterone system [edematous states], nephron adapatation [prolonged diuretic therapy], use of NSAIDS like celebrax, aspirin, brufen, etc.

2. To solve the problem of diuretic resistance, ensure that the dose is appropriate to the condition and patient takes a low salt diet with fluid restriction. Increase frequency of dosing to twice daily, though most patients prefer a morning dose so they do not have to wake up too often in the middle of the night to pass urine. Consider adding a thiazide diuretic to a loop diuretic or a loop to a distal potassium sparing diuretic for synergistic effects. For patients with eGFR <30 ml/min one would have to use larger doses of oral loop diuretic or consider the more potent ones like bumetamide.

Problem of Hyponatremia induced by diuretics

1. In general diuretics should not cause a decrease in eGFR unless the patient is severely volume depleted. Vigorous diuresis induced by diuretics can of course induce renal failure if the effects of diuretic use are not monitored by a physical examination of the patient to assess the fluid status including the checking for postural hypotension due to excessive loss of ECF volume. This is especially so if vigorous diuresis is induced in patients with impaired renal function, severe edema in nephrotic syndrome, cardiac failure or cirrhosis of the liver.

2. One of the reasons why diuretics cause hyponatremia is that initially the loss of the first 2 litres due to diuretics is isotonic [loss of both salt and water], but **after this the loss of salt is no longer accompanied by loss of water and this leads to progressive hyponatremia** in the patient.

3. Another reason for hyponatremia occurs in older people given thiazide diuretics **where free water excretion is impaired following a water load.** This problem occurs more commonly with thiazide diuretic compared to loop diuretic. Thiazide induced hyponatremia usually occurs in situations where patients drink excess water resulting in an expanded total body water.

Problem of Hypokalaemia induced by diuretics

1. Thiazide and loop diuretics both increase renal K^+ excretion and inhibit the coupled reabsorption of Na^+, K^+ and Cl^-. Several mechanisms have been identified, among them are flow dependent K^+ secretion by the distal tubule. In the distal tubules, Calcium mediated channels induce K^+ secretion through distinct channels.
2. Diuretic induced aldosterone secretion also promotes distal K^+ secretion thus promoting more K^+ loss causing hypokalaemia.
3. Finally, the alkalosis induced by diuretics also causes loss of K^+ enhanced secretion of K^+ in the distal tubule. All these mechanisms would account for the diuretic induced Hypokalaemia.

REFERENCE

1. Rovin BH and Herbert LA. Thiazide diuretic monotherapy for hypertension: diuretic's dark side just got darker. *Kidney Int* 2007, **72**:1423–1426.

CHAPTER 16

Kidney Stones

THE INCIDENCE OF STONE DISEASE

In Britain and Scandinavia, the incidence of stone disease is 0.2 to 0.5 per 1000 in the population. In Thailand it is 8 per 1000. The Central and South American Indians, Bantus and Black races in the United States are somehow protected from stone disease. Stone disease is commoner in dry climates and where people sweat a lot, especially among individuals who allow themselves to get dehydrated and not drink enough water to replace the fluid loss.

In Singapore, stones are twice as common in males than in females. It seems to be commoner among doctors. Location wise, 42% of stones are found in the kidney, 49% in the ureters, 7% in the bladder and 2% in the urethra. The peak incidence is from 20 to 40 years. 12.5% of patients experience recurrences and about one-third lose a kidney. (Data by courtesy of K.T. Foo)

FACTORS WHICH PREDISPOSE TO STONE FORMATION

1. The pH of urine affects stone formation. Eg. uric acid stones form in acidic urine.
2. Stones form when there is a high concentration of certain stone forming substances in the urine. If the concentration of these substances rises to a certain level stones are formed. If there is a lot of water in the urine to dilute these substances there is a lesser chance of stones forming. This explains why

people who sweat a lot and do not drink enough water have a tendency to form stones.

3. We have certain naturally occurring inhibitors in the urine which prevent stones from forming. Some people have less of these substances and are therefore more prone to stones.
4. Other factors such as obstruction to the free flow of urine causing stasis predisposes a person to stone formation. Infection by certain urea splitting bacteria can also cause stone formation.

THE DIFFERENT TYPES OF STONES

90% of renal stones are principally of calcium salts (calcium oxalate, calcium phosphate). A small proportion of these are composed of calcium, magnesium ammonium phosphate or triple phosphates which have a tendency to form 'Staghom' stones. These Staghorn calculi predisposes to infection and obstruction.

The remaining 10% of renal stones are uric stones. People living in hot climate who sweat a lot and drink little water tend to form uric acid stones.

35% of all stones among Singaporeans contain uric acid; 10% as urates alone and 25% in association with triple phosphates.

SYMPTOMS OF STONES IN THE URINARY TRACT

Many people have kidney stones but are often not aware of it until they develop symptoms. 75% of patients may complain of pain or backache, others may pass blood in the urine (31%) or have urinary tract infections (14%) and yet others may have the stones diagnosed on X-ray for some unrelated complaint (5%).

Pain due to kidney stone is called "renal colic". Actually this pain is felt only when the stone is moving down the ureter. The colic or pain results from contraction of the muscles in the ureter as it tries to force the stone lower down the ureter in an attempt to expel it. The pain usually starts in the left or right side of the abdomen and travels towards the groin and may radiate to the testicle in the case of males. It can be a very severe pain causing the patient to double up in bed or toss about in agony.

Large stones that are too big to be passed down the ureter can cause obstruction (7%) giving rise to a dull ache in the back. Bladder stones can sometimes cause a dragging sensation. When passing urine the stone may act like a ball valve causing urine to start, stop and start again. In addition there may be pain in the penis, bloody urine or bladder infection causing the patient frequent pain on passing urine.

Loin Pain Haematuria Syndrome (LPHS)

1. Patients present with loin pain and passage of blood in the urine but investigations do not reveal the presence of renal stones. A few may have had a stone which has been passed out and the Xrays after the event do not show evidence of stone disease.

2. Typically the patient with LPHS is often young to middle age complaining of loin pain often with gross haematuria and persistent microscopic haematuria. The diagnosis is one of exclusion of other causes of hamaturia like stones, urinary infection or renal tumour.

3. It is mandatory that an intravenous pyelogram or ultrasound of the kidneys and bladder be performed to exclude a tumour. Renal angiograms have been performed in some of these patients but they have usually been normal.

4. Some patients have had renal biopsies performed and in a few patients they have been found to have IgA nephritis and in others Thin Membrane Disease (TMD). Among those with TMD, it has been postulated that rupture of the glomerular capillary walls may have occurred resulting in haemorrhage into the renal tubules causing obstruction and edema with stretching of the renal capsule resulting in loin pain.

5. The long term prognosis is excellent with normal renal function even years after. The therapeutic goal should be symptomatic management with analgesics, including opiates and psychiatric evaluation and counselling as well as referral to a pain clinic. About 30% have a spontaneous resolution after a mean period of 3.5 years.

6. In my opinion patients should not have active intervention like autotransplantion or denvervation apart from reassurance and judicious use of analgesics when necessary. Autotransplantation and renal denervation should only be procedures of last resort. Pain can recur in the autotransplanted kidney and usually within a year. In some cases who had uninephrectomy, pain has recurred in the contralateral kidney. However, Shiel *et al.* compared the outcomes in 40 renal autotransplants with 24 renal denervation procedures performed in Australia over a 13 year period. Among those who had renal autotransplant, 76% remained pain free after a mean period of 8.4 years follow up compared with 33% from the renal denervation group who were pain free after a mean follow up of 8 years. [Sheila AG, Chui AK, Verran DJ *et al.*, Evaluation of the loin pain/haematuria syndrome treated by autotransplantation or radical nerve neurectomy. Am J Kidney Disease, 1998, 32:215–220].

INVESTIGATION OF PATIENTS WITH STONES

1. Urine is examined for presence of blood or infection caused by stones.

2. Blood tests are performed to check kidney function (blood urea and creatinine). Blood calcium and uric acid levels are also checked as high blood calcium or blood uric acid forms stones.

3. X-rays of the abdomen or intravenous pyelogram (IVP) are done to determine the site and number of stones. An ultrasound investigation is also useful to identify the site of the stone and exclude obstruction.

4. If it is suspected that the stone has caused obstruction to the flow of urine, a tube is passed into the bladder (cystoscopy) and through it fine catheters are passed up to the ureters. Contrast dye is injected and X-ray pictures are taken to demonstrate the site of obstruction.

5. 24 hours' urine is collected to measure calcium and uric acid in the urine. Excessive amounts of calcium and uric acid in the urine can cause kidney stones.

6. Stones passed out should be sent for stone analysis to determine the type of stone.

TREATMENT OF PATIENT WITH RENAL STONES

1. There are certain medical conditions which cause stones to form in the kidney. If these conditions are treated or removed then further stones will not form.

2. It is important that patients who have stones in the kidney should drink plenty of water to maintain a high urine volume as this will lower the concentration of substances which cause stones to form or even dissolve existing stones. Patients should drink enough water to pass at least 2 to 2.5 litres of urine per day.

   The patient should drink water before going to bed so that he would get up in the night to pass urine. After passing, he should drink (from the tumbler of water by the bedlocker) before lying in bed so that he would wake again to pass urine. Initially he may be apprehensive of broken or lost sleep but after a while he will get used to the waking process and having no difficulty in automatically falling asleep again. He will not therefore suffer from insomnia.

3. Stones that are less than 0.5 cm in diameter can be passed out but those more than 0.5 cm will require surgical intervention.

4. If the patient has severe pain he can be given an injection to relieve the pain.

5. Urinary infection can be treated with antibiotics.

6.   Recurrent stones due to excessive amounts of calcium in the urine can be treated with chlorothiazide (a diuretic). This will decrease the incidence of recurrence. In addition the patient should avoid high calcium food like dairy products (milk and cheese). Those who have stones due to too much uric acid in the urine can be treated with allopurinol which is also used for the treatment of gout. In addition, these patients also require alkalinisation of their urine by taking sodium bicarbonate solution and avoidance of food containing high urate content (liver, kidney and other organ meat).

7.   Stones that cannot be passed out and give rise to severe pain, urine infection or bleeding into the urine will require surgery.

Newer Techniques of Stone Removal

1.   **Percutaneous Nephrolithotomy (PCN)**
     This involves making a tract (tunnel) from the skin to the kidney. An instrument called a nephroscope is introduced to view the stone in the kidney. A small stone is removed by means of a pair of forceps passed through the nephroscope. A large stone is broken up by means of ultrasound and then removed with forceps or sucked out.

2.   **Extracorporeal Shock Wave Lithotripsy (ESWL)**
     The patient is immersed in a water bath and an external source of shock waves, generated by means of an electrode and a generator, is focussed on the stone in the kidney to cause it to break up. The fragments of stone are then passed out in the urine.

3.   **Transurethral Urethroscopy**
     Preliminary dilatation of the vesico-ureteric junction with ureteric bougies or balloon catheter is made. A ureteroscope is then introduced to view the stone which is then removed. Larger stones are disintegrated by ultrasound before removal.

GOUT

Gout is a condition due to excess uric acid in the blood which occasionally crystallises out into the joints giving rise to very severe pain, usually in the big toe. The toe becomes red, swollen and acutely tender. Attacks of gout often come on at night or in the early hours of the morning. See Chapter on Systemic Disease and the Kidney.

What Triggers Off an Attack of Gout?

A heavy meal containing too much offal (liver, kidneys, fish roe), heavy wine, undue exertion, an operation or severe illness; anything which suddenly changes the patient's lifestyle can precipitate an attack of gout. Such attacks may therefore occur more commonly on holidays or during travel overseas.

Treatment of Gout

The acute attack can be treated with either colchicine or Indocid. Two or three weeks after the acute attack has subsided the patient should take Allopurinol (Zyloric) or Probenecid (Benemid) to lower the uric acid in the blood. These two drugs should not be taken during the acute attack or just after an attack of gout as they may bring on the attack again. Patients should also avoid taking offal and wines.

1. **Treatment of the acute episode of gout**
   Apart from the use of colchicine other effective options for treatment include using NSAIDS, intra articular steroids and systemic steroid therapy. The rapidity with which treatment is commenced is important. Caution must be exercised in use of NSAIDS and steroids in those with renal, cardiac disease and peptic ulcers. After the intra -articular aspiration, the synovial

fluid is sent off for analysis and systemic prednisolone can be started in a dose of 20 to 40 mg a day, reducing to zero dosage after 10 to 14 days. Despite the popularity of using steroids, there is not much support on efficacy and effectiveness from the Cochrane review [Janssens HJ *et al*. Systemic corticosteroids for acute gout. Cochrane database Syst Rev 2008: CD005521]. However, some are of the view that the use of colchicine is associated with high GI side effects which may not be acceptable by many. Care should be exercised in patients with renal failure and those on cyclosporine therapy [Eleftheriou G *et al*. Colchicine induced toxicity in a heart transplant patient with chronic renal failure. Clin Toxicol 2008, 46:827–830].

The IL-1 receptor antagonist, **anakinra** has been used to treat refractory gout with apparent benefit. It is an NALP3 **inflamasome** leading to release of IL-1 in the pathogenesis of gouty inflammation [McGonagle D *et al*. Management of treatment resistant inflammation of acute on chronic tophaceous gout with anakinra. Ann Rheum Dis, 2007, 66:1683–1684]. Anti TNF has also been reported to be of benefit.

2. **Prophylactic therapy**

   Such therapy helps to prevent acute attacks as well as prevent joint damage and formation of tophi on tendons. The aim of prophylaxis is also to ensure that serum urate levels are kept at a sufficiently low level. How low should one keep serum uric acid [SUA] levels. In SGH the normal range is from 140 to 340 micromol/l. The British Society of Rheumatology guidelines recommends less than 300 micromol/l. The European league and the USA recommend <360 micromol/l. In Australia, <360 micromol/l is acceptable and <300 micromol/l is even better.

3. **Non Drug interventions**

   Weight and alcohol reduction are of great value but rarely lead to >15% reduction in SUA levels. Benefits may be obtained from low fat milk and yoghurt, soya bean and vegetable sources of protein. Restrict intake of high purine foods like liver, kidneys, shellfish, yeast extract, high protein foodstuff like red meat [Jordan KM *et al*. Brit Soc for Rheum and Brit Health Professionals in Rheumatology guideline for the management of gout, 2007, 46:1372–4].

4. **Drug Interventions**

   (i) Probenecid a uricosuric drug is a useful alternative for those sensitive to allopurinol which is the traditional drug used.

   (ii) Benzbromarone is a potent uricosuric drug useful for those who are allergic to allopurinol and do not have enough renal function for probenecid to be useful.

   (iii) Fenofibrate and Losartan have weak uricosuric effects.

   (iv) Allopurinol remains the most useful drug and accounts for 98% prescriptions for urate lowering therapy in Australia and worldwide. Using a hypouricemic drug often causes a temporary increase in the risk of a gouty flare. This can be reduced if we increase the allopurinol in low doses. Most patients are on 300 mg does. Start at 100 mg dose and progressively increase the dose. However, only about 24% of those on 300 mg a day of allopurionl achieve a target lowering of SUA to <300 micromol/l. For patients with renal impairment, the dose of allopurinol should be even lower, about 100 to 200 mg/day. This should be enough to inhibit uric acid production. In those with renal impairment the risk of allopurinol hypersensitivity is much higher, about 18% mortality [Lee HY, Ariyasinghe JT, Thirumoorthy T. Allopurinol hypersensitivity syndrome: a preventable severe cutaneous adverse reaction? Sing Med Journal 2008, 49:384–7].

   Among patients starting allopurinol, the appearance of a rash within the first 12 weeks should alert one to the possibility of hypersensitivity to allopurinol. Always check to make sure the patient is not on aza-thioprine before starting allopurinol as in the case of renal transplant or lupus nephritic patients. Allopurinol being a xanthine oxidase inhibitor will interfere with the metabolism of azathioprine via the purine pathway, thus potentiating the effect of azathioprine and causing bone marrow suppression.

Start with a small dose of 100 mg for the first 6 weeks and be alert for side effects before increasing the dose of allopurinol. Monitor the level of SUA to see if there is a need to increase the dose of allopurinol to achieve a level <360 micromol/l. For some patients with frequent attacks, it may be useful to put them on colchicine 0.5 mg BD or low dose prednisolone may be used initially to prevent a gouty flare. For those intolerant to allopurinol, use probenecid unless eGFR is <30–40 ml/min.

(v)   Febuxostat is a major advance for patients intolerant to allopurinol and have renal impairment. **Febuxostat inhibits the same enzyme as allopurinol (xanthine oxidase)** but unlike allopurinol is not a purine analogue. After administration it is rapidly absorbed and has a half life of 4 to 18 hours. No modification is required in relation to renal function and age. It is very effective and 93% of patients who tolerated the medication and continued for 5 years achieved a maintenance SUA of <360 micromol/l in a 28 day study, 0% for placebo, 56% for those on 40 mg, 76% for those on 80 mg and 94% for those on 120 mg/day. Gouty flares occur more commonly among those on 80 mg (43%) and on 120 mg (55%) groups without any prophylaxis but only in 8% and 13% among those on colchicine prophylaxis at 0.6 mg twice daily. In SGH, the colchicine tabs come as 500 mcg per tab.

In a study of patients with serum creatinine <133 micromol/l or eGFR <50ml/min on treatment for 1 year, with a SUA target <360 micromol/l, 53% were on 80 mg/day Febuxostat, 62% on 120 mg/day Febuxostat and only 21% on allopurinol 300 mg/day.

Safety of Febuxostat appears good but it should be avoided in those with CVS events like atherosclerosis, myocardial infarction and CHF. Elevation of hepatic tranaminases were uncommon, similar to allopurinol. Liver function tests should be reviewed. This drug may be an alternative to the use of allopurinol in the future but it is expensive. In Australia it costs about $240 (A$) a month.

(vi) **Uricase** (Urate oxidase) catalyses the conversion of urate to allantoin which is 5 times more soluble than urate and is easily excreted by the kidneys. This enzyme is active in most fish, amphibians and non primate mammals but not in man and higher primates.

Infusion of recombinant Aspergillus uricase (rasburicase) leads to a rapid reduction of SUA and is most useful for patients on chemotherapy for cancers where there is chemotherapy induced hyperuricemia.

The conjugation of uricase to polyethylene glycol (pegloticase) offers a more sustained action. In a dose of 8 mg every 2 weeks to 4 weeks, target SUA levels can be maintained for over 6 months. However gouty flares, infusion reactions and reduction of pegloticase half life in association with development of pegloticase antibodies were all common. Despite these difficulties pegloticase does have a place in patients intolerant of allopurinol or have renal insufficiency.

In Conclusion: If we were to manage our patients well we must monitor SUA levels and maintain target of SUA <360 micromol (but in SGH our upper limit of normal SUA is now at 340 micromol). Allopurinol hypersensitivity is uncommon, unless the patient has renal insufficiency. It is wise to begin with a small dose of 100 mg. Side effects occur usually within 3 months. We should monitor SUA levels and increase the dose of allopurinol to achieve target SUA levels. Febuxostat is a useful drug for those who have problems with allopurinol.

Reference: McGill NW. Management of Gout: beyond allopurinol. *Internal Medicine Journal*, 2010,40:545–553.

Renal Complications of Gout

In patients with gout, renal disease is the most common and serious complication. There are two types of renal involvement in gout:

1. **Kidney Stones**
   Patients with gout may pass 3 types of stones: uric acid stones, calcium oxalate stones and mixed urate-calcium stones.

   Uric acid stones are formed in the presence of acidic urine which contains plenty of uric acid. These stones are easy to treat and prevent. The patient should drink enough water to produce 3 litres of urine daily. In addition he has to take sodium bicarbonate solution to make the urine alkaline as uric acid stones form in an acidic urine. So if the urine is alkaline, stones are less likely to form. Allopurinol can also be prescribed to lower the uric acid level in the blood and urine.

   Calcium oxalate stones are more commonly formed in patients with gout than in the normal population. This is because uric acid in the urine forms a nidus for the deposition and growth of calcium oxalate crystals.

   Uric acid stones account for about 10% of kidney stones in the USA. In the Middle East, Japan and Asia the incidence is even higher. Type 2 Diabetics have a 3 fold higher incidence of uric acid stones, pure as well as mixed with calcium, both about 3 fold higher. Obesity is another factor as about 60% of stones in obese people have uric acid. There is a relationship between uric acid stone formation and insulin resistance. Patients with uric acid stone also have many of the features of the metabolic syndrome [Daudon M *et al.* High prevalence of uric acid calculi in diabetic stone formers. Nephrol Dial Transpl 2005, 20:468–469].

2. **Gouty** *Nephropathy*

Passage of protein in the urine is the first clinical sign. Sometimes there may be pus cells or blood in the urine if the patient also has kidney stones and urine infection. With time, "very rarely" some patients with gouty nephropathy may slowly develop mild renal impairment. Histologically there is microtophi and chronic interstitial inflammation in the kidney. Several investigators question the existence of specific gouty nephropathy as a primary event in patients with clinical gout. This is because these patients often have hypertension, diabetes mellitus or hyperlipemia, all of which can cause nephrosclerosis with accompanying azotemia. Treatment consists of liberal intake of fluid, with avoidance of offal and wines. Allopurinol should also be prescribed as it will reduce the formation of uric acid and may arrest the renal deterioration.

Struvite Stones

1. Struvite ($MgNH_4PO_4 6H_2O$) account for 10 to 15% of all kidney stones. These stones grow rapidly and enlarge filling up the whole renal pelvis giving the appearance of a staghorn, hence the term staghorn calculus. These stones form in urine infected by urea spiltting bacteria. They are difficult to treat and often recur causing significant morbidity and mortality even, hence the term "stone cancer". These stones are also called triple phosphate stones as they are composed of magnesium ammonium phosphate. They are also known as "infective stones".

2. Struvite stones are more common in females than males as females have more UTI than males. Chronic urinary stasis and infection also predispose. Hence it is more common in

     those with neurogenic bladders, elderly, indwelling catheters, cord lesions and those with abnormal urinary tract.

3. This is result of urease from urea splitting organisms which hydrolyses the conversion of urea to ammonia. Phosphate and magnesium combines with ammonia to form struvite and the calcium and phosphate with the carbonate form carbonite apatite. Ammonium can bind to the charged sulphates on the glycosaminoglycans that line the uroepithelium.

4. The majority of urease producing infections are caused by Proteus mirabilis although many types of gram positive and negative organisms including Mycoplasma and yeast can do so. Corynebacterium and Ureaplasma are also common culprits causing struvite stomes. They can use urease to split urea and supply their need for nitrogen in the form of ammonia.

5. In the past, staghorn calculi require surgical removal and if not treated properly, 50% can end up with nephrectomy. About 25% have recurrence and 50% have recurrent UTI. If aggressive lavage with hemiacidrin [mixture of citric acid, gluconic acid, magnesium hydrocarbonate and magnesium acid citrate at acidic pH of 3.9 for chemolysis] is used following open nephrectomy, the recurrence can be as low as 2%.

6. Nowadays, using percutaneous nephrolithotomy, up to 90% of struvite stones can be removed with 10% recurrence rate. Using extracorporeal shock wave lithotripsy with ureteral stenting, stone free rates of 50% to 75% can be achieved. In 1994, the American Urologic Association recommended a combination of percutaneous nephrolithotomy with shock wave litotripsy [Segura JW *et al.* Nephrolithiasis clinical guidelines panel summary report on the management of staghorn calculi. J Urol 1994, 151:1648–1651]. In the latest series by Grasso, using retrograde ureteroscopy with hominium: YAG laser stone disruption there was a reported fragmentation of all minor staghorn calculi with a recurrence rate of 60% at 6 months [Grasso M *et al.* Retrograde ureteropyeloscopic

treatment of 2 mm or greater upper urinary tract and minor staghorn calculi. J Urol 1998, 160:346–351].

DIETARY FACTORS AND CALCIUM NEPHROLITHIASIS[1]

1. Upper urinary tract stones correlate with economic affluence (high protein diet).
2. Bladder stones in Southern Asia and India — related to protein malnutrition,
3. Vegetarianism protects against stones though increases urinary oxalate excretion.
4. Protein load increases urinary calcium, oxalate and uric acid. A diet rich in animal protein results in increased urine calcium excretion into urine in which the calcium is less soluble because of the excess sulphate and reduced citrate thus promoting stone formation. Reduction of dietary protein in conjunction with a low salt diet and adequate dietary protein will reduce stone formation.
5. Traditionally, patients with calcium containing stones are told to refrain from taking calcium. However it has been found that a low calcium diet may increase the rate of stone formation. Hence taking adequate calcium in the diet is important. Increasing dietary calcium may increase urinary calcium. Post menopausal women given calcium supplements and Vitamin D may have an increased risk of stone formation if they are not deficient in calcium from their diet. Compared to women given a free choice diet, those on calcium supplements had increased risk of stone formation [Jackson RD, La Croix AZ, Gass M *et al.*, Calcium plus - Vit D supplementation and the risk of fractures. N Engl J Med, 2006, 354:669–683]. Based on evidence, one should have enough calcium from a balanced diet. It is not advisable to take calcium and Vit D supplements as it is now believed that such supplements will cause vascular calcification in

the coronary blood vessels resulting in a high incidence of ischemic heart disease.

High Level of Dietary Protein

1. Population studies — high consumption of animal protein increases prevalence of upper tract stones.
2. High dietary protein increases urinary calcium, uric acid and oxalate. High intake of animal protein increases endogenous production of oxalate.
3. Dietary protein restriction has citraturic and hypocalciuric effect.
4. Low incidence of stones in vegetarians.
5. Prophylactic effect of dietary protein reduction in hypercalciurics, hyperuricosurics.

Other Factors

1. Increase in dietary **sodium** causes inhibition of Ca^{++} and Na^+ reabsorption at proximal tubule and loop of Henle.
2. Increased ingestion of **oxalate** in diet (spinach, rhubarb, peanuts, strawberries, chocolates, tea) causes recurrent stones.
3. Dietary **calcium** restriction is detrimental because negative Ca^{++} balance leads to bone resorption. It also causes secondary hyperoxaluria.
4. **Fluid** therapy is good. But no carbohydrate or oxalate (fruit juice) should be taken or benefit will be negated by increased excretion of lithogenic components.

Dietary Therapy

1. Patients whose dietary Na^+, protein, oxalate and calcium are excessive, OR urinary volume low, require dietary modification.

2. Reduce: <100 mEq/day Na⁺, 1 gm/kg protein, 1000–1500 mg Ca⁺⁺, avoid oxalate-rich food, at least 3 litres urine per day.
3. High dietary fibre lowers dietary Ca⁺⁺ and oxalate absorption.
4. Assess: 24-hour urinary Na⁺ excretion, 24-hour urinary urea excretion (protein intake), 24-hour urine volume (fluid intake).

REFERENCES

1. Kidney Int. *Infection stones*, 1988, **34**: 544–555.
2. Nakagawa T *et al.* Unearthing Uric Acid: an ancient factor with recently found significance in renal and cardiovascular disease. *Kidney Int* 2006, **69**:1722–1725.
3. McGill NW. Management of Gout: beyond allopurinol. *Internal Medicine Journal*, 2010, **40**:545–553.
4. Dube GK *et al.* Loin pain haematuria syndrome. *Kidney Int* 2006, **70**:2152–2155.
5. Sheila AG, Chui AK, Verran DJ *et al.*, Evaluation of the loin pain/haematuria syndrome treated by autotransplantation or radical nerve neurectomy. *Am J Kidney Disease*, 1998, **32**:215–220.
6. Segura JW *et al.* Nephrolithiasis clinical guidelines panel summary report on the management of staghorn calculi. *J Urol* 1994, **151**:1648–1651.
7. Grasso M *et al.* Retrograde ureteropyeloscopic treatment of 2 mm or greater upper urinary tract and minor staghorn calculi. *J Urol* 1998, **160**:346–351.
8. Daudon M *et al.* High prevalence of uric acid calculi in diabetic stone formers. *Nephrol Dial Transpl* 2005, **20**:468–469.

CHAPTER 17

Diabetes Mellitus and the Kidney

Diabetes is the major cause of ESRF throughout the world. It is the primary diagnosis in 20% to 40% of people starting treatment for ESRF worldwide. In Australia, the number of new Type 2 Diabetics has increased 5 fold between 1993 and 2007. In Japan it has increased 7 fold from 1983 to 2005. In the UK prospective study (UKPDS), about 30% of the cohort develop renal impairment, of whom about 50% did not have preceding albuminuria. In Singapore, Diabetic Nephropathy accounts for about 52% of patients with ESRF every year and it is the commonest cause of ESRF.

There is evidence that early therapy in those with CKD can delay progression. The use of ACEI and ARB have been shown to delay the progression from normoalbuminuria to microalbuminuria and from microalbuminuria to macroalbuminuria and slow progression to ESRF. Use of ACEI/ARB is now standard therapy together with good control of glucose, lipids and BP. The latest step is developing new therapies to reduce renal damage and renal fibrosis including agents that block the formation of advanced glycation end products and other signalling pathways [Atkins RC and Zimmet P. Diabetic kidney disease. Act now or pay later. Kidney Int 2010, 77:375–377]. We should also be using the renin inhibitor Aliskiren and perhaps less of ACEI/ARBs in view of long term usage causing renofibrosis with ACEI/ARBs.

The Nephrology of Diabetes Mellitus (DM) embraces a broad spectrum of clinical renal entities ranging from diabetic nephropathy, urinary tract infections, papillary necrosis to autonomic bladder with all its complications. Diabetic Nephropathy

(DiabNx) however, is by far the predominant clinical entity accounting for more than 90% of the renal problems associated with DM. This chapter focuses on the treatment of DiabNx which is the commonest cause of end stage renal failure (ESRF) in Singapore accounting for 52% of new end stage renal failure seen every year.[1] In the USA, DiabNx is the commonest cause of ESRF (40%), Sweden 20% and Australia 12%. The trend for increasing incidence of DM should be a cause for concern for everyone. Previously chronic glomerulonephritis used to be the leading cause in Singapore.

DiabNx rarely develops before 10 years duration of Type I DM whereas 3% of Type II DM (NIDDM) already have overt nephropathy. About 30% to 40% of patients with Type I and II DM will develop DiabNx but those patients who survive 35 years of DM without developing DiabNx are at extremely low risk of doing so in future.[2] In the last two decades several interventional strategies have resulted in slowing the decline of renal function and the 10 year mortality rate of patients with DiabNx has been reduced from 70% to 20%.[3] Therapeutic strategies in DiabNx nowadays include strict glycemic control, strict control of hypertension, use of angiotensin converting enzyme (ACE) inhibitors or ARBs, dietary protein restriction and control of hypercholesterolaemia.

Natural History of Diabetic Nephropathy

There are 5 stages in the natural history. Stage I: Here there is glomerular hyperfiltration and renal enlargement. Albuminuria may be present. Stage II: Normoalbuminuria. With control of hyperglycemia, microalbuminuria disappears. Stage III: Incipient Diabetic Nephropathy. After 5 to 7 years, especially in patients where blood sugar is not well controlled, microalbuminuria appears again. If blood sugar is well controlled again, microalbuminuria may disappear. Stage IV: Overt or Established Diabetic Nephropathy. There is now persistent macroalbuminuria (dipstix for protein is positive, total urinary protein excretion more than 150 mg/day). Overt Diabetic Nephropathy is no longer reversible. With time there is accompanying decline in GFR with rise in blood pressure. Stage V: End Stage Renal Failure.

MICROALBUMINURIA

Microalbuminuria is a sign of endothelial cell damage and is correlated with damage to blood vessels in the kidneys, cardiovascular system and the brain accounting for higher incidence of kidney failure, ischemic heart disease and strokes. Diabetes Mellitus is a microangiopathy and the presence of abnormal amounts of microalbuminuria in patients with DM heralds the onset of nephropathy. The presence of persistent microalbuminuria in a patient with DM is therefore a predictor of the development of DiabNx later on. If one were to accept 20 mmol/l as the upper limit of microalbumin in the urine, it would mean that anyone with microalbumin >20 mmol/l would be at risk of increased renal and cardiac morbidity and mortality.[20] Indeed there is a positive correlation with renal and cardiac mortality with increasing microalbuminuria levels from 20 mmol/l and above. In a patient with DM, the presence of microalbuminuria 20–200 mmol/l equates with glomerular basement (GBM) thickening and mesangial expansion with development into overt proteinuria [macroalbuminuria], development of glomerular lesions of DiabNx, hypertension and progressive loss of eGFR with development of renal failure.

I. Role of Glycemic Control in Diabetic Nephropathy

Poor glycemic control initiates complications of DM and once established, DiabNx progresses inexorably. Metabolic control of DM is important for progression of DiabNx. Even if the blood pressure is controlled the impact of metabolic control of blood sugar is still obvious.[4] In the Diabetic Control and Complications Trial (DCCT)[5] from the DCCT Research Group, American Diabetes Research Association, 1993, a total of 1441 patients with IDDM (726 with no retinopathy and 715 with retinopathy) were randomly assigned to either (i) Intensive therapy with insulin pump or 3 or more times a day injections or (ii) conventional therapy on once or twice daily insulin injections. The goal was pre-parandial blood glucose of 3.9 to 6.7 mmol/litre, postparandial blood glucose less than 10 mmol/litre and HbA1C less than 6.05%. The mean duration of follow up was 6.5 years.

The conclusions were that strict glycemic control (i) in normoalbuminuric diabetics delays onset and slows progression of DiabNx (ii) in incipient DiabNx, it retards progression of nephropathy and (iii) in overt DiabNx, there were no beneficial effects in retardation of renal disease.

Therefore strict glycemic control in DiabNx is important for patients with normoalbuminuria and microalbuminuria (incipient DiabNx). Their HbA1C should be less than 7% but in those with overt or established DiabNx, that is, presence of macroalbuminuria (positive test for protein on dipstix) one should beware of hypoglycemia as renal failure progresses as insulin is metabolized by the proximal tubules of the kidney and the half life of insulin is prolonged as renal failure progresses. Blood glucose should be monitored regularly and insulin or oral hypoglycemics reduced accordingly.

II. Role of Hypertension in Diabetic Nephropathy

Hypertension aggravates underlying renal disease irrespective of the type of renal disease. Aggravation of the underlying renal disease itself also causes both hypertension and deterioration of renal function. In DiabNx, prospective studies have shown preservation of renal function by anti-hypertensive therapy. Mogensen in 1976[6] showed that improved blood pressure control in patients with DiabNx led to dramatic slowing on the rate of decline of the renal function. Hypertension is therefore a most important risk factor in DiabNx. In patients where the mean arterial blood pressure (MAP) is significantly reduced there is significant decrease in the rate of decline of the GFR. There is also a significant decrease in the rate of urinary albumin excretion. In a patient with DiabNx the optimum BP should be less than 130/80.

In the choice of an anti-hypertensive agent one should consider the metabolic and reno-protective effect. Thiazides and beta-blockers adversely affect glucose tolerance and lipid profile though they decrease proteinuria; whereas ACE Inhibitors, ARBs and calcium channel blockers decrease proteinuria without these adverse effects. In patients with DiabNx there is glomerular hyperfiltration where there is angiotensin II mediated vasoconstriction of the efferent glomerular arteriole. ACE Inhibitors and ARBs cause efferent arteriolar vasodilatation at the glomerulus thereby decreasing intra-glomerular hypertension and reducing proteinuria.

III. Role of Angiotensinogen Converting Enzyme Inhibitors

As early as 1934, Cambier[7] had already shown that GFR was increased in patients with DiabNx. Before insulin therapy, GFR was 40% above normal and with treatment there was a reduction to 25% above normal. The increase in GFR was related to glycemic control. Morgensen in 1976[6] demonstrated that patients with the highest GFR were those destined to develop overt DiabNx. Patients with DiabNx have activated renin-angiotensin system making ACE Inhibitors effective in influencing renal hemodynamics. Aurell in 1992[7] showed that captopril therapy (25 mg thrice daily) reduced the rate of decline of GFR by 50%. ACE Inhibitor also has reno-protective effect. Enalapril, a long acting ACE Inhibitor has anti-proteinuric effect compared to metoprolol.

In 1993, Lewis *et al.*[8] published the results of a collaborative study to determine if captopril, an ACE Inhibitor has reno-protective effects. It was a multicentre, randomised, double blind controlled trial with 207 patients on captopril and 202 patients on placebo. The primary study end point was a doubling of baseline creatinine to at least 2.0 mg/dl and the secondary analyses included the length of time to the combined end point of death, dialysis, transplantation and changes in renal function assessed in terms of serum creatinine concentration, 24 hour creatinine clearance and urinary protein excretion. The median follow up period was 3 years.

The results of the study showed that there were less patients in the captopril group who doubled their serum creatinine (n = 25) compared to 43 in the placebo group (p < 0.007). The mean rate of decline in creatinine clearance (11+/–21 ml/min) of the captopril group was slower than 17+/–21 ml/min in the placebo group (p < 0.03).

In the captopril group there was a 50% reduction in risk of death, dialysis and transplantation independent of the small disparity in BP between the 2 groups. The conclusion of the study was that captopril protects against deterioration in renal function in IDDM patients with nephropathy and is significantly more effective than BP control alone. The reno-protective effects were independent of its effect on BP. ACE Inhibitor therapy therefore should be recommended to diabetic patients with incipient DiabNx (presence of microalbuminuria) and those with overt or established DiabNx (dipstix positive or presence of macroalbuminuria).

However, there are certain precautions during use of ACE Inhibitor therapy. ACE Inhibitor is contraindicated in patients with renal artery stenosis and should be used with caution in patients with renal impairment as the drop in intraglomerular BP due to efferent arteriolar vasodilatation will cause further lowering of the GFR leading to further worsening of existing renal impairment. Since ACE Inhibitor is anti-aldosterone and anti-angiotensin it will cause retention of K^+, giving rise to hyperkalaemia and salt and water depletion as it counters the physiological functions of aldosterone and angiotensin to retain salt and water.

IV. The role of Angiotensin Receptor Blockers (ARBs)

Recently[16] in a randomized multicentre control trial, RENAAL (Reduction of End points in NIDDM with Angiotensin II Receptor Antagonist, Losartan), involving 1513 patients from 29 countries with NIDDM of which 751 patients in the treatment group were on Losartan 50 mg to 100 mg daily compared to 762 patients given placebo, both groups also continuing treatment for hypertension with conventional BP medicine, excluding ACE inhibitors and other Angiotensin Receptor Blocker (ARBs) there was a 28% reduction in development of End Stage Renal Disease among the patients treated with Losartan. Proteinuria in the Losartan treated group decreased by 35% compared to those on placebo. The trial was conducted over a 3 and a half years period. In a subsequent follow up study it was found that patients with the D allele of the ACE I/D polymorphism tend to have an unfavourable renal prognosis which could be mitigated by Losartan.[17] Parving *et al.* demonstrated that the optimal renoprotective dose for losartan was 100 mg/day, for Candesartan was 16 mg/day and for Irbesartan was 900 mg/day.[18] The American Diabetes Association has now recommended that in hypertensive Type 2 Diabetic patients with microalbuminuria, ARBs are the initial agents of choice.[19]

V. The Role of Dietary Protein Restriction in DiabNx

In 1981, Brenner[9] demonstrated that increased dietary protein accentuated the decline in renal function of one and two-thirds nephrectomised rats. Walker[10] in 1989 showed that protein restriction on the other hand could retard the progression of renal failure in patients with renal failure. Zeller in 1991[11] reported that dietary protein restriction slowed the rate of decline of GFR in IDDM patients (3 ml/min compared to 12 ml/min in controls).

Our current practice for patients with DiabNx is to recommend a 0.8 gm/Kg BW protein diet. A 50 kg weight patient will be prescribed a 40 gm protein diet. The American Diabetic Association recommends a 0.6 gm/Kg BW protein diet but such zealous dieting only leads to malnutrition by the time the patient requires dialysis. We would advise the patient to stop dieting when serum creatinine is about 400 micromol/litre to avoid the dangers of malnutrition.

VI. The Role of Hyperlipidemia in Diabetic Nephropathy

Hyperlipidemia is an important factor accelerating loss of kidney function in renal disease. In patients with any form of renal disease, hyperlipidemia is a significant risk factor. As early as 1967, French[12] and later Kasiske in 1970[13] demonstrated that the experimental rat model developed accelerated glomerulosclerosis when fed a high cholesterol diet. Mulec in 1990[14] showed that patients with DiabNx with serum cholesterol less than 7.0 mmol/litre had a slower decline of GFR (2.3 ml/min) compared to those with serum cholesterol more than 7 mmol/litre (GFR 8.4 ml/min) ($p < 0.01$).

Control of serum lipids is important, especially LDL-cholesterol. Oxidised LDL-cholesterol causes mesangial cell proliferation at a low dose and is cytotoxic at a high dose.[15]

Lipoprotein also binds to GBM altering its filtration property adversely leading to proteinuria. One should aim to decrease LDL-cholesterol to less than 3 mmol/litre, ideally around 2.6 mmol/l. Treatment for hypercholesterolaemia includes dietary control as well as cholesterol lowering drugs.

VII. Indications for Referral of a Patient with Diabetes Mellitus to a Nephrologist

The question of when to refer the patient to a nephrologist has often been asked.

1. Ideally, the patient should be referred when there is microalbuminuria (albumin excretion rate more 20 mg/day). At this stage the patient already has incipient diabetic nephropathy which may still be reversible.

2. When the patient has proteinuria on dipstix (macroalbuminuria or proteinuria more than 150 mg/day) or when the patient has the nephrotic syndrome he should be referred. At this stage it means that the patient already has overt or established diabetic nephropathy.

3. A patient with microscopic haematuria or other urinary abnormality (pyuria) needs referral as this may indicate that he has non diabetic nephropathy and such a patient should be referred to exclude other types of renal disease.

4. Presence of hypertension may indicate a patient with incipient or overt diabetic nephropathy.

5. Patients with renal impairment, indicating overt or established diabetic nephropathy.

SUMMARY

For the patient with Diabetes Mellitus with no proteinuria (normoalbuminuria) intensive blood glucose control as well as cholesterol control is mandatory. For those with incipient diabetic nephropathy (microalbuminuria excretion rate more than 20 mg/day, dipstix negative), intensive blood glucose control, control of hypertension, ACEI/ATRA therapy, dietary protein restriction and cholesterol control is necessary. For patients who do not respond to ACEI/ARB due to aldosterone breakthrough, one could use spironolactone. Eplerenone, a new drug which antagonises the deleterious effects of aldosterone shows much promise [See Chap on Hypertension]. I would recommend that we use Aliskiren if patients do not respond to ACEI/ARBs or if they have Aldosterone Breakthrough with the use of ARBs. It may also be a good idea to start treatment with Aliskiren instead of the traditional ACEI/ARBs in view of renofibrosis with these agents.

In patients with overt or established diabetic nephropathy one should monitor for decline in renal function and decrease the dose of insulin or oral hypoglycemics accordingly to prevent hypoglycemia. Control of hypertension, use of Angiotensin Receptor Blockers (ARB) to reduce proteinuria and retard progression of renal impairment, dietary protein restriction and treatment of hypercholesterolaemia and hypertriglyceridemia is necessary. The goals in the management of a patient with Diabetes Mellitus is to prevent the development of Diabetic Nephropathy. If the patient already has overt or established Diabetic Nephropathy one should still attempt to retard the progression of renal disease to prevent renal failure.

Aldosterone Breakthrough in patients on ACEI/ARBs

References: (1) Nakagawa T. Aldosterone breakthrough in patients on ACEI. *Kidney Int* 2010, **6**:194–195. (2) Weinberger MN. Comprehensive suppression of the RAS in CKD: Covering all bases. *Kidney Int* 2006, **70**:2051–2052.

1. Blockade of the renin angiotensin system (RAS), though beneficial in patients with Diabetic Nephropathy [DiabNx] can induce aldosterone breakthrough and become ineffective. Not all patients with DiabNx benefit from aldosterone blockade as about 20–40% develop aldosterone breakthrough due to prolonged ACEI/ARB therapy which leads to increase in plasma aldosterone levels which in turn causes deleterious effects of aldosterone.

2. Mehdi *et al.* [*Nature Reviews Nephrology*, 2010, **6**:194–195] reported a randomised trial of 128 patients with DiabNx. These patients had previous treatment with ACEI/ARB without reduction in proteinuria for 3 months. The ACEI/ARB were replaced by lisinopril in a daily dose of 20–40 mg and gradually increased to 80 mg daily. Antihypertensive drugs apart from ACEI and ARB, mineralocorticoid receptor

antagonists and calcium channel blockers were added to maintain systolic BP <130 mm Hg. This run in period lasted 4 weeks, thereafter 81 were assigned to receive placebo, losartan or spironolactone in addition to lisinopril for 48 weeks. It was found that spironolactone induced a reduction of Urinary Albumin Creatinine Ratio [UACR] by 34% compared to placebo. The decrease in proteinuria between losartan and placebo arm was not different though it was lower in the losartan group. Creatinine clearance and BP were not different in the 3 arms. Only 2 patients in the spironolactone arm discontinued the study because serum K was >6 mmol/l. The study lasted 2 years. The conclusion was that addition of spironolactone improved kidney protection in patients with DiabNx independent of BP control. Apart from improvement in proteinuria , there was no improvement in kidney function, perhaps due to the short trial duration.

3. In a diabetic mice model [Kosugi T *et al.*, Amer J Patho, 2010, 176:619–629], treatment with ACEI enalapril did not block disease progression. Serum aldosterone concentration was not suppressed but paradoxically increased despite ACE inhibition. Treatment with spironolactone lowered BP and blocked renal injury. It has been suggested that endothelial dysfunction due to lack of endothelial NO synthetase could contribute to the failure of enalapril to provide renal protection and to the development of aldosterone breakthrough. Aldosterone inhibits NO release to endothelial cells and lack of NO accelerates aldosterone synthesis. Aldosterone directly causes afferent renal arteriolar vasoconstriction. Aldosterone also mediates inflammation and renal fibrosis in rats. [Ikeda H *et al.* Kidney Int 2009, 75:147–155].

4. It is my belief that in patients with DiabNX, if RAS inhibition is no longer effective and one suspects aldosterone breakthrough, it would be wise to stop ACEi/ARB therapy and switch to the use of spironolactone [caution for hyperkalaemia] or eplerenome. The use of Aliskiren is another alternative.

REFERENCES

1. Woo KT. Renal Replacement Therapy in Singapore. In: Dialysis Therapy in the 1990s. Editor: H Tanaka. Contributions to Nephrology, Karger, Basel, 1990, **82**:6–14.
2. Breyer JA. Diabetic Nephropathy in Insulin Dependent patients. *Amer J Kid Disease*, 1992, **20**:533–547.
3. Parving HH, Hommel E. Prognosis in Diabetic Nephropathy. *Br Med J* 1989, **299**:230–233.
4. Mogensen CE. Prevention and Treatment of Renal Disease in Insulin Dependent Diabetes Mellitus. *Semin Nephrol* 1990, **10**:261–273.
5. The Diabetes Control and Complications Trial (DCCT) Research Group. The effect of intensive treatment of Diabetes on the development and progression of long term complications in Insulin Dependent Diabetes mellitus. *New Engl J Med* 1993, **329**:977–986.
6. Mogensen CE. Progression of nephropathy in long term diabetics with proteinuria and effect of initial antihypertensive treatment. *Scand J Clin Lab Invest* 1976: **36**:383–388.
7. Aurell M, Bjorck S. Determinants of progressive renal disease in diabetes mellitus. *Kid Int* 1992, **41**:S38-S42.
8. Lewis EJ, Hunsicker LG, Bain RP, Rohde RD for the collaborative study group. The effect of angiotensin converting enzyme inhibition on Diabetic Nephropathy. *New Engl J Med* 1993, **329**:456–462.
9. Brenner BM, Meyer TW, Hostetter TH. Dietary protein and the progressive nature of kidney disease. *New Engl J Med* 1982, **307**:652–659.
10. Walker JD, Dodds R, Murrells TJ, Bending JJ, Keen H, Viberti GC. Restriction of dietary protein and progression of renal failure in diabetic nephropathy. *Lancet*, 1989, **2**:1411–1415.
11. Zeller K, Whittaker E, Sullivan L, Raskin P, Jacobson HR. Effect of restricting dietary protein on progression of renal failure in patients with insulin-dependent diabetes mellitus. *New Engl J Med* 1991, **324**:78–84.
12. French JW, Yamanaka BS, Ostwald R. Dietary induced glomerulosclerosis in the guinea pig. *Arch Pathol* 1967, **83**:204–220.
13. Kasiske BL, O'Donell MP, Schmitz PG, Kim Y. Renal injury of diet induced hypercholesterolaemia in rats. *Kid Int* 1990, **37**:880–891.
14. Mulec H, Johnson SA, Bjorck S. Relation between serum cholesterol and diabetic nephropathy. *Lancet*, 1990, **335**:1537–1538.
15. Diamond JR, Karnovsky MJ. Focal and Segmental Glomerulosclerosis: Analogies to Atherosclerosis. *Kid Int* 1988, **33**:917–924.

16. Brenner BM, Cooper ME, de Zeeuw D, Keanne WF, Mitch WE, Parving HH, Remuzgi G, Snapinn SM, Zhang ZX, Shahinfar S for the RENALL Study Investigators. Effects of Losartan on Renal and cardiovascular outcome in patients with Type 2 Diabetes and Nephropathy. *N Engl J Med* 2001, **345**(12):861–869.
17. Parving HH, de Zeeuw D, Cooper ME *et al.*, Pharmacologic association of the angiotensin-converting enzyme insertion/deletion polymorphism on renal outcome and death in relation to Losartan treatment in patients with type 2 diabetes and nephropathy. *N Engl J Med* 2006.
18. Rossing K, Schjoedt KJ, Jensen BR *et al.*, Enhanced renoprotective effects of ultrahigh doses of irbesartan inpatients with type 2 diabetes and microalbuminuria. *Kidney Int* 2005, **68**:1190–1198.
19. American Diabetes Association. Diabetic nephropathy. *Diabetes care*, 2002, **25**:585–589.
20. Winocour PH, Microalbuminuria. *Br Med J* 1992, **304**:1196–1197.
21. Nakagawa T. Aldosterone breakthrough in patients on ACEI. *Kidney Int* 2010, **6**:194–195.
22. Weinberger MN. Comprehensive suppression of the RAS in CKD: Covering all bases. *Kidney Int* 2006, **70**:2051–2052.
23. Atkins RC and Zimmet P. Diabetic kidney disease. Act now or pay later. *Kidney Int* 2010, **77**:375–377.
24. Nakagawa T. Aldosterone breakthrough in patients on ACEI. *Kidney Int* 2010, **6**:194–195.
25. Weinberger MN. Comprehensive suppression of the RAS in CKD: Covering all bases. *Kidney Int* 2006, **70**:2051–2052.

CHAPTER 18

Fluid and Electrolytes

SODIUM AND WATER

1. Regulation of serum Na^+ concentration effected via thirst-neurohypophyseal-renal axis.
2. Osmolality of solution refers to concentration in solution of osmotically active solute.
   Serum Osmolality = (Na + K)2 + Glucose ÷ 18 + Urea ÷ 6
   Normal = 285 ± 5 mOsmol/l. If SI units used, not necessary to divide by 18 and 6.
3. Changes in serum osmolality will cause osmoreceptors to increase or decrease the release of ADH to conserve or excrete water.
4. SIADH: Normal control of ADH release is lost. Secretion of hormone is independent of body's needs to conserve water.

SODIUM (Na⁺)

Na^+ is the osmotic stuffing of the body. It has little metabolic activity per se. In contrast to K^+ which is an intracellular cation, Na^+ is an extracellular cation.

Distribution

Plasma 11%, interstitial lymph 30%, cartilage and connective tissue 12%, bone 42%, transcellular and intracellular 2.5% each.

Body Na^+ : Bone 2 600 mEq, muscle 420 mEq, ECF 2 500 mEq, others 135 mEq.

Symptoms of Hyponatraemia

Lack of concentration, apathy, headache, anorexia, nausea, vomiting. In severe cases there will be fits and patients may be comatose. Reflexes are depressed and temperature may be subnormal.

Symptoms of Hypernatraemia

Irritability, confusion, hyper-reflexia, variable pyrexia and coma.

Hyponatraemia

1. Dilutional Hyponatraemia (Expansion of body fluids)

    i.   Hysterical polydipsia
    ii. Inappropriate ADH (SIADH)
    iii. Renal failure
    iv. Cirrhosis
    v.   Nephrotic Syndrome
    Treatment: Water restriction.

2. Absolute salt depletion (Contraction of body fluids)

    i.   Gastrointestinal loss: Vomit, diarrhoea
    ii. Renal loss: Addison's disease, uraemia, recovery from acute tubular necrosis (ATN) Treatment: Hypertonic fluids (normal saline, 3% saline).

Hypernatraemia with Expansion of Body Fluids

Infusion of normal saline in excess will cause hypernatraemia with salt and water overload.

Treatment: Salt and water restriction; diuretic therapy.

Hypernatremia with Contraction of Body Fluids

1. Inadequate Water Intake (Patients in coma, palsy, hypothalamic lesions)

    i.   Amount of water required conditioned by diet and concentration ability of kidneys.
    ii. Progressive hypernatraemia in unconscious patients fed high protein and high calorie diets through Ryle's tube.
    iii. Or I.V. infusion of aminoacids and hyperosmolar fluids.
    iv. Patients require more water for excretion of end products of metabolism. Provision of adequate supply of water is important.
    v.   Treatment: Body fluid expansion with hyponatraemic infusions.

2. Renal Water Wasting
    Either due to:

    i.   Diabetes insipidus (neurohypophyseal, nephrogenic).
    ii. OR: Intrinsic Renal Disease like Pyelonephritis, Medullary Disease, Advanced Glomerular Disease (renal impairment), Hypercalcaemia and Hypokalaemia.

3. Given normal thirst mechanism, polyuria rarely causes hypernatraemia because of polydipsia induced by the thirst.
4. However if water intake is restricted or impairs consciousness, hypernatraemic contraction develops.

Oedema

1. Cardiac, hepatic and renal cause due to retention of salt and water resulting from hypoperfusion of kidney and increased ADH.
2. Excess infusion of saline.
3. Toxaemia of pregnancy due to intense Na^+ reabsorption and altered renal haemodynamics.

4. Idiopathic oedema of women. Oestrogens have been implicated as they promote Na⁺ retention by renal tubules. Another
   theory postulates capillary leakage.
5. Mineralocorticoid excess. Aldosterone causes Na⁺ and water
   retention.
6. Hypothyroidism due to myxoedema.
7. Diabetes mellitus due to capillary microangiopathy.
8. Chronic hypokalaemia increases tubular reabsorption of Na⁺.
9. Drugs like oestrogens, vasodilators (diazoxide, hydrallazine,
   clonidine, lithium carbonate) cause Na⁺ retention by renal
   tubule.
10. Arteriovenous fistula increases cardiac output and Na⁺ retention.

Idiopathic (Cyclical) Oedema

1. Disorder of women where there is weight gain and oedema,
   often in obese females.
2. There is Na⁺ and water retention in the upright position.
   Diuresis occurs with recumbency.
3. Exclude diabetes mellitus, hypothyroidism and premenstrual
   oedema.
4. Aetiology: Oestrogen, diuretic induced stimulation of the
   renin angiotensin aldosterone system, inability to decrease
   ADH, capillary leakiness, inability to increase natriuretic
   hormone.
5. Treatment: Stop diuretics, maximum weight gain is evident
   by 10 days of stopping diuretics, and spontaneous diuresis
   subsequently ensues. Sodium restriction may be required
   initially to control oedema formation.

Natriuretic Hormone (NH)

1. Saline expansion in dogs produces a brisk natriuresis because
   of humoral substance inhibiting Na⁺ reabsorption at renal
   tubule (HE de Wardener).

2. In congestive heart failure, advanced cirrhosis and nephrotic syndrome, there is relentless Na^+ retention. This could be due to a lack of natriuretic hormone.
3. Natriuretic hormone may be the cause of certain forms of essential hypertension.
4. A Hypothalamic Factor (HF) has been isolated which promotes Na^+ and water excretion in renal tubule but inhibits Na/K ATPase in other tissues (vasoconstriction).

Atrial Natriuretic Peptide (ANP)

1. A potent natriuretic and vasorelaxant 24-amino acid peptide found in granules of the heart's atria.
2. It does not inhibit Na/K ATPase. It causes greater natriuresis and diuresis.
3. Effects:

   i. Vasorelaxant on vascular smooth muscles.
   ii. Renal haemodynamics: ANP causes increased GFR, Na^+ and fluid excretion.
   iii. On BP: ANP causes a dose dependent reduction.
   iv. On the Renin-Angiotensin System: ANP is anti-Renin. It decreases its secretion and opposes vasoconstriction.
   v. On Aldosterone: ANP opposes its action and decreases Na^+ retention.

Syndrome of Inappropriate Secretion of ADH

1. Normal control of ADH release is lost. The hormone is secreted independently of the body's needs to conserve water.
2. Urine is concentrated and water retention occurs.
3. There is expansion of body fluids and circulating blood volume.
4. This is accompanied by increased renal perfusion and GFR with decreased Na^+ reabsorption as Aldosterone production is shut off.

5. Hyponatraemia is a consequence of water retention and Na^+ wastage.
6. With time, a new steady state develops where intake and excretion of water and Na^+ are in balance; but serum Na^+ is now set at a new level.
7. In a patient with hyponatraemia and normal rate of Na^+ excretion, SIADH should be suspected. In other words, the patient is in Na^+ balance when Urinary Output = Intake of Na^+.
8. If sodium is infused, sodium diuresis will result with no change in serum Na^+.

Causes of SIADH

1. By the neurohypophysis

   1. CNS disorders: Head injury, meningitis, encephalitis, brain tumour and subarachnoid haemorrhage.
   2. Lung disorders: TB, pneumonia.
   3. Endocrine diseases: Addison's disease, myxoedema and hypopituitarism.

II. By tumours
    Cancer of the lungs, duodenum and pancreas. Thymoma.

Cerebral Salt Wasting (CSW)

1. One of the most difficult causes to diagnose owing to frequent confusion with SIADH. This is because both syndromes share common key features: low serum sodium, low serum osmolality, a higher urine osmolality than serum osmolality and elevated urinary sodium concentration. What distinguishes CSW from SIADH is ECF contraction and inappropriately negative sodium balance which an SIADH patient does not have.
2. The principal features of CSW include hyponatremia and ECF contraction owing to renal salt wasting in the setting of

intracranial disease. These are subarachnoid haemorrhage, encephalitis, poliomyelitis, TB meningitis, craniotomy and brain tumours.

3. Disruption of neuronal control of renal sodium handling is the postulated cause.

4. The patient is truly volume contracted due to inappropriate natriuresis to distinguish CSW from non renal sodium depletion and SIADH.

5. The combination of physical signs and symptoms suggesting volume depletion, urinary sodium losses that were inappropriately elevated, hyponatremia and radiologic imaging demonstrating cerebral lesions will suggest CSW as the diagnosis. There is no necessicity to do tests like PRA and aldosterone levels, etc. as these will not help.

6. Management includes treatment of underlying cerebral disorder, volume resuscitation and sodium replacement. The key to diagnosis lies in demonstrating that hyponatremia is secondary to inappropriately high urinary sodium excretion in a patient who is volume contracted. Once diagnosis is established, treatment includes addressing underlying cerebral disorder, sodium loading, hydration and use of mineralocorticoids like fludrocortisone acetate if necessary. [Gutierrez OM, Kidney Int, 2007, 71:79–82].

Asymptomatic Hyponatremia: A clinical syndrome which should be treated

1. Hyponatremia is characterised by the equilibrium of water across cell membrane into cells which leads to their swelling.

2. If chronic hyponatremia is corrected rapidly (with increases of sodium more than 10–12 mmol/l over 24hrs), brain damage and even death can occur.

3. The term "asymptomatic hyponatremia" refers to symptoms of mild or moderate hyponatremia (< 125–135 mmol/l) like lethargy, restlessness, disorientation, headache, nausea and

vomiting, cramps and depressed reflexes. When hyponatremia is <125 mmol/l the condition becomes more severe
and patients manifest with seizures, coma and cardiopulmonary arrest.

4. In a study of patients with hip fractures [Renneboog B *et al.*
    Amer J Med, 2006, 119:71.e1 –71.e8], it was found that these
    patients had a 67 fold higher risk of being hyponatremic than
    being normonatremic and they had associated gait distur-
    bances, decreased reaction time like people with alcohol
    excess.

5. In another study, mild hyponatremia defined as serum sodium
    about 131 mmol/l was associated with the risk of bone
    fracture (odds ratio 4.16) in elderly patients [Gankam K *et al.*
    Q J Med, 2008, 101:583–588].

6. Another placebo controlled study of 448 patients with
    hyponatremia it was reported that there was a significant rise
    of serum sodium after 30 days of vasopressin V2 receptor
    with improvement in mental ability [Schrier RW *et al.* N Engl
    Med 2006, 355:2099–2112].

7. Schrier contends that with the growing elderly population,
    including those with subclinical and clinical dementia,
    about 30% have been reported to have asymptomatic
    hyponatremia. Some are on thiazide diuretics, yet others
    are on anti-depressants, all these making them prone to
    hyponatremia. He is of the opinion that in individuals with
    a range of serum sodium 130–135 mmol/l, we should offer
    treatment for hyponatremia the same way we treat patients
    with hypokalaemia. We should consider hyponatremia as a
    serious clinical issue like hypokalaemia. The following
    options in therapy should be considered: fluid restriction,
    frusemide, hypertonic saline, demeclocycline or V2 receptor
    antagonists.

Reference: Robert W Schrier. Does "asymptomatic hyponatremia" exist? Editorial, *Kidney Int* 2010, 6:185.

Treatment of Salt Loss

1. Infuse normal saline or 3% saline. Sometimes salt tablets may be sufficient. Free salt diet.
2. Measure 24-hour urinary excretion of Na^+ to determine urinary salt loss.
3. 1 gm oral NaCl = 17 mEq of Na^+, 1 litre of normal saline = 154 mEq, 1 litre of 3% saline = 513 mEq of Na^+.

Calculation of Sodium Deficit

If Body Weight is 65 kg and serum Na^+ 120 mEq/l,
  Na^+ deficit = 140–120 = 20 mEq/l
  Body Water = 60% of Body Weight
  Hence Na^+ deficit = $\dfrac{65 \times 60 \times 20}{100}$ = 780 mEq/l
                              = 5 litres 0.9% NaCI
Give 1/2 the calculated Na^+ deficit in 12–24 hours. Check serum Na^+ the next day and using same calculation see how much more Na^+ is needed.

POTASSIUM

1. Body K^+ Distribution:

   Plasma-0.4%
   Interstitial Lymph-1.0%
   Dense Connective Tissue and Cartilage-0.4%
   Bone-7.6%
   Intracellular-89.6%
   Transcellular-1.0%
   Note that most of the K^+ stays intracellularly in contrast to Na^+ which is mainly extracellular.

2. Total Body K^+ (TBK$^+$)
   — measured by K^{42} or K^{40}

Muscle cells-3 000 mEq
Extracellular fluid-65 mEq
Liver-200 mEq
RBC-235 mEq
Urine-92 mEq/day
Stool-8 mEq/day

3. K^+ is excreted in the urine via the distal tubule at a rate proportional to the reabsorption of Na^+.
4. In Acidosis, H^+ goes into the cell and K^+ comes out of the cell. Hence serum K^+ becomes high (Hyperkalaemia).
5. In Alkalosis, K^+ stays in the cell; so serum K^+ is low (Hypokalaemia). H^+ comes out of the cell to compensate.
6. K^+ is responsible for Enzyme Action in the cell. Conduction of nerve and muscle impulses (transmembrane potential difference) requires K^+.

K$^+$ Depletion

1. Increased loss in urine

    i. In Hyperaldosteronism, Na^+ is retained while K^+ is lost into the urine.
    ii. Cortisol excess (Cushing's) too causes retention of Na^+ and loss of K^+ giving rise to Hypokalaemic Alkalosis.
    iii. Diuretics (Frusemide, Chlorothiazide) cause loss of Na^+ and K^+ into the urine, resulting in Hypokalaemic Alkalosis.
    iv. Renal Tubular Acidosis is associated with K^+ loss in the urine since the excretion of H^+ into the urine is impaired.
    v. Alkalosis is associated with K^+ loss in the urine.
    vi. Bartter's syndrome where there is hyper-renin hyperaldosteronism resulting in hypokalaemia.

2. Loss in gastrointestinal tract
   — Vomiting, diarrhoea, Ryle's tube aspiration and fistulae all result in K^+ loss.

3. Decreased intake
   Patients who are starved have low K^+ due to decreased intake.

Effects of K^+ Depletion

K^+ depletion may cause:

1. Hypokalaemia.
2. Renal Tubular Necrosis with Nephrogenic Diabetes Insipidus.
3. Treatment: Administer KCI. Never give KCI intravenously in a bolus dose for it will kill the patient. Intravenous K^+ must be given gradually by I.V. drip infusion slowly over 1 hour, if necessary under ECG monitoring. Give oral KCI if patient can take orally and urgent correction is not necessary. 1 gm KCI = 13.3 mEq/I.

Hyperkalaemia

Causes:

1. Fever, trauma and infection will cause cell damage with release of K^+.
2. Any catabolic or hypercatabolic states; conditions associated with acidosis except in states where there is urinary loss of K^+ (renal tubular acidosis, ureterosigmoidostomy, ileo-conduit).
3. Renal failure is a very common cause.

Treatment of Hyperkalaemia

1. Stop all sources of K^+ (fruits and juices).
2. Administer I.V. calcium gluconate or calcium chloride (10 ml slowly) to combat the effects of hyperkalaemia on the heart.

3. Give I.V. insulin 12 units together with 50 ml of 50% dextrose either as a bolus dose or over I hour in a drip.
4. I.V. $NaHCO_3$ 8.4% (10 ml) to combat acidosis which is often present.
5. Commence Oral Resonium A 15 gm 6 hourly if patient can take orally. If patient cannot take orally, give Resonium Retention Enema, 30 gm 8 hourly instead.
6. Check the serum electrolytes and repeat bolus doses of insulin and dextrose 4 hourly.
7. If hyperkalaemia persists, dialysis would have to be considered.
8. Treat the cause of hyperkalaemia wherever possible.
9. For patients with renal impairment and need to take ARBs for renoprotection one could prescribe Oral Resonium 15 gm every other day to help control the tendency towards hyperkalaemia. This way they can still have the renoprotective effects of the ARBs which would help retard the progression to ESRF. Otherwise if the ARBs have to be withdrawn, they will soon end up on dialysis which is a far worse scenario.

Effects of Hyperkalaemia

1. Early phase: No signs are present.
2. Late Phase: Flaccid palsy, shallow respiration, anxiety, anaesthetic.
   ECG: Tented T, ST depressed, Bradycardia, Prolong PR, Prolong QRS, Nodal Rhythm, Ventricular Arrhythmias, Cardiac Arrest in Dilatation.

MAGNESIUM

Total Body Mg = 2 400 mEq
Bone contains 2/3, soft tissue 1/3 and ECF 1%.

Function

1. Enzymes require it for their function.
2. Stabilisation of membrane potential.
3. Permissive action for Parathyroid Hormone.

Mg Deficiency

1. Fatigue, lethargy, weakness, tremors, fits, arrhythmia, paresthesia, psychosis, Chovstek and Trousseau's sign.
2. May be associated with Hypo Ca^{++}, Hypo K^+, Hypo Na^+.
3. Causes: Diarrhoea, alcohol, diuretics, aldosteronism, hypoparathyroidism.
4. Treat with $MgCl_2$ (40–50 mEq/day).
   1 gm $MgSO_4$ $7H_2O$ = 8.13 mEq/l Magnesium
   1 gm $MgCl_2$ $6H_2O$ = 9.15 mEq/l Magnesium

Hypermagnesaemia: Associated with hyporeflexia, coma and cardiac arrest.

REFERENCES

1. Gutierrez OM and Lin HY. Refractory Hyponatremia due to Cerebral Salt Wasting. *Kidney Int* 2007, **71**:79–82.
2. Schrier RW. Does "asymptomatic hyponatremia" exist? Editorial, *Kidney Int* 2010, **6**:185.

CHAPTER 19

Acid-Base Balance

PATHOGENESIS OF METABOLIC ACIDOSIS

Non-carbonic acid-base equilibrium in the ECF compartment of the body is modulated by 3 processes: (1) cellular metabolism, (2) intestinal absorption and secretion, and (3) renal acidification.

The net renal input of bicarbonate into the ECF and the net endogenous acid production are approximately equal, so that the plasma bicarbonate and blood pH are kept constant.

NET ENDOGENOUS ACID PRODUCTION

Net endogenous acid production increases because of:

1. Disordered cellular metabolic processes, e.g. ketoacidosis, hypoxia (lactic acidosis).
2. Loading of the normal metabolic pathway with ingested non-carbonic precursors, e.g. ammonium chloride.
3. External losses of abnormally large amounts of gastrointestinal secretions containing bicarbonate, e.g. diarrhoea; external drainage of pancreatic, biliary or small bowel secretions; ureterosigmoidostomy; ingestion of calcium chloride, magnesium sulphate, cholestyramine.

PHYSIOLOGICAL RESPONSE TO METABOLIC ACIDOSIS OF EXTERNAL ORIGIN

1. In the Pulmonary Response to metabolic acidosis, the CO_2 tension of body fluid decreases and as a consequence the

concentrations of carbonic acid and H⁺, which are in equilibrium with CO_2 decreases concomitantly.

2. In the Renal Response, the net renal input of bicarbonate into the ECF of the body increases.
3. With increasing degrees of acidosis (low plasma bicarbonate), hyperventilation increases, but this is insufficient to prevent lowering of blood pH.
4. Hence respiratory compensation offers little protection in severe metabolic acidosis.

RENAL RESPONSE TO METABOLIC ACIDOSIS OF EXTRARENAL ORIGIN

1. When endogenous acid production becomes great, the amount of bicarbonate delivered to the ECF by the kidneys (via renal venous blood) begins to exceed the amount delivered to the kidneys (in renal artery) by a greater amount than normal (i.e. 1.0 mEq/kg body weight per day).
2. If the rate of endogenous acid production remains abnormal for several days, net renal input of bicarbonate progressively increases till it becomes adequate.
3. In persisting metabolic acidosis, bone supplies additional base.
4. The kidney's ability to correct metabolic acidosis depends on excretion of buffered H⁺ (Titratable Acid and NH_4^+)

CONSEQUENCES OF METABOLIC ACIDOSIS

1. Acidosis leads to circulatory collapse.
2. Decreases cardiac response to catecholamines.
3. Depresses myocardial contractile force.
4. Increases pulmonary arteriolar resistance.
5. Venous constriction causes redistribution of large amounts of blood into the central circulation, leading to heart failure.

6. Circulatory insufficiency leads to tissue hypoxia and increased lactic production.
7. Movement of potassium out of somatic muscle cells causes hyperkalaemia.

CAUSES OF METABOLIC ACIDOSIS

I. Hyperchloraemic, Normal Anion Gap Acidosis

1. Acid load: Ammonium chloride, hyperalimentation.
2. Bicarbonate losses: diarrhoea, fistulae, ureterosigmoidostomy.
3. Defects in urinary acidification: Proximal renal tubular acidosis, distal renal tubular acidosis.
4. Renal impairment.

II. Normochloraemic, High Anion Gap Acidosis

1. Causes: Lactic acidosis; diabetic, alcoholic and starvation acidosis; drug and toxin induced acidosis; advanced uraemic acidosis.
2. Addition to body of non-chloride acid load will cause high anion gap acidosis.
3. Anion gap = $Na^+ - (Cl^- + HCO_3^-)$.
   Normally this is about 12 mEq/l (range: 8 to 16 mEq/l).
4. In practice: $(Na^+ + K^+) - (Cl^- + HCO_3) \geq 20$ (abnormal).
5. Occurs if anion does not undergo glomerular filtration (uraemic acid anions) OR anion filtered but readily absorbed (ketoacids, lactate).

LACTIC ACIDOSIS (COHEN AND WOODS)

1. Lactic acid in blood causes decreased bicarbonate and elevation in lactate concentration and anion gap.

2. Considered abnormal if blood lactate >4 mEq/l (normal is 1 mEq/l).

    Type A: Poor tissue perfusion
      i.   Shock (cardiogenic, haemorrhagic, septic)
      ii. Acute hypoxaemia
      iii. Carbon monoxide poisoning

    Type B:
      i.   Common diseases like diabetes mellitus, renal failure, liver disease, infection.
      ii. Drugs, toxins like phenformin, metformin, ethanol methanol, salicylates.
      iii. Hereditary disorders like pyruvate dehydrogenase deficiency, methylmalonic aciduria.

SYMPTOMS OF LACTIC ACIDOSIS

Hyperventilation, abdominal pain, disturbed consciousness, inadequate cardiopulmonary function (Type A), leukocytosis, hypoglycaemia, hyperkalaemia.

TREATMENT OF LACTIC ACIDOSIS

1. Treat underlying cause.
2. Vasodilator nitroprusside improves hypoperfusion by enhancing cardiac output, liver and renal blood flow. This will augment lactate removal.
3. Alkali therapy advocated if blood pH < 7.1. Danger of fluid overload because of large amounts of bicarbonate required.
4. Diuretics, ultrafiltration and bicarbonate haemodialysis can be used to remove lactic acid.
5. In treating acidosis, "overshoot alkalosis" may occur because of lactate conversion to bicarbonate by the liver, renal generation of bicarbonate and bicarbonate load from therapy.

TREATMENT OF METABOLIC ACIDOSIS

1. Mitigate severity of acidaemia and/or hyperkalaemia by reversal of pathogenetic processes. Give $NaHCO_3$ Correct if serum bicarbonate less than 15 mEq/l e.g. if Serum Bicarbonate = 10 mEq/l

   1/3 Body Weight × Bicarbonate Deficit = x ml 8.4% $NaHCO_3$

   1/3 60 kg × (25 − 10) = 20 × 15 = 300 ml 8.4% $NaHCO_3$
2. Prevent recurrence of acidaemia by maintenance therapy.
3. It is not necessary to correct acidosis completely within minutes or hours as hyperventilation continues for hours after correction of acidaemia.
4. Rapid normalisation of plasma bicarbonate concentration is associated with inappropriate increase in arterial blood pH with occurrence of respiratory alkalosis.
5. Hypokalaemia is a complication of bicarbonate treatment. If serum K^+ is less than 4 mEq/l give KCl.

METABOLIC ALKALOSIS

The pH of blood is given by ratio of the bicarbonate concentration to dissolved CO_2:

$$pH = 6.1 + \log \frac{HCO_3^-}{CO_2}$$

1. Plasma CO_2 tension maintained within very narrow limits through regulated excretion of CO_2 by lungs.
2. Kidney stabilises the concentration of serum bicarbonate.

Under certain circumstances, the kidney far exceeds its homeostatic responsibility. It operates to sustain a high serum bicarbonate concentration by:

I. **Generating Alkalosis:** Large amounts of $NaHCO_3$ are added to the blood.

2. The kidney's **capacity to reabsorb** $NaHCO_3$ may be greatly **augmented**, so that new $NaHCO_3$ whether generated by renal or extra-renal factors, is not lost into the urine.

SYMPTOMS OF METABOLIC ALKALOSIS

1. Like hypocalcaemia.
2. Mental confusion, obtundation, seizures, paraesthesia, cramps, tetany, arrhythmias.
3. Hypokalaeinia is often an associated feature.

CAUSES OF METABOLIC ALKALOSIS

1. Exogenous bicarbonate loads like acute alkali administration, milk alkali syndrome.
2. Gastrointestinal origin: Vomiting, gastric aspiration, villous adenoma.
3. Renal origin: Diuretics, potassium depletion, Bartter's syndrome.
4. Mineralocorticoids: Primary aldosteronism, Cushing's syndrome, liquorice ingestion.

PATHOGENESIS OF METABOLIC ALKALOSIS

1. Bicarbonate Generation
   i. Renal: Excretion of NH_4^+ plus titratable acidity must exceed that required to neutralise acid load (dietary, metabolic acid production, alkaline faecal loss).
   ii. Dietary NaCl furnishes Na^+ which is returned to the blood as $NaHCO_3$; the anion Cl^- is excreted into urine as NH_4Cl.
   iii. Extra-Renal: Acid loss due to vomiting; or alkaline gain, e.g. milk-alkaline syndrome.

2. Maintenance of Metabolic Alkalosis

   Capacity of the kidney to reclaim bicarbonate must be enhanced by a rise in tubular reabsorption commensurate with the filtered load, i.e. **augmentation** in capacity of kidney to reclaim filtered bicarbonate.

GENERATION OF METABOLIC ALKALOSIS

1. Three features are usually present before this can occur:

   i. Relatively high distal delivery of Na^+ salts.

   ii. Persistent mineralocorticoid excess.

   iii. K^+ deficiency occurring simultaneously.

2. Enhanced bicarbonate reclamation is also necessary.

3. Na^+ reabsorption results in H^+ secretion, urine pH falls, buffers are titrated; NH_3 diffuses into acid urine and is trapped as NH_4^+. For every mole of Na^+ reabsorbed, one mole of bicarbonate is reclaimed and this represents $NaHCO_3$ regeneration.

4. Giving diuretics to oedematous patient may result in increased Na^+ delivery distally. The resulting bicarbonate generation allows an increased capacity for bicarbonate reclamation.

5. Vomiting leads to loss of HCl associated with K^+ deficiency. The extra-renal generation of bicarbonate may be reclaimed by virtue of increased H^+ secretion in the proximal tubule.

MAINTENANCE OF METABOLIC ALKALOSIS

1. In situations where there is increased "proximal" bicarbonate reabsorption because of increasing H^+ secretion, e.g. as in patients with K^+ deficiency. Though expansion of volume can override the effect of K^+ deficiency, if K^+ depletion is severe, it will still maintain alkalosis.

2. K^+ deficiency also augments "distal" H^+ secretion. In K^+ depletion, Na^+ is preferentially exchanged for H^+. This serves to reclaim bicarbonate.

3. Shrinkage in effective arterial blood volume causes a reduction in back-leak of bicarbonate into the proximal tubular lumen; thereby enhancing bicarbonate reclamation.

4. Mineralocorticoids (aldosterone) stimulate Na^+/H^+ process in cortical collecting tubule. This augments bicarbonate reclamation in the distal tubule. A necessary condition is K^+ deficiency.

5. In Summary: Bicarbonate reclamation is increased by contraction of Effective Arterial Blood Volume, K^+ deficiency and excess aldosterone.

TREATMENT OF METABOLIC ALKALOSIS

1. Remove stimulus to bicarbonate generation (excess mineralocorticoid, intragastric suck, diuretics).

2. Remove factors maintaining bicarbonate reabsorption like extracellular volume (ECV) contraction, low K^+.

3. For "saline responsive alkalosis" like those due to vomiting, nasogastric suction, diuretics, K^+ deficiency, alkalosis following bicarbonate therapy for organic acidosis, post hypercapnia alkalosis (because of high aldosterone), NaCl infusion and KCl replacement are usually sufficient.

4. In "saline resistant alkalosis" like Bartter's, Conn's, Cushing's and renal artery stenosis (RAS), magnesium deficiency and severe K^+ deficiency, saline infusion is of no use. Treatment is aimed at the underlying cause. In RAS, alkalosis is due to non-oedematous aldosteronism (high aldosterone, low ECV).

5. For severe cases of alkalosis, titrate plasma bicarbonate with arginine HCl, NH_4Cl or dilute HCl and increase bicarbonate excretion with acetazolamide.

THE ROLE OF CHLORIDE DEFICIENCY
IN METABOLIC ALKALOSIS

1. NaCl and $NaHCO_3$ are the only two salts whose reabsorption is readily regulated by the kidney that can function to maintain the extracellular volume.
2. The extracellular volume will contract with chloride (Cl^-) restriction, unless alkalosis is produced by giving $NaHCO_3$
3. The role of Cl^- in metabolic alkalosis is due to its capacity to permit expansion or contraction of EC volume.
4. Cl^- restriction reduces EC volume, stimulates Na^+ retention and aldosterone secretion. The urine is free of Cl^- as the kidneys retain all filtered Na^+ salts, with Cl^- and bicarbonate reabsorbed.
5. If metabolic alkalosis is produced by extra-renal means, e.g. gastric aspirate, the contraction of effective EC volume will maintain it.
6. Giving NaCl restores EC volume and relieves stimulus to Na^+ retention, Cl^- and bicarbonate are delivered distally and excreted in the urine and this corrects the alkalosis. The volume expanding effect of NaCl overcomes the effect of K^+ deficiency.

BARTTER'S SYNDROME

1. Metabolic alkalosis with hypokalaemia, juxta-glomerular apparatus (JGA) hyperplasia, hyper-renin hyperaldosteronism.
2. These patients have no oedema. They are normotensive, have elevated serum prostaglandins and prostacycline, polycythaemia, hypercalciuria and normal GFR.
3. In the differential diagnosis, consider vomiting, diuretics and laxatives. These conditions are associated with low urinary chloride and saline responsive alkalosis whereas Bartter's syndrome is associated with high urinary chloride and saline resistant alkalosis.

4. The underlying causation may be a defect in the reabsorption of NaCl at the ascending limb of Henle. This leads to ECV contraction which causes raised renin and aldosterone, which in turn causes alkalosis and hypokalaemia.

5. Prostaglandins have been found to inhibit NaCl reabsorption by the cortical ascending limb of Henle; hence the use of indocid, a prostaglandin synthetase inhibitor in the treatment of Bartter's syndrome.

6. Treatment: Potassium replacement, inhibition of renin-angiotensin aldosterone and prostaglandin systems using captopril and indocid. These measures are still empirical.

CHAPTER 20

Clinical Problems on Fluids, Electrolytes and Acid-Base Balance

QUESTION 1

A 53 year-old-man presents with a duodenal ulcer, bronchopneumonia and diabetes mellitus.

Serum				
	Glucose	238	mg/dl	(13.2 mmol/l)
	Urea	360	mg/dl	(60 mmol/l)
	Creatinine	5.9	mg/dl	(522 umol/l)
	Na	157	mmol/l	
	K	2.3	mmol/L	
	Cl	116	mmol/L	
Arterial	pH	7.5		
	Base Excess	10.2		
	SBC	34	mmol/L	
	Oxygen Sat	95.9	%	

1. Why is he hypernatraemic?
2. Calculate serum osmolality.
3. What is the acid-base disturbance?
4. Treatment?

QUESTION 2

A 23-year-old woman presents with severe diarrhoea and laboured respiration. Her body weight is 65 kg.

Serum			
	Na	120	mmol/l
	K	5.5	mmol/l
	Cl	86	mmol/l
	Urea	184	mg/dl	(30.7 mmol/l)
	Creatinine	5.1	mg/dl	(451 umol/l)
	SBC	10	mmol/l
Arterial	pH	7.21	

1. What is the acid-base and electrolyte disorder?
2. Why are serum creatinine and urea raised?
3. Calculate sodium deficit.
4. Calculate bicarbonate deficit.

QUESTION 3

A 43-year-old female has an ileal conduit because of tuberculous cystitis. Her body weight is 60 kg.

Serum			
	Na	137	mmol/l
	K	2.9	mmol/l
	Cl	115	mmol/l
	SBC	15	mmol/l
Arterial	pH	7.124	

1. What is the acid-base disorder?
2. Explain hypokalaemia in this condition.
3. Calculate bicarbonate deficit.
4. What are long-term complications?

QUESTION 4

A 13-year-old girl presents with vomiting and palsy. X-ray of the abdomen shows bilateral renal calcification.

Serum	Na	125	mmol/l
	K	2.3	mmol/l
	Cl	118	mmol/l
	SBC	12	mmol/l
Arterial	pH	7.20	
Urine	pH	6.80	

1. What is the acid-base disorder?
2. What is the clinical diagnosis?
3. How do you treat?
4. After treatment of acid-base disorder, what test can be performed to confirm diagnosis?

QUESTION 5

An 18-year-old girl was admitted for diarrhoea.

Serum	Na	128	mmol/l	
	K	3.2	mmol/l	
	Cl	98	mmol/l	
	SBC	20	mmol/l	
	Creatinine	1.8	mg/dl	(159 umol/l)
	Urea	126	mg/dl	(21 mmol/l)
Urine	Na	3	mmol/l	
	K	25	mmol/l	
	Osmolality	850	mOsmol/l	
	Creatinine	180	mg/dl	(159 umol/l)

1. What is the status of patient's body water?
2. Why are plasma creatinine and urea elevated?
3. Would you give patient 3% saline?
4. Why is serum K^+ low?

QUESTION 6

A 40-year-old man was admitted for dyspnoea, oedema and mitral valve disease.

Serum	A	B	Urine	A	B	
Na	123	135 mmol/l	Na	2	40	mmol/l
K	3.4	2.7 mmol/l	K	2.8	65	mmol/l
Cl	96	87 mmol/l	Creatinine	280	70	mg/dl
Creatinine	2.8	1.0 mg/dl	Osmolality	490	200	mOsmol/kg
Urea	120	40 mg/dl	24 hr vol	400	2000	ml
Osmolality	257	285 mOsmol/kg				

1. Does hyponatraernia at A indicate total body Na^+ deficit?
2. Why is the biochemistry different in A and B?
3. Why does he have hypokalaemia at A and why is it worse at B?
4. Why are serum creatinine and urea elevated?

QUESTION 7

A 60-year-old man presents with cough and weight loss. Skin turgor is normal, neck veins are not distended and there is no oedema. Chest X-ray shows a right upper lobe density.

Serum				
	Na	124	mmol/l	
	K	3.7	mmol/l	
	Cl	88	mmol/l	
	SBC	24	mmol/l	
	Urea	8	mg/dl	(1.3 mmol/l)
	Creatinine	0.6	mg/dl	(53 umol/l)
Urine	Na	39	mmol/l	
	Osmolality	340	mOsmol/kg	

1. What is his state of hydration?
2. Explain urinary Na^+ excretion and urine osmolality.
3. How do you treat this condition?
4. If serum urea was 160 mg/dl and creative 7.0 mg/dl would you change your diagnosis?

QUESTION 8

A 48-year-old female had a hypophysectomy done to remove a pituitary adenoma. 72 hours later, she is confused and has lost 5 kg in weight (65 to 60 kg).

Serum	Na	165	mmol/l	
	K	4.3	mmol/l	
	Cl	132	mmol/l	
	SBC	24	mmol/l	
	Urea	56	mg/dl	(9.3 mmol/l)
	Creatinine	1.8	mg/dl	(159 umol/l)
	Calcium	10.4	mg/dl	(2.6 mmol/l)
Urine	Na	4	mmol/l	
	Osmolality	90	mOsmol/kg	

1. Why is she hypernatraemic?
2. Explain increased creatinine, urine Na^+ and urine osmolality.
3. Calculate fluid deficit if there is no gain or loss of total body Na^+.
4. Treatment?

QUESTION 9

A 23-year-old male had severe diarrhoea and fever. His weight is 50 kg.

Serum	Na	162	mmol/l
	K	4.0	mmol/l
	Cl	133	mmol/l
	SBC	18	mmol/l
	Hct	48	%
	Osmolality	327	mOsmol/l

1. How much saline do you give?
2. How much water to correct hypernatraemia?
3. What are the dangers of giving this as 5% dextrose and water very rapidly? Very slowly?
4. What fluid therapy would be best?

QUESTION 10

A 57-year-old woman was admitted for syncopal attack and vomiting. She had a previous history of duodenal ulcer.

		Day 1	Day 5	
Arterial	pH	7.62	7.48	
	$PaCO_2$	75	36	mm Hg
	PaO_2	52	82	mm Hg
	SBC	75	26	mmol/l
Serum	Na	141	142	mmol/l
	K	1.8	4.3	mmol/l
	Cl	51	103	mmol/l

1. What is the acid-base disorder present?
2. Is compensation adequate?
3. What would you expect urine Cl^- to have been on Day 1?
4. Discuss treatment.

QUESTION 11

A 50-year-old man was admitted in coma. He was cyanotic and febrile, barrel-chested and had finger clubbing. Chest X-ray showed a right lower lobe consolidation.

Arterial	pH	7.24	
	$PaCO_2$	91	mm Hg
	PaO_2	38	mm Hg
	SBC	38	mmol/l
Serum	Na	138	mmol/l
	K	5.0	mmol/l
	Cl	85	mmol/l

1. What is the acid-base disturbance present?
2. Is compensation adequate?
3. Comment on underlying disorder?
4. Treatment?

QUESTION 12

An 18-year-old model was admitted for hyperventilation and confusion. She had been taking an unknown medication for 6 months to maintain her curvaceous figure.

		0 hours	6 hours	12 hours	
Arterial	pH	6.78	7.33	7.44	
	PaCO$_2$	14	19	28	mm Hg
	SBC	2	10	19	mmol/l
Serum	Na	144	146	151	mmol/l
	K	5.2	2.1	2.7	mmol/l
	Cl	137	118	119	mmol/l

1. What is the acid-base disorder at Time Zero?
2. Discuss differential diagnosis and treatment.
3. Explain lab values.
4. What happened to plasma K$^+$?

ANSWERS

Answer 1

1. He is dehydrated (salt depleted).

2. Serum osmolality $= (Na^+K)2 + \dfrac{glucose}{18} + \dfrac{urea}{8}$

$$= (157 + 2.3)2 + \frac{238}{18} + \frac{360}{6}$$

$$= 392 \text{ mOsmol/kg}$$

NB: If glucose, urea expressed as mmol/l it is not necessary to divide by 18 and 6.

Diagnosis: Hyperosmolar non-ketotic diabetes.

Normal serum osmolality $= 285 \pm 5$ mOsmol/kg

3. Hypokalaemic metabolic alkalosis.
4. Treatment consists of normal saline infusion with potassium chloride replacement.

Answer 2

1. Metabolic Acidosis with salt depletion.
2. This is due to pre-renal failure resulting from dehydration.
3. Calculation of sodium deficit:
   (Normal serum Na^+ – patient's serum Na^+) × 2/3 BW in kg
   Assuming normal serum Na^+ is 140 mEq/l,
   Sodium deficit = (140 – 120) × 2/3 × 65 = 867 mEq/l of sodium
4. Calculation of bicarbonate deficit:
   Assuming normal serum bicarbonate is 25 mEq/l,
   Deficit = (25 – 10) × 1/3 × 65 = 325 ml of 8.4% sodium
   bicarbonate.

Answer 3

1. Metabolic Acidosis.
2. Urine in bowels causes irritation inducing a villous diarrhoea.
3. Bicarbonate Deficit = (25 – 15) 1/3 × 60
   $$= 10 \times 20 = 200 \, ml \text{ of } 8.4\% \, NaHCO_3$$
4. Long-term complications are urinary infection and ureteric stenosis due to stricture at site of ureteric implantation into bowels. The stenosis can cause obstructive uropathy.

Answer 4

1. Hyperchloraemic metabolic acidosis.
2. Type I Renal Tubular Acidosis (RTA), also known as Distal or Classic Renal Tubular Acidosis (RTA). These patients have nephrocalcinosis and are still unable to acidify the urine in spite of severe metabolic acidosis, in contrast to patients with Type II or Proximal RTA.
3. Treatment consists of sodium bicarbonate together with potassium replacement.
4. Ammonium Chloride Loading Test can be performed.

Clinical Problems on Fluids, Electrolytes and Acid-Base Balance 337

Answer 5

1. Patient is dehydrated (salt and water depletion) as evidenced by history of watery diarrhoea and low serum sodium.
2. This is due to pre-renal failure resulting from diarrhoea.
3. No, this patient requires water as well as sodium, hence normal saline infusion is better than 3% saline.
4. Potassium is low because of secondary hyperaldosteronism. Dehydration stimulates increased aldosterone secretion. This causes increased sodium absorption and potassium excretion.

Answer 6

1. No, patient has dilutional hyponatraemia due to excess body water.
2. He was treated with diuretics.
3. He has diuretic induced hypokalaemia.
4. This is due to pre-renal failure.

Answer 7

1. The patient has excess water due to inappropriate secretion of antidiuretic hormone (SIADH).
   Excess water:
   Weight = 65 kg × 0.6 = 39 litres total body water
   Serum sodium = 124 mEq/l
   $$\frac{124}{140} \times 39 = 34.5 \text{ litres}$$
   39 − 34.5 = 4.5 litres excess water
2. In SIADH, the urine is concentrated, urine sodium is more than 20 mEq/l, hence urine osmolality is high (340 mOsmol/kg).
3. Treatment:
   i) Excretion of excess water:
   Use diuretics, replace electrolytes with IV hypertonic saline.

ii) Oedematous hyponatraemic patient:
     Treat with sodium and water restriction. Agents that antago-
     nise renal action of arginine vasopressin (AVP) like lithium
     and demeclochlorcycline can also be used. Recently, antago-
     nist of water diuresis with no solute excretion.
4.   Patient has renal failure with salt losing nephropathy.

Answer 8

1.   She has no ADH and has lost much body water.
2.   The patient has little sodium and low urinary osmolarity. This
     is due to a lack of ADH. ADH enables one to produce con-
     centrated urine. A lack of it will cause the passage of very
     dilute urine.
3.   Fluid deficit:
     Weight = 60 kg × 0.6 = 36 litres total body water.
     Water needed to lower serum sodium to 140 meq/l:

$$\frac{165}{140} \times 36 = 42.4 \text{ litres}$$

     42.4 − 36 = 6.4 litres (water deficit).
4.   Treatment consists of water or 5% dextrose.

Answer 9

1.   No saline as patient has hypernatraemia.
2.   Water required to correct hypernatraemia:
     Weight = 50 kg × 0.6 = 30 litres total body water
     Water needed to lower serum sodium to 140 mEq/l:

$$\frac{162}{140} \times 30 = 34.7 \text{ litres}$$

     34.7 − 30 = 4.7 litres water.

3. If water or 5% dextrose is given too rapidly, patient may develop cerebral oedema. Given slowly, idiogenic osmoles have time to dissipate.
4. The best form of fluid therapy is ½ strength saline.

Answer 10

1. Respiratory acidosis and metabolic alkalosis.
2. Compensation:
   Rise in standard bicarbonate $= 4 \times$ (rise in $PaCO_2$) ± 4 mmol/l $= 4 \times (35/10) \pm 4 = 14$ mmol/l.
   But patient's SBC is 75 mmol/l, compensation is more than adequate.
3. Urine chloride is expected to be high because of paradoxical aciduria.
4. Treatment consists of oxygen and I.V. normal saline.

Answer 11

1. Chronic respiratory acidosis with acute hypercapnia.
2. Compensation:
   Compensation of SBC should rise above 24 mmol/l by 4 mmol/l per 10 mm Hg increment in $paCO_2$ above 40 mm Hg within a range of ± 4 mmol/l.

   i.e. Rise in SBC $= 4 \times \dfrac{\text{rise in } PaCO_2}{10}$

   $$= (4 \times 50/10) \pm 4 = 16 \text{ mmol/l}$$

   Patient's SBC is 18 mmol/l. Compensation is therefore adequate.

   In Respiratory Acidosis:

   There is increased $PaCO_2$ (> 40 mm Hg)
   Arterial pH is decreased (Acidaemia)
   SBC is high (compensation)

Low Serum Chloride
Serum K is normal or low.
3. This patient has chronic obstructive airway disease with pneumonia and respiratory failure.
4. Adequate oxygen and treatment of underlying cause.

Answer 12

1. Severe Metabolic Acidosis with Compensatory Respiratory Alkalosis.
2. The patient may have taken aspirin, inducing metabolic acidosis and treated with forced alkaline diuresis using bicarbonate, normal saline infusion and frusemide.
3. Explanation of lab values:
    This is the result of above treatment as well as correction by respiratory compensation.
    Compensation:
    $PaCO_2 = 14$, SBC = 2
    $PaCO_2 = (1.5 \times SBC) + 8 \pm 2$
    $\quad\quad = 11 \pm 2$ mm Hg
    Value for $PaCO_2$ below 9 or above 13 defines mixed disturbance.
4. Plasma K is low because of loss in the urine due to forced diuresis. As acidosis is corrected, patient tends towards alkalosis, and plasma K also falls.

ADDITIONAL NOTES

Respiratory Alkalosis accounts for 46% of all acid-base disorders.

There is decreased $PaCO_2$ (< 40 mm Hg)
Arterial pH is high (alkalaemia)
SBC is low (compensation)
High serum chloride

In Respiratory Alkalosis:

$PaCO_2$ is seldom below 14 mmol/l (range 14 to 24) and SBC seldom less than 18 mmol/l.

Normal: $PaCO_2$ = 40 mm Hg

SBC = 25 mmol/l

Treatment:

i. Oxygen if hypoxaemic.
ii. Treat volume depletion, hypotension, sepsis.
iii. If pH > 7.55, anaesthetise, ventilate and paralyse patient. This is the best means of raising $PaCO_2$ and decreasing pH in severe alkalaemia.

+ **Table 16.1** Simple acid-base disorders*

Type of Disorder	pH	$PaCO_2$	$[HCO_3^-]$
Metabolic acidosis	↓	↓	↓
Metabolic alkalosis	↑	↑	↑
Acute respiratory acidosis	↓	↑	↑
Chronic respiratory acidosis	↓	↑	↑
Acute respiratory alkalosis	↑	↓	↓
Chronic respiratory alkalosis	↑	↓	↓

* Note that the metabolic $[HCO_3^-]$ and respiratory ($PaCO_2$) components of the "acid-base equation" always change in the same direction in simple acid-base disorders.
+ Courtesy of R. Schrier.

+ **Table 16.2** Rules of thumb for bedside interpretation of Acid-Base Disorders

Metabolic acidosis	$PaCO_2$ should fall by 1.0 to 1.5 × the fall in plasma HCO_3^- concentration.
Metabolic alkalosis	$PaCO_2$ should rise by 0.25 to 1.0 × the rise in plasma HCO_3^- concentration.
Acute respiratory acidosis	Plasma HCO_3^- concentration should rise by about 1 mmol/l for each 10 mm Hg increment in $PaCO_2$ (± 3 mmol/l)
Chronic respiratory acidosis	Plasma HCO_3^- concentration should rise by about 4 mmol/l for each 10 mm Hg increment in $PaCO_2$ (± 4 mmol/l)

(Continued)

342   *Clinical Nephrology*

+ **Table 16.2**   (*Continued*)

| Acute respiratory alkalosis | Plasma HCO_3^- concentration should fall by about 1–3 mmol/l for each 10 mm Hg decrement in the $PaCO_2$ usually not to less than 18 mmol/l. |
| Chronic respiratory alkalosis | Plasma HCO_3^- concentration should fall by about 2–5 mmol/l per 10 mm Hg decrement in $PaCO_2$ but usually not to less than 14 mmol/l. |

+ Courtesy of R. Schrier.

CHAPTER 21
Renal Tubular Acidosis

Renal tubular acidosis (RTA) is a clinical syndrome of disordered renal acidification characterised by minimal or no azotaemia, hyperchloracmic acidosis, inappropriately high urinary pH, bicarbonaturia and reduced urinary excretion of titratable acid (TA) and ammonium (NH_4^+). The syndrome reflects a disorder of renal acidification that can cause acidosis with little or no apparent reduction in renal mass as measured by the glomerular filtration rate (GFR).

Renal tubular acidosis was first described by Lightwood and Butler in children and by Baines *et al.* in the adult. Two main types of RTA have been described (Types I and II), though at least four types have now been recognised (Types III and IV).

TYPE I RTA

Type I RTA, also known as Distal or Classic RTA is due to an inability of the distal tubule to establish an adequate pH gradient between the blood and the distal tubular fluid. There is a defect in the luminal membrane causing a limitation of tubular cell lumen H^+ gradient. Type I RTA per se is not associated with impaired tubular reabsorption of amino acids or glucose. Even during severe degrees of acidosis the urine pH does not drop below 5.4, in contrast to Type II RTA. Furthermore tubular reabsorption of bicarbonate in the proximal tubule is not greatly reduced. The defect is due to an inability to generate or maintain normally steep lumen-peritubular H^+ gradients. A significant disposal of H^+ ions as titratable acid and ammonium is possible provided the distal tubule can achieve a large H^+ ion gradient. When the distal tubule is incapable of transporting H^+ ion efficiently the urine

343

pH remains more alkaline than would be expected and the plasma bicarbonate falls. Characteristically, these patients have hyperchloraemic acidosis, often accompanied by hypokalaemia, normal glomerular filtration rates and a tendency to develop nephrocalcinosis and renal calculi.

Type I RTA, like Type II RTA, can be primary (idiopathic) or secondary, ie. due to exogenous causes or associated with other renal or generalised disorder. In a series of 10 cases, Type I RTA seems to be the one we encounter. Six of the 10 cases had secondary RTA: 2 due to medullary sponge kidney, 2 associated with gout, 1 with idiopathic hypercalciuria and hyperuricosuria and the remaining associated with systemic lupus erythematosus. Other causes of secondary Type I RTA are described in association with hypercalcaemia, light chain proteinuria, amphotericin toxicity, toluene toxicity (glue or paint sniffing), lithium toxicity and transplant rejection. Primary RTA can be genetically transmitted as an autosomal dominant trait or it can occur sporadically.

Medullary sponge kidney is a disease characterised by collecting ductular ectasia. It affects primarily the papillary portion of the medulla. Disorder of tubular function has been described with medullary sponge kidney and it consists of an inability of the kidney to concentrate and acidify the urine maximally, i.e. a distal or Type I RTA.

The occurrence of RTA in patients with medullary sponge kidney and Ehlers-Danlos syndrome has led workers to suggest that the acidification defect reflects a structural rather than a metabolic defect. The acidification defect might of course result from a metabolic abnormality of the epithelial membrane. In medullary sponge disease the impairment in renal acidification may be the result of structural alterations of the renal tubule initiated by deposition of calcium salts in the renal parenchyma. This possibility is suggested by the association of Type I RTA and nephrocalcinosis in a variety of clinical conditions in which Type I RTA is not a characteristic complication in the absence of nephrocalcinosis: primary hyperparathyroidism, vitamin D intoxication, hyperthyroidism, idiopathic hypercalciuria and medullary sponge kidney.

In 1959 Wrong and Davis described a form of RTA without overt metabolic acidosis. They suggested that such patients had an incomplete RTA which could be preacidotic. In our series we had 2 patients who initially presented with nephrocalcinosis, normal plasma bicarbonate, a marked acidification defect and a normal production of ammonia. It is important to detect this type of Incomplete Type I RTA because like the complete form, renal calcification and osteomalacia may disappear with long-term alkali therapy.

TYPE II RTA

The other main type of RTA is Type II RTA which is also referred to as Proximal RTA. These patients have a defect in the reabsorption of bicarbonate by the proximal tubule that causes the distal tubule to be flooded with bicarbonate. If the plasma bicarbonate is low or lowered by the prolonged use of ammonium chloride, the reduced filtered load of bicarbonate can be reabsorbed, allowing the final urine to fall to normal acid levels. This group of patients who often have other evidence of proximal tubular involvement such as aminoaciduria, phosphaturia and glycosuria usually require larger amounts of alkali to correct their acidosis than do those who have the distal tubular defect (Type I RTA). Type II RTA is associated with certain errors of metabolism (cystinosis, Wilson's disease) or it can be a consequence of heavy metal toxicity, outdated tetracycline, multiple myeloma, dysproteinaemia, nephrotic syndrome or transplant rejection. A mild form may be seen in primary or secondary hyperparathyroidism.

Type II RTA also exists in an incomplete form. These are patients with Fanconi's Syndrome who are not acidotic, i.e. net renal secretion of H^+ at normal plasma bicarbonate was not subnormal. They resemble Incomplete Type I RTA, except urinary pH decreases to appropriate low values during Ammonium Chloride Loading.

TYPE III RTA

Type III RTA has been referred to as a Dislocation or Bicarbonate Wasting "Classic" RTA which presents as a bicarbonate wasting

RTA that is not Fanconi's syndrome (triad of proximal tubular dysfunction of renal glycosuria, aminoaciduria and increased phosphate clearance).

TYPE IV RTA

In this type of RTA, patients with Chronic Renal Insufficiency become acidotic before the GFR becomes greatly reduced (i.e. before 30 ml/min). The pathology in this group of patients does not affect the glomeruli principally, rather it is associated with tubulo-interstitial diseases like reflux nephropathy, polycystic kidney and analgesic nephropathy. These patients have hyporeni-naemia and hypoaldosteronism, while their acidosis is usually associated with hyperchloraemia, hyperkalaemia and acidic urine. Their physiology is like those of Type II (Proximal) RTA with 2–17% bicarbonaturia. However they do not have features of Fanconi's syndrome. It is postulated that they have a combined defect in secretion of H^+ and K^+ in the distal tubule and the cause could be a deficiency or a resistance to the action of aldosterone.

There were 2 patients in our series who initially presented with Incomplete Type I RTA as evidenced by impaired urinary acidification in the absence of systemic acidosis. Their plasma bicarbonate levels were 24 and 25 mEq/l. In these patients, systemic acidosis is not present and net acid excretion does not appear to be frankly subnormal, although urinary pH is clearly inappropriately high when measured during ammonium chloride induced acidosis.

INVESTIGATIONS

1. Blood urea, serum creatinine, electrolytes, serum bicarbonate
2. Blood gases
3. Urine pH
4. Ammonium Chloride Loading Test
5. Maximal Osmolar Concentration

6. 24-hour urinary calcium, uric acid
7. 24-hour urinary amino acids, phosphate; glycosuria
8. Serum calcium, phosphate and serum alkaline phosphatase, serum uric acid
9. Urinary protein, Creatinine Clearance Test
10. Radiological: X-ray abdomen, intravenous pyelogram, tomogram, skeletal survey
11. Collagen work-up: ESR, ANF, anti-DNA, serum immunoglobulins, serum complement

Ammonium Chloride Loading Test

Patients were allowed to have a light breakfast before onset of test and at 8 am, oral NH_4 CI was given in a dose of 0.1 gm/kg BW with a cup of orange juice or plain water. Urine was voided at 8 am and discarded, following which all urine passed from 8 am till 10 am was collected and labelled as First Specimen. At 10 am a blood gas was done. Urine from 1 pm to 3 pm was again collected and this was labelled as Second Specimen. A specimen of arterial blood was again collected for blood gas analysis.

Patients who were unable to acidify the urine to a pH of 5.3 at the Second Specimen were considered to have impairment of urinary acidification. Urinary specimens were estimated for the following:

	Ist specimen	2nd specimen
○ pH of urine	4.75–5.5	4.5–5.2
○ Titratable Acid	14.4–39 mEq/min	14.6–34.4 mEq/min
○ Ammonium (NH4⁺)	39–154 mEq/min	39–58 mEq/min

Maximal Osmolar Concentration

Patients were put on a fast from midnight and on arrival at the ward the next day a subcutaneous injection of pitressin tannate in oil (5 units) was administered at 8 am. Urine was then collected at hourly intervals from 9 am onwards, both the volume as well as the osmolarity being measured at the same time. The test was terminated after 6 to 8 samples of urine had been collected or if the urine osmolarity had already exceeded 800 mOsmol/l, whichever occurred first. The highest concentration reached during this period would be the Maximal Osmolar Concentration (MOC) and a concentration defect was said to be present if the MOC was less than 800 mOsmol/l at the end of the test period.

The normal ranges for some of the indices measured above are as follows:

1. 24-hour urinary amino acid
    normal adult male = 2.9 – 12.5 mmol/day   40–175 mg/day
    normal adult female = 2.1 – 9.5 mmol/day   29–133 mg/day
2. 24-hour urinary inorganic phosphate
    adult male = 6.5 – 32.3 mmol/day   0.2–1.0 gm/day
    adult female = 8.1 – 22.6 mmol/day   0.25–0.7 gm/day
3. 24-hour urinary calcium
    adult male = 0.41 – 3.38 mmol/day   33–270 mg/day
    adult female = 0.33 – 3.13 mmol/day   26–250 mg/day
4. 24-hour urinary uric acid = up to 4.2 mmol/day
                                                              700 mg/day

TYPE I OR DISTAL RTA

(Classic or Gradient RTA)

This is due to a defect in the distal tubule whereby it is unable to generate a sufficient hydrogen ion gradient to cause its secretion into the distal tubular lumen. The excretion of titratable acid (TA) and ammonium (NH_4^+) therefore will be low and the urine pH remains alkaline (above 5.3). The patient will not be able to acidify the urine despite severe metabolic acidosis (serum bicarbonate < 15 mEq/1) unlike Type II RTA.

Clinical Features of Type I RTA

1. The commonest mode of presentation is muscular weakness or paralysis due to hypokalaemia. Some patients present with haematuria or renal colic due to renal calculi. Urinary tract infection may complicate renal stones and occasionally, obstructive uropathy with renal failure may result. Properly treated, these patients should not develop renal failure.

2. A low serum K^+ associated with hyperchloraemia and metabolic acidosis should alert one to the possibility of the patient having RTA. The differential diagnosis is a patient with an ileal conduit or ureterosigmoidostomy. If the patient has renal failure, then RTA cannot be diagnosed and the acidosis is likely to be due to uraemic acidosis in which case the serum K^+ is usually high.

   Urine pH and blood gases should be performed when RTA is suspected. In the presence of severe acidosis and urine pH more than 5.3 with hypokalaemia and hyperchloraemia, a diagnosis of Type I RTA is fairly certain. The presence of nephrocalcinosis on plain X-ray of the abdomen confirms the diagnosis of Type I RTA as patients with Type II RTA do not usually have nephrocalcinosis. Patients with Type II RTA are able to acidify the urine (pH less than 5.3) when acidosis is severe (serum bicarbonate less than 15 mEq/l).

3. A skeletal survey should be performed in patients with RTA as children may have rickets and adults osteomalacia. Rickets is due to low serum calcium resulting from failure of the renal tubules to produce adequate amounts of 1,25-dihydroxycholecalciferol. Some patients have osteomalacia because of low serum phosphate. This occurs in those with Type II RTA because of associated phosphaturia.

TYPE II OR PROXIMAL RTA

(Bicarbonate Wasting or Rate RTA)

The defect is in the proximal tubule whereby there is an inability to reabsorb filtered bicarbonate. Normally, the proximal tubule reabsorbs up to 85% of filtered bicarbonate, the distal tubule about 10 to 15% and the collecting duct about 5%. In Type II RTA only about 65% of bicarbonate is reabsorbed. The excess bicarbonate (about 35%) is now presented at the distal tubule. But this is much more than what the distal tubule can absorb. Excess bicarbonate therefore remains in the urine and keeps it alkaline (urine pH > 5.3).

However, when the patient is severely acidotic, the little bicarbonate presented at the proximal tubule is almost completely reabsorbed. Only a little filters into the distal tubule. Since the distal tubular mechanism is intact in Proximal RTA and there is now no excess bicarbonate to compete for excretion of titratable acid and ammonium, the distal tubular acidification proceeds normally and urine is acidified with urine *pH* of less than 5.3.

The patient with Proximal RTA also has associated features of glycosuria, aminoaciduria, hypophosphataemia and hypouricaemia in addition to the usual features of RTA like hypokalaemia, hyperchloraemic acidosis and alkaline urine as in Type I RTA.

Each time bicarbonate is reabsorbed, whether by the proximal or distal tubule, it is accompanied by the reabsorption of sodium (Na^+). The reabsorption of Na^+ is accompanied by excretion of either H^+ or K^+. Normally H^+ is excreted in the form of titratable acid and ammonium. If bicarbonate is not reabsorbed, Na^+ is not absorbed and H^+ is not excreted. The result is metabolic acidosis. In addition, patients with Type II RTA also have a reduction in the rate of H^+ secretion into the tubular lumen. K^+ is therefore excreted in exchange for reabsorbed Na^+ and hence patients become hypokalaemic.

In Type I or distal RTA, since H^+ cannot be secreted, K^+ is exchanged with Na^+ absorption and the patient develops hypokalaemic acidosis.

In many patients with Proximal RTA due to Fanconi's syndrome, renal acidification defect involves both the proximal and the distal tubule.

Clinical Features of Type II or Proximal RTA

1. The clinical manifestations of hypokalaemic paralysis and metabolic acidosis are the same as those of Type I RTA. Patients with Type II RTA have a triad of proximal tubular dysfunction of renal glycosuria, aminoaciduria and increased phosphate clearance (low serum phosphate). Serum uric acid is often low (less than 2 mg/dl) because of associated hypouricaemia. If they have associated distal tubular defects (Type I RTA) as many patients with Fanconi's syndrome do, they will also have nephrocalcinosis with renal stones, colic and haematuria with occasional urinary infection due to stones.

2. These patients are able to acidify the urine when acidosis is severe (serum bicarbonate <15 mEq/l) because the distal tubule is intact. The urine pH will then be <5.3 instead of about 7 or 8.

3. Skeletal survey may show rickets or osteomalacia.

TREATMENT OF RTA

1. Treatment will vary with the type of RTA and the underlying cause. Patients with Type I RTA require less bicarbonate than those with Type II RTA who may require as much as 10 to 20 gm of bicarbonate, hence the term "bicarbonate wasting RTA". Patients with Type II RTA usually require more than 6 mEq/kg/day of bicarbonate in contrast to those with Type I where they require much less (about 1.5 mEq/kg/day).

2. Hypokalaemia will require potassium chloride replacement. KCl should be given slowly in a continuous intravenous drip. Oral supplements can also be given. Patients with Type II

RTA usually require much more KCl for correction of hypokalaemia and they usually require maintenance KCl supplements even when acidosis has been corrected.

3. Patients should be encouraged to drink a lot of fluids as this has been shown to be helpful in reducing nephrocalcinosis. Their fluid regime should be the same as for anyone with stones, ie. to drink especially before retiring to bed so that he would wake up in the night to pass urine and thereafter to drink again to pass once more in the early morning. Patients should drink enough to pass at least 3 litres of urine a day.

4. Vitamin D therapy (1,25 dihydroxycholecalciferol) and calcium supplements are necessary if they have rickets or osteomalacia.

5. A 24-hour urinary estimate of calcium and uric acid should be performed to exclude idiopathic hypercalciuria and hyperuricosuria as such patients may require treatment with thiazides and allopurinol if they do not respond to dietary counselling.

6. Finally, energetic treatment should be promptly instituted for those who develop obstructive uropathy (due to calculus disease) and urinary infections.

7. With proper management, renal failure should never occur in patients with RTA.

PRACTICE POINTS

1. If nephrocalcinosis is present the patient is likely to have Type I RTA.

2. If the patient has severe acidosis (serum bicarbonate <15 mEq/l) and cannot acidify the urine (urine pH > 5.3) he has Type I RTA. There is no necessity in performing the ammonium chloride test.

3. A patient with Type I RTA cannot acidify the urine, ie. bring the urine pH down to < 5.3, no matter how acidotic he is, unlike one with Type II RTA where the distal tubule is intact and can secrete H^+ into the urine.

4. The ammonium chloride loading test should not be performed when the patient is acidotic.

5. In performing the ammonium chloride loading test, it is necessary to do a blood gas and confirm that the patient has systemic acidosis. If he is not acidotic it may mean that he has vomited the ammonium chloride which would render the test useless unless he takes another dose.

CHAPTER 22

Renal Tubular Disorders

The following conditions can cause renal tubular disorders:

1. Renal Tubular Acidosis (RTA): Type I or Distal RTA
2. Fanconi's syndrome: Type II or Proximal RTA
3. Cystinuria
4. Cystinosis
5. Medullary sponge kidney
6. Medullary cystic kidney
7. Diabetes insipidus
8. Pseudohypoparathyroidism
9. Uraemic acidosis
10. Interstitial nephritis

Renal Tubular Acidosis and Fanconi's Syndrome have been covered in the chapter on Renal Tubular Acidosis.

CYSTINURIA

1. This is a proximal tubular lesion. It is usually inherited in an autosomal recessive manner but can occasionally be autosomal dominant.
2. Patients are unable to reabsorb cystine, ornithine, lysine and arginine. These 4 amino acids can be remembered by C.O.L.A.
3. It is associated with small bowel disturbance where the same amino acids are also not absorbed. There may be a common transport disorder.
4. Renal calculi is the usual manifestation. These stones are radio opaque as they contain sulphur.

355

5. Treatment consists of alkalinisation of the urine, diuretics and in severe cases, penicillamine. Penicillamine itself causes side effects like gastrointestinal upset, liver dysfunction and nephrotic syndrome.

CYSTINOSIS

1. This condition is due to an accumulation of cystine in the reticuloendothelial system, leukocytes, fibroblasts, kidneys and eyes.
2. One should look for crystals in the lymph node, leukocyte, bone marrow, cornea (using slit lamp), and kidneys.
3. It is a cause of Fanconi's syndrome causing Type II or proximal RTA. The childhood form is associated with growth failure and renal failure because of its severity.
4. Retinopathy due to cystine deposits in the retina may cause blindness.
5. The adult type is more benign as the kidneys can be spared. However, a variant exists which occurs as a late onset juvenile type and such patients may have slow progressive renal failure.
6. Patients with cystinosis with Fanconi's syndrome have aminoaciduria, glycosuria and rickets. Cystine stones are rare.

MEDULLARY SPONGE KIDNEY

1. This is a congenital condition related to an abnormality of the collecting duct of the kidney where there is dilatation of the renal tubules (tubuloectasia), sometimes "cystic", which communicates with the calyces.
2. Patients may present with haematuria, urinary tract infection related to stones or nephrocalcinosis. They may also present as Type I RTA with nephrocalcinosis.

3. The diagnosis may be suspected by the pattern of nephrocal-cinosis and stones on a plain film of the abdomen. An IVP confirms the diagnosis.
4. An ammonium chloride loading test and maximal osmolar concentration are usually performed to exclude RTA and assess tubular function. It is also useful to measure the 24-hour urinary excretion of calcium and uric acid as there is an association with idiopathic hypercalciuria and hyperuricosuria.
5. Treatment consists of drinking enough fluids to pass at least 3 litres of urine a day. Urinary infections and stones should be treated.

MEDULLARY CYSTIC KIDNEYS

1. This disease is inherited in an autosomal recessive fashion.
2. Patients have a congenital cystic dilatation of the tubules.
3. They may present with cramps and hypotension due to salt loss resulting from impaired tubular function.
4. Anaemia, polyuria and acidosis are common presentations related to chronic renal failure which most would have by the time they become juveniles. They are also stunted because of renal bone disease.
5. A non-specific aminoaciduria may also be associated as a manifestation of Type II RTA which can be diagnosed only when the patient still has normal renal function.
6. This is a condition with a poor prognosis unlike medullary sponge kidneys which have a good prognosis and is compat-ible with normal life expectancy.

DIABETES INSIPIDUS (DI)

1. May be neurogenic (Pituitary DI) or nephrogenic (Nephrogenic DI) in origin.

In Pit Dl the renal tubules are normal but the pituitary fails to produce antidiuretic hormone (ADH) and the urine therefore is not concentrated and the patient has frequency of micturition associated with polyuria.

In Nephrogenic DI there is ADH but the tubules are not capable of responding to ADH and therefore the urine is always hypotonic to plasma. Patients also have increased frequency of micturition and polyuria.

2. In Pit DI the onset is often acute with increased frequency of micturition, especially at night, every half to one hour; whereas in Nephrogenic DI the onset is more gradual. Cerebrovascular disease is a common cause of Pit DI, especially in elderly patients. In about 30% of Pit DI the cause is unknown.

   Nephrogenic DI may be congenital or drug induced, e.g. lithium given for depression. Other causes include hypokalaemia, hypercalcaemia as well as hydronephrosis and pyelonephritis where damage to the distal tubules results in their failure to respond to ADH.

3. A Pitressin Test (Maximal Osmolar Concentration) can help to differentiate Pit DI from Nephrogenic DI. In Pit DI there will be a response to pitressin and one of the urine specimens will show an osmolarity >800 mosmol/l but in Nephrogenic DI there will be no response to pitressin. In a patient with normal plasma osmolarity of 285 mosmol/l and urine osmolarity of 140 to 180 mosmol/l not responding to pitressin, the diagnosis is Nephrogenic DI.

   One should be very very cautious in performing the Pitressin test in the elderly as there is the risk of inducing a stroke or a myocardial infarction. Do a baseline ECG and assess for cerebrovascular insufficiency before proceeding if one must perform the test in an elderly patient.

4. Treatment consists of removal of the underlying cause. In Nephrogenic DI thiazides are useful. They cause increased excretion of Na^+ at the distal tubule. This stimulates proximal tubular reabsorption of Na^+ and water, and less fluid is

delivered to the distal tubule to be excreted. The electrolytes and renal function must be monitored, especially in the elderly. In Pit DI chlorpropamide may be useful as it has a "pitressin-like effect" on cyclic AMP on the distal tubule. The blood sugar must be monitored because of the risk of hypoglycaemia. Desmopressin or intranasal pitressin can also be used, but with caution in the elderly.

PSEUDOHYPOPARATHYROIDISM

1. These patients have the characteristic shortened 4th metacarpal.
2. The biochemical features consist of low serum calcium due to decreased absorption from the bowels. They have a high serum phosphate.
3. Hypocalciuria and hypophosphaturia are additional features of the condition.

URAEMIC ACIDOSIS

1. Irrespective of the cause, Chronic Progressive Renal Disease results in some degree of systemic acidosis when the GFR is less than 25 ml/min. This is due to:
   i.   impaired reabsorption of bicarbonate
   ii. impaired production of ammonia so that excretion of H^+ in the urine in the form of ammonium is decreased.
2. In some patients, there is a large amount of bicarbonate loss (ranging from 15% to as much as 50%) resembling bicarbonate wastage in Type II or Proximal RTA.
3. Part of the cause of the acidosis is related to the renal disease which reduces the activity of renal carbonic anhydrase. This enzyme is responsible for the generation of bicarbonate:

$$CO_2 + H_2O \rightarrow H_2CO_3$$
Carbonic Anhydrase

4. Seldin and Rector suggested that the impairment of bicarbon-
    ate reabsorption was a consequence of reduction in the
    number of functioning nephrons leading to reduced bicarbon-
    ate level.

5. Muldowny designated uraemic acidosis as parathyroid acido-
    sis as he found the plasma concentration of parathormone was
    inversely correlated with plasma concentration of bicarbonate
    and hence the degree of systemic acidosis; i.e. the higher the
    PTH levels the lower the serum bicarbonate level.

INTERSTITIAL NEPHRITIS

This is a term given to conditions where the main reaction of the
kidney occurs in the interstitium. There is cellular reaction (usually lymphocytic) in the interstitium and tubular damage (atrophy
and necrosis).

There are two types of Interstitial Nephritis:

I. Acute Interstitial Nephritis

1. Sudden onset usually due to:

    i.   Drugs like non-steroidal anti-inflammatory drugs
         (NSAID), methicillin, ampicillin, sulphonamides, sep-
         trin, dilantin, dindevan, gentamicin, cephaloridine,
         allopurinol.

    ii. Septicaemia from any cause: leptospirosis, streptococcal
         and staphylococcal infection, cytomegalo-virus (CMV)
         infection.

    iii. Other causes include lupus nephritis, transplant rejec-
         tion, beestings, toxins and poisons.

2. Antibiotics like methicillin, or even ampicillin can cause an
    acute allergic interstitial nephritis where the patient presents
    with fever, rash, haematuria (even gross haematuria), pyuria,
    proteinuria and acute renal failure with eosinophils in the
    urine.

In a patient with acute allergic interstitial nephritis a renal biopsy would show interstitial oedema with infiltration of lymphocytes, plasma cells, polymorphs, eosinophils and varying degree of tubular atrophy and necrosis. The glomeruli are norrnal.

3. Treatment of acute interstitial nephritis consists of removal of the offending drug and treating the infection. In the case of patients with acute renal failure they will require dialysis to tide them over the acute episode. For patients with acute allergic interstitial nephritis, prednisolone may be required.

II. Chronic Interstitial Nephritis

1. For this category of interstitial nephritis there is more interstitial fibrosis associated with chronic lymphocytic infiltrates and tubular atrophy.

2. The causes are:

    i.   analgesic nephropathy, reflux nephropathy, polycystic kidneys.
    ii. chronic transplant rejection, lupus nephritis and chronic conditions like sarcoidosis
    iii. Sjogren's syndrome, irradiation, gout
    iv. lead and cadmium nephrotoxicity
    v.   obstructive uropathy, heat stroke and medullary cystic kidneys

3. Treatment consists of removal or treatment of the underlying cause. A patient with analgesic nephropathy who stops taking analgesics will arrest the progression of the interstitial lesions.

CHAPTER 23

Systemic Disease and the Kidney

Considering that the kidneys receive about one quarter of the cardiac output and the glomeruli act as filters for blood constituents, it is not surprising that the kidneys are involved in various kinds of systemic diseases.

This chapter discusses the renal aspects of different types of systemic diseases.

RENAL VASCULITIS[1]

Vasculitis refers to necrotising inflammation of the blood vessels and is seen in a large spectrum of diseases. It could be due to any one of the following causes: some are systemic vasculitis and others predominantly renal vasculitis with a high incidence of end stage renal failure.

1. SLE
2. Polyarteritis nodosa (PAN)
3. Wegener's granulomatosis
4. Dermatomyositis
5. Henoch-Schonlein purpura
6. Cryoglobulinaemia
7. Rheumatoid arthritis
8. Hypersensitivity vasculitis
9. Behcet's disease
10. Infections: Hepatitis B antigen (positive in 6–40% of PAN), Beta-haemolytic strep, otitis media, post-infectious GN

11. Drugs: Sulphonamides, septrin, penicillin, iodine
12. Cancer: Leukaemia, lymphoma

Clinical Features

1. The peak age is between 40 to 50 years.
2. Patients often have a prodrome consisting of a flu-like illness. Some may have sores or history of drug ingestion.
3. Renal presentation could be haematuria, proteinuria, nephrotic syndrome, oliguria with acute renal failure or renal impairment.
4. Skin lesions such as purpura and cutaneous vasculitis.
5. Ocular lesions such as conjunctivitis, iritis.
6. Hypertension occurs in 25% of patients.
7. Liver, pancreas and gastrointestinal involvement with gastrointestinal bleeding and pain. These occur in 50% of patients.
8. CNS involvement occurs in 25% of patients: peripheral neuropathy is not uncommon.
9. Cardiovascular complications such as myocardial ischaemia and congestive heart failure.
10. Respiratory involvement may be in the form of bronchial asthma.

Investigation

1. ESR, FBC, Eosinophilia
2. LE cell, ANF, Anti-DNA, ANCA
3. Serum complements, circulating immune complexes (CIC)
4. Cryoglobulinaemia
5. ASOT, Hepatitis B screening
6. Splanchnic or renal arteriogram to detect aneurysms

Renal Lesions

1. Glomerular
   i. Segmental necrotising glomerulitis, ischaemic shrinkage of glomeruli, glomerular fibrinoid necrosis, "segmental crescents".
   ii. Associated with mesangial proliferative GN, membranous GN, mesangiocapillary GN, endocapillary GN.
2. Tubular
   i. Acute tubular necrosis, interstitial lesions, infiltrate of plasma cells, lymphocytes, polymorphs.
   ii. Eosinophils present if vasculitis due to allergic angiitis and granulomatosis.
3. Renal blood vessels
   i. Fibrinoid necrosis with infiltration of polymorphs, eosinophils, lymphocytes.
   ii. Irregular intimal thickening, aneurysms, involving arcuate or interlobular arterial lesions.
4. IMF: Look for fibrin + +. Immunoglobulin staining depends on underlying cause.
5. EM features: Features depend on underlying cause.

Treatment

1. Prednisolone (1 mg/kg BW per day).
2. Cyclosphosphamide (1.5 mg/kg BW per day).
3. Pulse therapy with methylprednisolone (0.5 gm I.V. daily for 3 days).
4. Plasmapheresis has been shown to be useful in patients with rapidly progressive GN.
5. Dialysis is necessary in patients with oliguria, especially when they have more than 70% crescents on biopsy.
6. After renal transplantation, these patients have a low recurrence rate.

SYSTEMIC LUPUS ERYTHEMATOSUS

This has been dealt with separately in the chapter on Lupus Nephritis.

POLYARTERITIS NODOSA

This is a disease associated with fever, symptoms referrable to the muscles, gastrointestinal tract, lungs, heart and the kidneys. It is characterised by nodular swellings of medium-sized arteries.

Like SLE it has protean manifestations. Males are more commonly affected than females. All ages are affected. There is fever, leukocytosis, eosinophilia especially among patients with respiratory involvement, and is associated with weakness and weight loss. Patients may have arthritis, abdominal pain, polyneuritis, cardiac failure, asthma and pneumonia.

Renal involvement occurs in 70% of patients. They may present with acute nephritis with haematuria and proteinuria, sometimes with rapidly progressive glomerulonephritis. Others have only haematuria or proteinuria with rising serum creatinine. Some may develop malignant hypertension due to renal infarction and may have hypertensive cardiac failure. Death could result from cerebral haemorrhage or renal failure.

Renal arteriogram may show aneurysms affecting the larger arteries of the kidneys. Hepatitis B antigen has been associated with this condition.

The kidneys may be normal or reduced in size. There may be evidence of infarction. Petichial haemorrhages are associated with malignant hypertension. Small localised swellings may be seen on the main divisions of the renal artery in 70% of patients.

The renal biopsy changes include fibrinoid necrosis within the glomeruli. Epithelial crescents may be present. Part of the circumference of the blood vessels or the whole circumference may be replaced by fibrinoid necrosis. Plasma cells and sometimes eosinophils are found in the interstitium.

Treatment consists of prednisolone and cyclophosphamide. Plasmapheresis or methylprednisolone pulsing is usually prescribed for patients with rapidly progressive glomerulonephritis.

WEGENER'S GRANULOMATOSIS

Clinically, this condition is characterised by the presence of a granulomatous process in the upper respiratory tract and the lungs. The process is associated with necrosed blood vessels and a florid form of renal lesion in which the glomeruli show necrosis. About two-thirds of patients have purulent rhinorrhoea with nasal obstruction and crusting, antral pain, epistaxis while one-third has cough, haemoptysis and pleurisy.

The renal lesions are the same as for the microscopic form of polyarteritis nodosa, except that "granulomas" may form in relation to blood vessels, glomeruli and tubulo-interstitium. Rapidly progressive glomerulonephritis is associated with acute renal failure and the presence of crescents in the renal biopsy (pauci-immune crescenteric GN).

80% to 90% of patients are positive for cytoplasmic — anti neutrophilic cytoplasmic antibody (c-ANCA), which is highly specific and sensitive in the diagnosis. If untreated there is 80–90% mortality. Those treated with Cyclophosphamide have 80–90% remission. There is a high incidence of Cancer of the Bladder 10 years later in those treated with Cyclophosphamide. Prednisolone is used as adjunctive therapy especially for severe renal pulmonary, skin or cerebral vasculitis. In place of Cyclophosphamide, newer immunosuppressants like Cyclosporine A and even Mycophenolate Mofetil can be used. However, at this point in time there are no controlled trials to show that these agents are as good as or better than Cyclophosphamide.

SCLERODERMA

This is also known as progressive systemic sclerosis. Males are more commonly affected than females with a predominance in the age group of 30 to 50 years.

Patients have calcinosis of the finger pulps on X-rays, Raynaud's phenomenon, sclerodactyly and telangiectasia (CRST syndrome).

Renal involvement occurs in about 45% of patients manifesting as proteinuria, hypertension, renal failure and oliguria to complete anuria, sometimes with malignant hypertension.

In the acute form with death in renal failure, the kidneys look normal or slightly increased in size. Sometimes there may be areas of scarring due to preexisting arterial narrowing. Petechial haemorrhages may be present. In the chronic form with a slow progression the kidneys are reduced in size.

On renal biopsy, some glomeruli may show ischaemic changes with segmental sclerosis. Others may reveal mesangial and endothelial hypercellularity and thickening of capillary tufts with tubular atrophy. Blood vessels show intimal hyperplasia.

Treatment consists of maintenance of renal perfusion and avoidance of dehydration. In the treatment of hypertension, do not cause hypotension as this will reduce renal blood flow.

RHEUMATOID ARTHRITIS

This condition has now been shown to be associated with non-specific mesangial proliferative glomerulonephritis with IgG on immunofluorescence. It is likely to be an immune complex GN.

Amyloidosis has also been associated with RA.

As a result of arteritis, some patients have a non-specific thickening of the small blood vessels in the kidneys which can lead to renal deterioration.

Chronic interstitial nephritis and papillary necrosis due to analgesics are other renal complications of the disease.

Therapy with gold and penicillamine also induces a nephrotic syndrome associated with membranous glomerulonephritis.

MULTIPLE MYELOMA

Patients affected by this condition may have nephrotic syndrome due to myeloma kidney and amyloidosis. Renal failure may be the first presenting feature of the disease. Others have the Fanconi's syndrome or nephrogenic diabetes insipidus due to hypercalcaemia.

Renal lesions of the myeloma kidney consist of tubules filled with myeloma casts surrounded by giant cells. The casts contain Bence Jones protein or amyloid. Amyloidosis and nephrocalcinosis should be looked for.

As a result of hypercalcaemia, patients may have depression, itch, constipation, thirst and confusion. Treatment of hypercalcaemia will require rehydration with saline and diuresis with frusemide. Steroids, phosphates, EDTA, mitramycin and dialysis have all been used in the treatment of hypercalcaemia.

Beware of IVP in the investigation of renal failure as it is contraindicated.

Serum electrophoresis, skeletal survey, bone marrow and renal biopsy will confirm the diagnosis.

Treatment is with steroids and cytotoxic drugs. Recently, patients with Multiple Myeloma have been offered stem cell bone marrow transplant with good results. It can induce remission in some patients and improve the quality of life, even though the disease can recur a few years later.

AMYLOIDOSIS

Nephrotic syndrome is a usual presentation. It can be due to primary amyloidosis or secondary to rheumatoid arthritis, tuberculosis, leprosy, osteomyelitis, chronic infection and myeloma.

The glomeruli show the characteristic deposits in thick lines round the blood vessels and tubules. Special staining using Congo Red and Thioflavine T will confirm amyloidosis. Electron microscopy will reveal the amyloid fibrils.

Renal vein thrombosis is a known complication in these patients.

Some patients have responded well to stem cell bone marrow transplant with good results.

CRYOGLOBULINAEMIA

It tends to affect females. They have arthralgia, haemolysis, Raynaud's phenomenon and nephrotic syndrome. Rheumatoid arthritis factor and anti-nuclear factor may be positive.

Some may present for the first time in chronic renal failure.

The presence of purpura and nephrotic syndrome should alert one to the possibility of the condition.

A renal biopsy will show intracapillary deposits of proteinaceous material. There is a non-specific mesangial proliferation with IgG and IgM on immunofiuorescence.

MACROGLOBULINAEMIA

Males are more commonly affected. They have a bleeding tendency and purpura. Examine the fundi and look for evidence of hyperviscosity.

Treatment consists of massive fluid infusion to get rid of proteins.

A renal biopsy will show PAS deposits inside the capillaries

RENAL TUBULAR ACIDOSIS

This has been dealt with in the chapter on Renal Tubular Acidosis.

SARCOIDOSIS

This condition is associated with direct infiltration of the kidneys causing renal failure. It also causes RTA.

Hypercalcaemia may cause the "red eye syndrome".

A chest X-ray will show enlarged lymph nodes.

Treatment consists of steroids. This will reduce the hypercalcaemia and improve renal function.

NEPHROTIC SYNDROME AND MALIGNANCY

Immune complex glomerulonephritis has been associated with cancers of the breast, colon, lymphoma and leukaemia.

Renal vein thrombosis, amyloidosis and neoplastic infiltration are often associated. Renal vein thrombosis is not a cause of nephrotic syndrome but a complication of the nephrotic syndrome.

Treatment directed at the underlying condition will result in a regression of the nephrotic syndrome.

RENAL COMPLICATIONS OF LYMPHOMA

May occur as a result of direct involvement like primary renal lymphoma, metastatic invasion of the parenchyma, hydronephrosis due to compression by lymph nodes and finally compression of the renal pedicel. All these are known causes of renal failure in this condition.

Hypercalcaemia induces nephrogenic diabetes insipidus.

Renal complications of therapy include conditions like uric acid nephropathy and radiation nephritis.

Immunological reactions may manifest as nephrotic syndrome and amyloidosis.

GOUT

See chapter on Kidney Stones.

Uric acid is strongly associated with cardiovascular and renal disease. Recent evidence suggests that uric acid may contribute to the development of hypertension, the metabolic syndrome and kidney disease.

1. Uric acid can cause a wide variety of deleterious effects. It can enter vascular smooth muscle cells resulting in release of proinflammatory cytokines and platelet derived growth factor

and vasoactive substances. Uric acid is an independent predictor of hypertension.

2. It has a role in the development of insulin resistance through a urate induced inhibition of Nitric Oxide. Lowering uric acid improved the features of the metabolic syndrome.

3. It causes a range of kidney disease through the development of albuminuria, microvascular disease, glomerulosclerosis and tubulointerstitial fibrosis. The mechanisms involved are stimulation of intrarenal renin expression with renal hypertrophy, acceleration of intrarenal microvascular disease and development of glomerular hypertension. This is largely due to preglomerular vascular disease.

4. Hyperuricemia is common in renal transplant patients and is a consequence of calcineurin inhibition. Hyperuricemia itself mimics and exacerbates CyA nephrotoxicity. Of interest is that experimental hyperuricemia produces a model similating chronic allograft nephropathy.

5. Uric acid also has a contributory role in pre eclampsia. It is a cause of intra uterine growth retardation and congenital reduction in nephron numbers.

6. Nakagawa *et al.* also has unpublished data of the role of Uric Acid in acute renal failure through its vasoconstrictive and proinflammatory effects [Nakagawa T *et al.* Kidney Int 2006, 69:1722–1725].

SUBACUTE BACTERIAL ENDOCARDITIS

Renal failure is one of the causes of death in this condition. The patient presents with gross haematuria and proteinuria and casts in the urine.

Petechial haemorrhages and infarction give rise to the flea bitten kidney.

There are two types of lesions in the glomeruli:

i. Focal embolic glomerulonephritis where there are focal areas of fibrinoid necrosis or hyaline and intracapillary thrombosis.

ii. Diffuse proliferative glomerulonephritis due to an immunologically mediated immune complex glomerulonephritis.

One may sometimes visualise sub-epithelial humps as in post
infectious glomerulonephritis. Immunofiuorescence would reveal
IgG predominantly with IgA, IgM and C3.

Renal involvement takes a few weeks to develop.

XANTHOGRANULOMATOUS PYELONEPHRITIS

This is a rare condition which occurs when infection affects a
kidney which is partially obstructed by calculi.

Patients with this condition have fever with chronic urinary
tract infection and a mass in the loin which is seen on the IVP as
a tumour mass. Angiography however does not suggest a tumour.

Urine cultures grow *Proteus* in 60% of the cases and *E. coli* in
the rest.

The gross pathology reveals large kidneys with adhesions and
abscesses. Histology reveals foam cells, foreign body giant cells
with necrotic debris and polymorphs. Some glomeruli will have
masses of clear cells like in a carcinoma but with no mitosis.
Nephrectomy may be needed if the kidney is non-functioning.

See chapter on UTI.

DIABETES MELLITUS

See chapter on Diabetes Mellitus.

All patients would have some degree of retinopathy with the onset
of proteinuria. Other manifestations include nephrotic syndrome,
hypertension, papillary necrosis and renal failure.

The glomerular lesions are:

i. Nodular Kimmelstiel-Wilson lesions which are pathog-
nomonic of diabetic nephropathy.

ii. Diffuse intercapillary glomerulosclerosis with marked
expansion of mesangial matrix. This is the commonest

renal lesion for a patient with diabetic nephropathy. It is related to glomerular hyperfiltration and is accompanied by hypertrophy of the kidneys. Control of hypergly-caemia reduces hyperfiltration.

iii. Capsular drops are waxy and eosinophilic. They occur between the basement membrane and parietal epithelium of Bowman's capsule.

iv. Fibrin cap or exudate correlates with vascular disease.

Tubular lesions are Armanni-Ebstein change (glycogen nephrosis) and tubular atrophy.

Both the efferent and afferent arterioles have sub-intimal hyaline thickening due to arteriosclerosis.

The interstitium is often fibrotic with chronic inflammatory cells.

Immunofiuorescence may show IgG in a linear pattern in the capillary wall. This is related to non-immunological and non-specific trapping or basement membrane dysfunction.

HENOCH-SCHONLEIN NEPHRITIS

Adults with this disease fare worse than children. There is a greater incidence of haematuria and proteinuria in adults (51%) compared to children (29%). Adults have a higher incidence of renal failure, 14% compared to 5%.

Nowadays, this condition is considered as part of the spectrum of IgA nephritis, hence the similarity in light microscopic and immunofluorescent findings with IgA nephritis.

Renal biopsy may show:

i. Minimal lesion with a good prognosis.

ii. Focal proliferative (mesangial) GN, sometimes with sclerosis and crescents.

iii. Diffuse mesangial proliferative GN like in IgA nephritis. There may be associated sclerosis and crescents.

Immunofiuorescence will show IgA predominantly with less intense staining for IgG. C3 is usually present.

The bad renal prognostic features are similar to IgA nephritis but patients with nephrotic syndrome usually do worse whatever the histology.

For those patients who present with the nephrotic syndrome they can be offered a course of prednisolone and failing that cyclophosphamide, cyclosporine A and mycophenolate mofetil [MMF].

FUNCTIONAL RENAL FAILURE ASSOCIATED WITH LIVER DYSFUNCTION

The term "Hepatorenal Syndrome" is specific for renal failure which occurs secondary to liver failure due to cirrhosis of the liver. All other conditions where there is simultaneous involvement of the liver and kidneys are termed "Functional Renal Failure". These conditions include septicaemia from any cause, cholangitis, leptospirosis (which can cause renal failure because of acute tubular necrosis or interstitial nephritis), toxins (certain mushrooms) and poisons (carbon tetrachloride). Liver failure from any cause apart from cirrhosis can also cause functional renal failure.

The cause of renal failure is due to a diversion or shunting of blood to the juxta-medullary nephron with underperfusion of the cortical nephrons resulting in oliguria, low urine sodium and proximal absorption of water. This shunting could be due to failure of the liver to deconjugate vasoactive amines leading to renal shutdown. In addition, bile acids are tubulotoxic and they increase vascular sensitivity to catecholamines.

The kidneys in this condition are in fact healthy and when transplanted to healthy persons regain normal renal function.

FALCIPARUM MALARIA

Acute renal failure in this infection results from acute tubular necrosis, haemolysis, disseminated intravascular coagulation and heavy parasitic infection which causes sludging of RBC in the capillaries. Intravascular haemolysis also gives rise to haemoglobinuria.

Glomerulonephritis can also occur because of associated immunological injury. The renal biopsy would show diffuse mesangial proliferative GN with IgM, IgG and C3 on IMF. The nephritis is mild and usually resolves in 4 to 6 weeks.

Hypertension and nephrotic syndrome may also occur.

QUARTAN MALARIA

The renal manifestations may be in the form of haematuria and proteinuria, nephrotic syndrome or hypertension. In a series of 115 patients in Uganda, 26% were protein free, 45% had urinary abnormalities and 29% had chronic renal failure.

Renal biopsy shows focal and segmental proliferation with mesangiocapillary changes and sclerosis. IMF reveals IgG, IgM and C3 in a coarse granularity in the capillary walls.

Treatment is symptomatic, consisting of diuretics and therapy for infection and anaemia. Prednisolone, cyclophosphamide and antimalarials do not help in arresting the progression to renal failure.

Plasmapheresis in the Therapy of Systemic Vasculitis

1. In patients with Vasculitis, plasmaphereis removes the acute phase proteins like CRP as well as pathologic autoantibodies and toxins including complements and other cytokines. For patients with acute renal failure, they will also require dialysis at the same time or in between plasmapheresis [P/P]. There are 2 types of P/P, centrifugation and membrane filtration. Venous access is necessary, either through a CVP, or through the I/J catheter or a femoral catheter.

2. In P/P, the blood components are separated from the plasma components. The plasma component is removed together with the acute phase proteins, antibodies, immune complexes and noxious cytokines. The cellular component of the blood is returned to the patient. In exchange for plasma stable plasma protein substitute or plasma in the form of fresh frozen plasma or fresh plasma is used as replacement fluid. Depending on the severity of the condition, P/P may be performed daily for the first 14 days and thereafter thrice weekly until the problem is resolved or the patient stable.

3. The indications for Plasmapheresis [P/P] include:

   (a) Renal Diseases with Anti-GBM antibodies

   (b) Rapidly Progressive Glomerulonephritis [RPGN].

   Here there are 3 subgroups [i] those with anti-GBM disease and Goodpasture's Syndrome [ii] those with immune complex mediated disease due to autoimmune disease like SLE, post infectious GN, mixed cryoglobulin and malignant IgA nephritis [iii] pauci immune diseases that are associated with anti-neutrophil cytoplasmic antibodies [ANCA] like Wegener's Granulomatosis and microscopic Polyarteritis Nodosa.

   Use of P/P in these conditions should be accompanied by intravenous methylprednisolone pulses as well as cyclophosphamide or cyclosporine A therapy with maintenance oral prednisolone. [i] and [ii] are more amenable to P/P, [iii] less amenable to P/P.

   (c) Lupus nephritis. Those patients with SLE complicated by RPGN (Crescenteric Lupus Nephritis) or those with Lupus Lung should have P/P as additional therapy. Euler *et al.* [Plasmapheresis and subsequent pulse cyclophosphamide in severe SLE. An interim report of the Lupus Plasmapheresis Study Group. Ann Med Intern (Paris) 1994, 145:296–302] in an uncontrolled study of 14 patients reported good response with P/P. However, in 1992, the Lupus Nephritis Collaborative Study Group in a larger randomised controlled trial of 46 patients with Class III, IV and V on P/P for 4 weeks showed no beneficial results [Lewis EJ *et al*. New Engl J Med 1992, 326:1373–1379]. Perhaps the duration of P/P was too short. In our Department our indications for P/P in SLE would be those with RPGN and Lupus Lung.

(d) Mixed Cryoglobulinemia — for severe cases, P/P thrice weekly for a month may be of help, plus cyclophosphamide, steroids and antiviral drug like ribavarine and interferon.

(e) Multiple Myeloma . Here renal impairment is related to several factors, namely precipitation of myeloma light chains in the renal tubules, hyperuricemia resulting from therapy, hypercalcemia, amyloidosis, infections, hyperviscosity, nephrotoxicity due to chemotherapy. There may be a role for removal of Bence Jones Protein via P/P and this could be renoprotective.

(f) Hemolytic Uremic Syndrome [HUS] and Thrombotic Thrombocytopenic Purpura [TTP] HUS is associated with severe renal failure, hemolysis due to microangiopathic haemolytic anemia and thrombocytopenia. If in addition to the above features, there are neurological features, then the condition is called TTP. The pathology is endothelial and microthrombi causing widespread organ injury. Among the underlying causes are autoimmune disease like SLE, antiphospholipid antibody syndrome, pregnancy and drugs including cyclosporine A and ticlopidine. If there is associated haemorrhagic diarrhoea caused by *E. coli*, the diagnosis is HUS due to *E. coli* toxins causing vascular injury to the colon thereby inducing endothelial and platelet injury with microthrombi. P/P is of benefit here and can be life saving as was shown in the outbreak of *E. coli* 0157:H7 in Scotland in 1996 [Dundas *et al*. Lancet 1999, 354:1327–1330].

(g) ABO Incompatible Kidney Transplant
Nowadays, using desensitising protocols consisting of intravenous immunoglobulin (IVIG) and P/P to remove IgG and IgM antibodies against the ABO group of the potential recipient, kidney transplantation can be done successfully. The recipient is also treated with the usual immunosuppressant

drugs consisting prednisolone, tacrolimus and mycophenolate mofetil. In Japan, ABO incompatible kidney transplant has gained popularity and good results of their outcome have been reported [Takahashi K *et al.* Amer J Transplant 2004, 4:1089–1096].

Rituximab versus cyclosphamide in ANCA associated renal vasculitis

To address the need to characterize the safety of rituximab, 44 patients from 8 centers with newly diagnosed ANCA related vasculitis were randomised to a 3:1 ratio of rituximab versus cyclophosphamide. After randomisation all patients received 1 gm methylprednisolone and 1 mg/kgBW of oral prednisolone daily. The steroids were reduced to 5 mg by end of 6 months. Those randomised to rituximab received 375 mg/m^2 per week of rituximab for 4 consecutive weeks and IV cyclophosphamide (15 mg/kg with the 1st and 3rd rituximab infusions) but did not receive azathioprine. Patients in the control group had IV cyclophosphamide for 3–6 months followed by azathioprine. Primary outcomes were sustained for remission and rates of severe adverse events at 12 months.

Sustained remission occurred in 76% of patients in the rituximab group and 82% of patients in the control group. Six patients in the rituximab group and 1 in the cyclophosphamide group died within the first 12 months. The median time to remission was 90 days in the rituximab and 94 days in the control groups. Forty two % of those in the rituximab and 36% of those in the control group had severe adverse events. 36% in the rituximab and 27% in the control group had infections. Mean eGFR increased from 20 to 39 ml/min in the rituximab and 12 to 27 ml/min in the control group at 12 months.

Though this trial may provide supportive evidence for the use of rituximab in ANCA associated renal disease, patients should be considered on a case by case basis as the risks of serious infections and even death are high [Lynda Szczech, Editorial, Kidney Int 2010, 78:631–632].

REFERENCES

1. Serra A, Cameron JS, A Review of Systemic Vasculitis. QJM, 1984, Llll, No. 210, pp. 181–207.
2. Nakagawa T *et al.* Unearthing Uric Acid: An ancient factor with recently found significance in renal and cardiovascular disease. *Kidney Int* 2006, **69**:1722–1725.
3. Lewis EJ *et al.* A controlled trial of plasmapheresis therapy in severe lupus nephritis. The Lupus Collaborative Study Group. *New Engl J Med* 1992, **326**:1373–1379.
4. Dundas *et al.* Effectiveness of therapeutic plasma exchange in the 1996 Lankashire E coli O157: H7 outbreak. *Lancet* 1999, **354**:1327–1330.
5. Takahashi K *et al.* Excellent long term outcome of ABO Incompatible living donor kidney transplant in Japan. *Amer J Transplant* 2004, **4**:1089–1096.
6. Jones *et al.* Rituximab versus cyclophosphamide in ANCA associated renal vasculitis. *New Engl J Med* 2010, **363**:211–220.

CHAPTER 24

Pregnancy and the Kidney

Patients with most forms of kidney diseases can become pregnant. Pregnancy however may cause the kidney function to become worse in patients with glomerulonephritis if there is already mild kidney failure before pregnancy and the blood pressure proves difficult to control. In general, regardless of the type of kidney disease, as long as the patient develops hypertension in pregnancy and as long as the blood pressure is uncontrolled, the patient is at great risk of developing kidney failure. In the case of patients who already have moderate renal failure, the stress of pregnancy may cause the patient to develop end stage renal failure sometimes within a few months of pregnancy.

PRECAUTIONS DURING PREGNANCY

A patient with kidney disease who becomes pregnant will require more intensive supervision. She has to visit not only the antenatal clinic but also the renal clinic very frequently. For example, she sees the nephrologist once a month or once in two months initially, but later, she may have to report once a fortnight or even weekly, depending on the progress of the pregnancy. This is because when patients with renal disease become pregnant, especially in cases of glomerulonephritis, they run a greater risk of developing pre-eclampsia, a condition in pregnant women associated with swelling of the legs, protein loss in the urine and hypertension. Pre-eclampsia can affect the kidneys and can cause kidney failure.

Regular and frequent visits to the nephrologist allows the monitoring of renal function. Blood tests (blood urea, creatinine and uric acid) and urine examination can detect worsening renal abnormalities including the presence of excess amounts of albumin in the urine. If the patient has pre-eclampsia it may precipitate kidney failure. This is especially when it is also associated with hypertension, and most of the time it is usually the uncontrolled hypertension in a patient with kidney disease and pregnancy which causes the patient to develop kidney failure. Hence the importance of frequent follow-ups to detect early kidney failure and uncontrolled hypertension. Hypertensive patients can be treated with methyldopa, labetalol, nifedipine LA. ACE inhibitors and ARBs should be avoided as they can cause renal dysfunction in the foetus. For severe hypertension intravenous labetalol, nicardipine and hydrallazine can be used. During breast feeding, methyldopa, labetalol, propranolol are preferred over atenolol and metoprolol which are concentrated in breast milk. ACE inhibitors are poorly excreted in breast milk and can be given. Diuretics cause poor production of milk and should be avoided.

If renal function progressively deteriorates in pregnancy and blood pressure becomes uncontrolled, the nephrologist may have to advise the termination of pregnancy.

In many pregnant patients with kidney disease prematurity appears more common. During pregnancy, a dialysis patient may have to increase the number of hemodialysis to 20 hours a week. Pregnant patients can also have Continuous Ambulatory Peritoneal Dialysis [CAPD]. They do just as well as on hemodialysis. ACE inhibitors should be avoided. The dose of Erythropoeitin should be adjusted to approximate physiological anemia of pregnancy. Exacerbation of hypertension is common during pregnancy. Measurement of volume status may prove difficult as the dry weight increases throughout pregnancy. For some mothers an early delivery may be necessary at 36 or 38 weeks. This is because in some cases the placenta cannot support the baby any longer and to persist with pregnancy may risk the health of the foetus.

PREGNANCY AND SYSTEMIC LUPUS ERYTHEMATOSUS (SLE)

This patient can become pregnant provided she has normal kidney function, blood pressure is well controlled and the disease is not active. However, she still runs the risk of developing renal failure as the disease is aggravated by pregnancy. The drugs the mother takes can also damage the foetus. (See chapter on Lupus Nephritis.) Those patients with active lupus, impaired renal function, hypertension and proteinuria during pregnancy would run the risk of fetal and maternal morbidity and mortality. Women with SLE with positive anti-phospholipid antibodies are at great risk of thrombosis with fetal loss and preeclampsia. Those with LN Class III and IV have higher risk of preeclampsia compared to LN Class II or V.

The drugs taken by a patient with SLE are prednisolone and azathioprine. These drugs are necessary if there is a lupus activation or uncontrolled lupus during pregnancy. In laboratory animals these drugs cause malformation of the offspring. But in practice the risk is small, i.e. 1 in 200 babies. About 25% of SLE patients who become pregnant will abort their foetus.

Immediately after pregnancy, the activity of the disease may become greater and some doctors raise the dosage of the drugs just before this stage as a precaution.

PREGNANCY IN A PATIENT ON DIALYSIS OR WITH A KIDNEY TRANSPLANT

The patient on regular dialysis can become pregnant. However, the incidence of pregnancy is low and when they do become pregnant it is important that the patient be dialysed more often in an attempt to improve the uraemic environment within the womb. The less uraemic the mother is, the better the foetus' chances of survival.

The patient who has undergone a kidney transplant can also become pregnant though the incidence is lower than in a normal woman because the prednisolone and azathioprine given to the patient may sometimes cause foetal abnormality. 90% of women regain fertility within 6 months of receiving a kidney transplant.

PREGNANCY IN A PATIENT WITH INHERITED RENAL DISORDERS

Patients with inherited disorders will need advice before contemplating pregnancy. In the case of a pregnant patient with polycystic kidneys, there is a possibility of the enlarged kidney causing obstruction to the passage of the baby during delivery.

Pregnancy in early Chronic Kidney Disease (CKD)

There is recent evidence that CKD even in the early stages of the disease increases the risk of adverse pregnancy related outcomes. Patients with stage 1 CKD had significantly worse outcomes than patients with low risk pregnancies. The early stages of CKD are frequently undetected due to the lack of symptoms. The diagnosis of this condition is even more challenging in pregnant women since the serum creatinine levels drop during early pregnancy. Researchers found that adverse pregnancy related outcomes, including caesarean section, pre term delivery, reduced foetal weight and need for neonatal intensive care were common in patients with CKD than in low risk individuals. The increased risks of adverse outcomes were significant even for patients with CKD stage 1. These findings suggest that a policy of early referral of CKD patients, preconception counselling and strict follow up of women with kidney disease even in the absence of renal impairment. The study also highlights the usefulness of pregnancy as a tool for the early diagnosis of CKD [McSharry C. Early CKD increases the risk of adverse outcomes in pregnancy. Nature Reviews Nephrology, 2010, 6:385.

REFERENCE

McSharry C. Early CKD increases the risk of adverse outcomes in pregnancy. *Nature Reviews Nephrology*, 2010, **6**:385.

Pregnancy in Renal Transplant Recipients

The voluntary National Transplantation Pregnancy Registry (NTPR) was established in the US in 1991 to collect information on pregnancy. They cautioned that specific immunosuppression therapies administered in pregnant transplant patients have not been addressed. Recent studies have shown that administration of mycophenolate mofetil to solid organ transplant recipients can cause increased risks of adverse outcomes in pregnancy and a specific pattern of birth defects. Also there is the risk of decreasing fertility rates in these patients.

REFERENCE

Coscia LA and Armenti VT. Pregnancy related outcomes in kidney transplant recipients: more data are needed. *Nature Reviews Nephrology*, 2010, **6**:131–132.

CHAPTER 25

Cancer and the Kidney

Cancers of the kidney are very uncommon. In fact, kidney tumours account for less than 1% of deaths from all forms of cancers. With the current treatment options for metastatic cancer which are sadly inadequate we have to evaluate new approaches to the therapy of cancer in order to make advances which will alleviate the plight of patients affected.

HYPERNEPHROMA

Cancer can occur in any organ and the kidney is no exception. When it arises in the kidney it is called renal carcinoma or hypernephroma. The cancer cells are actually cells in the renal tubules which have undergone a cancerous or malignant change. It is commoner in males and the peak age is from 60 to 70 years.

The patient may have blood in the urine, pain over the side of the abdomen or he may feel a weight or a mass in the side. Sometimes he may have fever associated with loss of weight and appetite.

Investigations

In the past the traditional investigation modalities consist of an intravenous pyelogram (IVP), ultrasound examination and renal arteriogram. Nowadays with the CT and MRI scans better morphological delineation can be obtained. The recent availability of the PET scan has enabled a greater accuracy in preoperative diagnosis as well as in detecting benign lesions differentiating malignant from benign cysts. The PET Scan can help to provide a high degree of specificity and sensitivity and is complementary to data obtained with the CT and MRI scans and can help affect management decisions.

Extent of involvement and Staging

Once a diagnosis of Renal Cell Carcinoma [RCC] is made, the next step is to stage the cancer. One has to assess the extent of involvement or spread of the tumour and whether the lymph nodes are affected and whether there any spread to distant organs or metastasis. The TNM staging is used for RCC where T refers to Primary Tumour [the size of the tumour, whether it is confined to the kidney or gone beyond the kidney capsule and extended to surrounding tissue or organs [T1 to T4]. N refers to involvement of Lymph Nodes [no metatasis to lymph nodes, whether it has involved a single regional lymph node or involved more than one regional lymph node [N0 to N2]. M refers to Distant Metastases, no distant metatases to presence of distant metatases [M0 to M1].

RCC can grow very large locally and spread to surrounding tissues, regional lymph nodes and other organs like the lungs, bones, liver, brain, adrenal glands and the contralateral kidney. A CT scan of the abdomen together with a CT of the chest and a bone scan usually would suffice, unless there are symptoms or signs to suggest other organ like the brain, in which a brain scan would be necessary. Finally a biopsy of the primary tumour or biopsy of a metastatic site is performed to obtain a tissue diagnosis and establish the type of cancer cell.

Surgical treatment

This can be radical nephrectomy or simple nephrectomy. Radical nephrectomy involved ligation of the renal artery and renal vein with en bloc excision of the kidney with surrounding fascia and the ipsilateral adrenal gland. This was practised in the 1960s. It offered a 5 year 66% survival rate compared to 48% for simple nephrectomy [Waters WB *et al*. Aggressive surgical approach to renal cell carcinoma, J Urol 1979, **122**(3):306–309]. Nowadays with better understanding of the process of metastasis and newer imaging technology, the role of radical nephrectomy is being debated, especially the removal of the ipsilateral adrenal gland. It may make subsequent therapy difficult if the tumour were to spread to the contralateral adrenal later on.

Today nephron sparing surgery or partial nephrectomy is being considered more frequently, especially for elective partial nephrectomy when the tumour is less than 4 to 5 cm in the polar region and the contralateral kidney is normal. Other reasons for nephron sparing surgery would be when both kidneys are involved, when there is only a solitary kidney or when there is already renal impairment or compromised renal function.

Radiofrequency Tissue ablation

In recent years, for patients with small tumours who are adverse to surgical removal, ablation of the tumour can be achieved with good results. However, some may consider this as not a total eradication of viable cancer cells especially since there is some evidence to suggest that the pathological analysis of tumour viability is between 90% to 100% tumour destruction. In other words, there is the remote possibility of small foci of tumour not eradicated and may pose problems in the future. Since the technique is relatively new compared to standard surgery, careful post procedure follow up is mandatory and hopefully with time such ablation techniques including cryoablation. These technique may in the longer term prove to be comparable to established surgical removal of the tumour [de Baere T *et al*. Radio frequency ablation of Renal Cell Carcinoma: Preliminary clinical experience. J Urol 2002, **167**(5):1961–1964].

Angioinfarction

This is a procedure to embolise the renal artery resulting in infarction of the renal tumour in situations where the tumour is very vascular and there is the risk of severe haemorrhage. It is also useful for large or difficult to resect tumours in order to control symptoms of bleeding and pain in patients where surgery is no so readily amenable. Patients may experience pain and nausea with fever for a few days following the procedure. The tumour will regress post procedure and in some cases distant metastases will also regress.

Radiation Therapy

Such therapy is useful for patients with metastases to organs like lungs, bone and brain. Radiation will shrink the metastatic lesions and provide relief of pain in kidney and bones. Cord compression can be relieved and the disability of the brain caused by the cerebral lesions may improve. Radiation is also useful for haemorrhage resulting from lesions in the bronchial mucosa.

Chemotherapy

The reponse to Chemotherapy have been disappointing. Vinblastine have response rates of less than 25%. Gemcitabine and 5 Flurouracil (5FU) have a response rate of about 15%. The poor response to chemotherapy could be due to the presence of markedly elevated mRNA for multidrug resistance protein found in the proximal tubules of the kidney, the source of renal cell carcinoma or the P-glycoprotein expression [Fojo AT *et al*. Intrinsic drug resistance in human kidney cancer is associated with expression of a human multidrug resistance gene. J Clin Oncol 1987, **5**(12):1922–1927].

Surgical removal of the tumour is the best form of treatment especially if the tumour has not spread beyond the capsule of the kidney. Radiotherapy to the tumour bed may be of some use but treatment with drugs (chemotherapy) is of little effect.

If the tumour is confined to the kidney during operation, a 60% 5-year survival rate can be expected. The overall survival is 40% at 5 years and 25% at 10 years. For patients with metastatic tumour, the survival is about 10 to 12 months [Motzer RJ *et al.* Survival and prognostic stratification of 670 patients with advanced renal cell carcinoma. J Clin Oncol 1999, **17**(8):2530–2540].

The mammalian target of rapamycin (mTOR) are new areas of therapy which could prove useful. Therapy with HIF inhibitors is another pathway involved in "success" and progression of RCC [Weiss RH and Lin PY. Kidney Cancer: Identification of novel targets for therapy. Kidney Int 2006, **69**:224–232].

WILMS' TUMOUR

This is a malignant tumour of the kidney which occurs in childhood, usually before the age of 5 years. The child is noticed to have a swollen abdomen and examination would reveal a mass on one side of the abdomen. The child may sometimes complain of pain in the abdomen. This tumour may also be associated with fever, high blood pressure or blood in the urine.

Surgery is usually performed to remove the tumour. This is followed by radiotherapy to the tumour bed and the surrounding areas. A drug called Actinomycin D is also given to destroy tumour cells. About 80% will survive 5 years. The outlook is poorer if the tumour has already spread to other areas.

ADENOMA OF THE KIDNEY

This is a benign tumour of the kidney. It is usually diagnosed during the investigation of some other unrelated complaint and the benign tumour shows up as a distortion of the kidney, usually as an abnormality on the IVP.

REFERENCES

1. Weiss RH and Lin PY. Kidney Cancer: Identification of novel targets for therapy. *Kidney Int* 2006, **69**:224–232.
2. De Baere T *et al.* Radio frequency ablation of Renal Cell Carcinoma: Preliminary clinical experience. *J Urol* 2002, **167**(5): 1961–1964.

CHAPTER 26

Inherited Kidney Diseases

Most forms of kidney diseases are not hereditary. Some however, can be inherited but these are rare and have a recessive pattern of inheritance. This is because in nature few individuals with dominant forms of disease would survive. Polycystic kidney disease in fact is the only common dominant form of kidney disease. It does not affect all individuals seriously and they can usually have a family.

PATTERNS OF INHERITANCE OF DISEASE

Dominant inheritance means that as long as the abnormal chromosome is passed to the offspring from one parent, the disease will appear in the offspring.

Recessive inheritance means that the individuals who carry the abnormal chromosomes are well. They are called carriers of the disease but are unaffected by it. Only if they marry another carrier will the disease appear in the offspring.

POLYCYSTIC KIDNEY

Polycystic kidney is the commonest form of inherited kidney disease. The kidneys are enlarged and replaced by cysts. Usually both kidneys are affected but one kidney may be larger than the other. It may appear at any age from infancy to old age but is usually diagnosed between 20 to 40 years. Polycystic kidney in an individual is usually diagnosed after an affected relative has been discovered and the other family members are called up for screening. Or the patient may present with high blood pressure, blood in the urine, chronic renal failure or urinary infections, and investigations for these manifestations lead to polycystic kidneys as the cause.

The most serious problem with this disease is chronic renal failure due to progressive loss of kidney function. The kidneys are slowly replaced by the enlarging cysts, and the patient usually develop end stage renal failure between the age of 45 and 65 years.

Renal failure begins in the 3rd and 4th decade of life when the GFR begins to decrease. Evolution of chronic renal failure is homogenous within families because genetic factors contribute to determining the age of onset of uraemia. The incidence of chronic renal failure is high amongst those with hypertension. The cause of chronic renal failure is attributed to:

(i) progressive arteriolar sclerosis resulting from activation of the renin angiotensin system (RAS). Patients have increased susceptibility determined by abnormal gene product and;

(ii) progressive interstitial fibrosis mediated by PDGF which causes increased proliferation of fibroblasts which in time leads to progressive fibrosis of the tubulo-interstitium. Hence ADPCK is considered a chronic tubulo-interstitial nephritis. PDGF is secreted by the epithelial cell of the cyst wall.

Hypertension is the most potent predictor of renal failure in ADPCK. The hypertension is caused by:

(i) impaired Sodium excretion and

(ii) increased production of renin from the parenchyma adjacent to expanding cysts giving rise to Angiotensin II medicated hypertension. Even normotensive ADPCK patients have been found to have increased renin activity (high PRA) suggesting a particular role of ACE inhibitor in the management of these patients.

In hypertensive ADPCK disease, treatment with ACE inhibitor or ARBs will control hypertension as well as ameliorate progressive arteriolar sclerosis resulting from activation of RAS, hence retarding progression of renal failure.

REFERENCE

Ritz E *et al*. Autosomal dominant PCK — mechanisms of cyst formation and renal failure. *Aust NZ J Mel*, 1993, **23**:35–41.

Inheritance of Polycystic Kidneys

Adult Polycystic Kidney Disease is due to an autosomal dominant trait with complete penetrance. There are 2 genes identified. In 85% of patients it is due to PKD1 due to an abnormality on the short arm of Chromosome 16 [chromosome region 16p13.3]. The other gene is PKD2 occurring in 15% [Chromosome region 4q21] of patients.

It is inherited in a dominant pattern which means that it has the potential to appear in every successive generation. Sometimes it may skip a whole generation. About 1 in 5 patients with polycystic kidneys has no known affected relative. Children of affected parents have a 1 in 2 chance [50%] of carrying the abnormal gene. Their children have a 1 in 4 chance of getting the disease.

Autosomal Dominant Polycystic Kidney Disease (ADPKD) is a common nephropathy caused by mutations in either PKD1 or PKD2. Mutations in PKD1 account for 85% of cases and cause more severe disease than mutations in PKD2. Diagnosis of ADPKD before the onset of symptoms is usually performed doing renal imaging by either ultrasonography, CT or MRI. In general these modalities are reliable for the diagnosis of ADPKD in older individuals. However, molecular testing can be valuable when a definite diagnosis is required in young individuals, in individuals with a negative history of ADPKD, and to facilitate preimplantation genetic diagnosis. Although linkage based diagnostic approaches are feasible in large families, direct mutation screening is generally more applicable. As ADPKD displays a high level of allelic heterogeneity, complete screening of both genes is required. Consequently, such screening approaches are expensive. Screening of individuals with ADPKD detects mutation in up to 91% of cases. However, only about 65% of patients have definite mutations with about 26% having nondefinite changes that require further evaluation.

Collation of known variants in the ADPKD mutation database and systemic scoring of nondefinite variants is increasing the diagnostic value of molecular screening. Genic information can be of prognostic value and recent investigations of hypomorphic PKD1 alleles suggests that allelic information may also be valuable in some atypical cases.

Nowadays various clinical trials are in progress for the treatment of PKD with a view to decreasing the growth of the cysts and preservation as well as retarding the progression of renal deterioration. This will shed a new light on a hitherto non treatable disease. With newer and more effective therapies developed for ADPKD, molecular testing will become more important and more widespread. In the foreseeable future the rapid developments in DNA sequencing will also revolutionise molecular testing for ADPKD [Harris PC and Rossetti S. Molecular diagnostics for ADPKD. Nature Reviews Nephrology, 2010, 6:197–206].

Patients with PKD1 have a more severe disease compared to those with PKD2. About 19% of PKD1 have adequate renal function at 60 years, compared to about 40% of those with PKD2. Those with PKD1 are also more likely to have intracranial aneurysms [Berry's aneurysm].

The cysts within the kidneys cause renal enlargement. Initially the kidneys are mild to moderately enlarged but with time, in advanced cases, the kidneys can be 20 times as enlarged. The cysts begin as outpouchings from preexisting renal tubules and as they grow larger they become detached from the tubule of origin. Int the end, the kidneys are usually several times larger than the normal kidneys, filled with numerous cysts full of fluid inside. There is little normal renal tissue between the cysts and the spaces between are occupied by fibrous tissues and sclerosed arterioles. About 90% of adults with ADPCK also have cysts within the liver. Liver cysts begin as outpouchings of the biliary ductules. They become detached as they grow and no longer communicate with the biliary tract.

Diagnosis

This condition is usually not detected on the intravenous pyelogram (IVP) until the child is in the late teens about 18 years or so. An IVP or ultrasound examination when the child is young may not detect the disease. However, even if cysts are seen, it does not mean that the child will always develop symptoms of the disease later on. A good number of people go through life without experiencing any clinical manifestations of the disease and majority do not have kidney failure. Once the disease is diagnosed the person should have an annual check of the blood pressure, and perform urine and blood tests once a year since the complications of these diseases are chronic renal failure, hypertension and urinary infections. The diagnosis is often made by renal ultrasound which is safe and inexpensive. The **criteria for diagnosis of PKD for individuals with 50% risk is at least 2 cysts which are unilateral or bilateral cysts in patients younger than 30 years**. For **those age between 30 years and 59 years, the criteria is 2 cysts in each kidney and for those above 60 years it is 4 cysts in each kidney**. For those with PKD1, aged 30 years and below, the sensitivity of these criteria is 100%. For PCK2, the sensitivity is about 67%. The **above criteria applies only for Ultrasound examination**. For more sensitive imaging like a CAT scan or an MRI, these techniques provide better anatomic definition as well as gives a better assessment with regards to severity and prognosis of the disease. This is also more easily applicable in individuals without family history or liver involvement.

The brother and sister of an individual with the disease will have a 1 in 2 chance of being affected. Sometimes new patients are found to have the disease without any known family history of the disease or any evidence of ADPKD in other family members despite ultrasound screening of siblings or parents. In these individuals, a change or mutation could have taken place causing a defect in the chromosome which gives rise to the disease. This could occur in about 5 to 20% of individuals and is due to spontaneous mutation of the gene.

Genetic Testing for ADPKD

One could resort to genetic testing for diagnosis when a child is young, when the results of imaging are inconclusive or when the person is being considered for living related kidney donation. Genetic testing is usually performed by linkage or sequence analysis. Linkage analysis uses highly informative microsatellite markers flanking PKD1 and PKD2. This method requires sufficient numbers of affected family members to be tested if it is going to be successful.

Another method is to do direct gene sequencing and a yield of up to 80% may be obtained. Some of the problems encountered however are that most mutations for PKD are unique and up to 1/3 of PKD1 changes are missense.

Clinical Features

One of the earliest features in the disease is the loss of the ability to concentrate the urine. The presence of haematuria may indicate infection in the cysts, rupture of the cyst with haemorrhage, stone formation within the cysts or even the presence of a renal cell carcinoma.

Urinary tract infection could be due to an infection in the urinary system, infection within the cysts, infected stones or an infection superimposed on a renal cell carcinoma.

Since ADPKD is a form of chronic tubulointerstitial nephritis with progressive fibrosis as glomeruli are lost, the surviving nephrons would be subject to Glomerular Hyperfiltration resulting in proteinuria and intraglomerular hypertension with further glomerulosclerosis leading eventually to chronic renal failure. ARBs are useful in reducing glomerular hyperfiltration and retarding the progression of renal failure.

Hypertension is due to the pressure and stretching of the renal vascular tree caused by the expanding cysts causing activation of the renin angiotensin system [RAS]. The RAS is also activated at the juxta glomerular apparatus [JGA] of the kidneys. In addition ectopic renin is also produced by the epithelial cells of the dilated renal tubules and the epithelium of the cyst walls. About 50% of patients have hypertension when they are in the late twenties and the thirties and as renal failure sets in almost 100% of patients eventually develop hypertension.

ARBs and if necessary, calcium channel blockers like amlodipine are useful agents in treating hypertension and retarding progression of renal failure. The target BP should be 130/80 mm Hg.

Pain in ADPKD could be due to haemorrhage within the cysts, rupture of cyst, infection, stones or presence of renal cell carcinoma which can be a rare cause of pain in ADPKD. Patients should be cautioned about excessive intake of NSAIDS causing deterioration of renal function.

Sometimes massive gross haematuria may occur associated with cyst rupture or haemorrhage within cysts, stones causing haemorrhage or burst vessel in the tumour. This may last from 2 to 3 days to a week. If the haemorrhage persists, imaging with ultrasound, CT or MRI would be necessary to exclude the underlying cause. If the ultrasound shows a solid mass, or if there is speckled calcifications on CT and regional lymphadenopathy on CT or MRI, the presence of a renal cell carcinoma is very likely and should be treated accordingly. For severe haemorrhage that persists, referral to a urologist for radiological imaging to elucidate the cause of the haemorrhage and if necessary surgery performed to remove the stone, infected cyst or tumour by means of a partial or total nephrectomy. In a patient already on dialysis, the treatment for cancer of the PKD would be total nephrectomy since there is no benefit derived from conserving the diseased kidney apart from its relatively small value of contributing towards erythropoietin [EPO] production since many patients with ADPKD do not require the use of human recombinant erythropoietin injections as the polycystic kidneys are still producing substantial amounts of EPO. Haemorrhage within cysts are usually self limiting. For severe haemorrhage, nephrectomy or segmental arterial embolisation may be necessary.

In the case of infected cysts, sometimes they are difficult to treat as the antibiotics may have difficulty penetrating into the cysts. One may have to resort to surgical drainage if antibiotics are unsuccessful. On some occasions, nephrectomy may have to be considered if the infection cannot be controlled.

Renal stone disease should be removed using percutaneous lithotripsy or extra corporeal shock wave lithotripsy. If stones cannot be removed, one would have to resort to alkalinisation of urine using sodium bicarbonate as well as long term prophylactic or suppressive antibiotics.

Chronic Renal failure usually occurs when the patients are in their 40's to 60's. By this time the kidneys would be fairly large and distorted and patients may feel discomfort in the abdomen. Those who have pain may need imaging to exclude some of the above causes described above. The following would be adverse risk factors for renal failure, PKD1 worse than PKD2. Males do worse than females. Those who are diagnosed before 30 years, those with proteinuria or hypertension before 30 years. For the patient with ESRF both hemodialysis and continuous ambulatory peritoneal dialysis [CAPD] or automatic peritoneal dialysis [APD] are all equally effective and there is no contraindication for PD despite the size of the kidneys. Renal transplantation is an acceptable modality of renal replacement therapy, either living related or cadaveric. There are no additional complications related to PKD and graft survival is comparable to the rest of the renal failure population not due to PKD. However, for patients with frequently infected cysts or haemorrhage, it may be advisable to perform pretransplant nephrectomy.

Polycystic liver is a common component of ADPKD. It is usually asymptomatic but with time as the cysts develop and grow larger complications like cyst haemorrhage, infection or rupture will occur. Cyst infection is associated with fever, pain and raised leukocyte counts. Cysts can occur also in the pancreas, arachnoid and seminal vesicles.

Apart from Intra Cranial Aneurysms [ICAs] or Berry's aneurysms, patients can develop coronary artery aneurysms and dissecting aneurysms in the thoraxic aorta. ICAs can be associated with focal seizures or facial palsy due to local compression. These aneurysms can rupture resulting in death. Once an aneurysm ruptures the patient should quickly have neurosurgery to clip the aneurysm as a life- saving procedure. Routine screening for ICAs is not recommended as the yields are usually small consisting of small aneurysms in the anterior communicating artery with small risk of rupture. However, screening in an individual is necessary if there is a family history of ICA rupture or subarachnoid haemorrhage or a patient in a high risk occupation like a pilot with ADPKD where the individual may have many lives depending on his fitness. CT angiography or MR angiography usually yield satisfactory results.

Another associated feature of the disease is the presence of mitral valve prolapse in about a quarter of the ADPKD population. Colonic diverticulosis is another associated feature.

Patients with this condition will require treatment for hypertension or urinary tract infection. Sometimes stones may form in the cysts and very rarely, a neoplastic change. Berry's aneurysm is another associated feature. Rupture of the aneurysm causes cerebral haemorrhage.

Clinical Trials

An important ongoing clinical trial in human ADPKD uses long acting octreotide which is a somatostatin analog which has been shown to arrest the growth of cysts in the kidneys and liver of rats with PKD [Masyuk TV, Masyuk AI, Torres VE *et al*. Octreotide inhibits hepatic cystogenesis *in vitro* and *in vivo*: a new therapeutic approach for treatment of polycystic liver disease. Gastroenterology 2006, 132:1104–1116]. Other drugs like rapamycin and everolimus, both mTOR inhibitors have also been shown to arrest cysts growth and clinical trials in human ADPKD are underway [Shillingford JM, Murcia NS, Larson CH *et al*. The mTOR pathway is regulated by polycystin-1, and its inhibition reverses renal cystogenesis in polycystic kidney disease. Proc Natl Acad Sci USA, 2006, 103:5466–5471]. However, recent reports have been disappointing, see below.

mTOR inhibitors and kidney growth in ADPKD

Walz [Walz *et al*. New Engl J Med advance on line publication, 26th June 2010, doi:10.1056/NEJMoa1003491] in a two year double blind trial randomly assigned 433 patients with ADPKD to receive either placebo or mTor inhibitor everolimus. Total kidney volume increased between baseline and 1 year by 102 ml in the everolimus group versus 157 ml in the placebo group and between baseline and 2 years it was 230 ml versus 301 ml respectively. Cyst volume increased by 76 ml in the everolimus group and 89 ml in the placebo group. At 2 years it was 181ml versus 215 ml respectively. The mean decrease in eGFR after 2 years was 8.9 ml/min in the everolimus group versus 7.7 mls in the placebo group. Therefore despite the slowing of cyst growth, there was no decline in progressive renal impairment.

In another study by Serra [Serra *et al*. New Eng J Med advance on line publication, 26th June 2010, doi:10.1056/NEJMoa0907419] with sirolimus, among 100 patients with ADPKD over 18 months, comparing those randomly assigned on sirolimus versus standard care, all patients with creatinine clearance of at least 70 ml/min. At randomisation, the median total kidney volume was 907 cc in the sirolimus group versus 1003 cc in the control group. The median increase at 18 months in the sirolimus group was 102% of that in the control group. The GFR was not different in the two groups but albumin excretion was higher in the sirolimus group.

These two studies therefore did not provide evidence of slowing the progression of renal insufficiency, though treatment may initially retard the growth of the cysts. The GFR did not improve. Stomatitis was a common side effect. The increase in proteinuria in the treatment group was also not encouraging.

REFERENCE

Detlef Schlondorff. *J Am Soc Nephrol* 2010, **21**:1031–1040.

AUTOSOMAL RECESSIVE POLYCYSTIC KIDNEY DISEASE (ARPKD)

ARPKD or Infantile polycystic kidney is another form of polycystic kidney that appears in infancy. The baby is born with enormous kidneys. The disease is different from the dominant adult form of polycystic kidney as it is inherited in a recessive fashion and has a very poor outlook compared to the adult form. ARPKD is due to mutation on chromosome 6p21.1-p12 (PKHD1). Parents who have an affected child have a 1 in 4 chance of having another child with the same disease in any subsequent pregnancy. Studies have shown that ARPKD Mutations are also responsible for Congestive Heart Failure and Caroli disease (non obstructive intrahepatic bile duct dilatation).

Both the kidneys and liver are affected in inverse proportions. There is a spectrum where the kidneys are severely affected and the liver mildly affected to one where the kidneys are mildly affected but liver severely affected. The form where the kidneys are more affected is more common and occurs at or near the time of birth. The kidneys are affected in the perinatal and neonatal forms that is manifested at or near the time of birth. Kidneys can be symmetrically and bilaterally affected up to 20 times normal and may cause difficulty at childbirth. Diagnosis is made by ultrasound in utero or shortly after birth which show enlarged kidneys with increased echogenecity in the cortex and medulla. The demand for prenatal diagnosis is high among couples with previous pregnancies affected by ARPKD.

Among the Clinical Features would be bilaterally enlarged kidneys which would be evident even in utero, sometimes associated with oligohydramnios due to decreased urine output. Other features include respiratory embarrassment at birth due to pulmonary hypoplasia or the enlarged kidneys . As a result about 30% of the neonates would perish at birth. Those infants who survive this period would usually survive to adulthood nowadays, compared to long ago when many more would have perished before reaching adulthood. These adult patients with ARPKD would usually have hypertension and renal insufficiency even from an early age. As a result many have growth retardation, anemia, renal osteodystrophy. Even as adolescents they would have portal hypertension presenting with bleeding oesophageal varices, splenomegaly and hypersplenism.

Treatment for those patients who survive the initial neonatal period consists of addressing the immediate problems associated with pulmonary embarrassment due to pulmonary hypoplasia, atelectasis, pneumothorax and pneumonia. They will require the expertise of the respiratory physician and thoraxic surgeon for assessment and corrective measures. For cases related mainly to the enlarged kidneys, bilateral nephrectomies may have to be considered followed by renal replacement therapy in the form of peritoneal dialysis, hemodialysis or renal transplant. Hypertension should be treated together with urinary infections when they occur. Portosystemic shunting would be required for severe bleeding oesphaageal varices.

MEDULLARY SPONGE KIDNEY

This is a condition where there are many tiny ductular cysts (tubular ectasia) in the medulla or inner portion of the kidneys. The outlook for patients with this condition is very good as they do not develop kidney failure compared to polycystic kidney disease. However they are prone to two complications. One is urinary infection and the other is very small stones forming in the kidney. It is not a hereditary disorder.

INHERITED RENAL STONES

Cystinuria is a condition that is inherited in an autosomal recessive fashion. It causes recurrent kidney stones in the patient because the patient excretes excessive amounts of the amino acid cystine in the urine. Patients usually respond well to treatment with a combination of high fluid intake, alkalinisation of urine and a drug called penicillamine. If the patient can be kept free of recurrent stones he should not develop kidney failure. This will require cooperation on the part of the patient to adhere to his medical treatment.

HEREDITARY GLOMERULONEPHRITIS

Most forrns of glomerulonephritis are not hereditary. However there are a few rare forms that run in families.

1. Alport's Syndrome

This is a form of glomerulonephritis where the patient passes blood in the urine and develops progressive deafness. It is a sex-linked disorder with males more severely affected than females. When a male is affected he is usually deaf by 10 years and has chronic renal failure by 15 years. But in the case of the affected female she only has some blood and protein in the urine and is none the worse even years afterwards.

2. Benign Familial Haematuria

This is a condition where individuals in a family pass blood in the urine, usually microscopic amounts, but they do not develop deafness or renal failure.

3. Congenital Nephrotic Syndrome

The affected child is born with the condition where he has swelling of the face and limbs, passes a lot of protein in the urine and has low serum albumin level because of the protein loss in the urine. It is inherited as a recessive disease and parents have a 1 in 4 chance of further having affected children with subsequent pregnancies. It is particularly common in Finland but is very rare here.

FABRY'S DISEASE (ANGIOKERATOMA CORPORIS DIFFUSUM)

1. This is an X-linked recessive disease. It is a glycosphingolipidosis affecting young adults which leads to renal failure.
2. Manifestations include peripheral neuropathy, cutaneous non-blanching angiectases, vascular occlusions of the cardiovascular and the central nervous system. The renal lesions are characterised by fat deposits.
3. An enzyme called trihexosyl ceramidase is deficient and this leads to deposition of fat in the tissues.
4. The patient requires a renal transplant to cure the condition as the donor kidney produces the deficient enzyme.

CONGENITAL MALFORMATION AND DEVELOPMENTAL ANOMALIES

These include horseshoe kidneys, duplex kidneys (duplication of the kidneys or the pelvis and ureter), bifid ureter and other malformations like agenesis and hypoplastic kidney as well as cysts, aberrant renal arteries and retrocaval ureter.

REFERENCES

1. Torres VE and Harris PC. Autosomal Dominant Polycystic Kidney Disease. *Kidney Int* 2009, **76**:149–168.
2. Chapman A. The cadence of kidney growth in ADPKD. *Nature Reviews Nephrology*, 2009, **5**:311–312.
3. Harris PC and Rossetti S. Molecular diagnostics for ADPKD. *Nature Reviews Nephrology*, 2010, **6**:197–206.
4. Detlef Schlondorff. mTOR inhibitors and kidney growth in ADPKD. *J Am Soc Nephrol* 2010, **21**:1031–1040.

CHAPTER 27

Drugs and the Kidney

Nowadays with the number of patients with Chronic Kidney Disease [CKD] with renal dysfunction it is important that the nephrologist is aware of the side effects of many of the drugs the patients with kidney disease require and also the precautions to be taken when administering various drugs to these patients because many drugs can cause a worsening of renal function. Another aspect is that many patients with cardiac disease also have renal impairment because of associated renal disease and many of the drugs taken by patients with hypertension or diabetes mellitus also affect the renal function. Likewise, renal patients also take many types of drugs and these classes of drugs are also the same ones used by cardiologists for various cardiac indications. Drugs like ACEI and ARBs as well as many types of other drugs used for hypertension are used by cardiologists and nephrologists for indications within their respective specialities. We must remember that the kidney is the organ which excretes many drugs and any change in renal function will affect the pharmacology of these drugs. Finally, existing or residual renal function of the patient will have to be taken into account during drug prescribing. This is just as important for the patient with CKD 4 and 5 as well as the patient on peritoneal dialysis as they tend to have better preservation of residual renal function compared to the hemodialysis patient. Nephrotoxic drugs including NSAIDS can very readily destroy whatever residual renal function they still have. Residual renal function is important to preserve as it contributes to less patient morbidity and mortality. Recently, there have been adverse reports of Zoledronic Acid [Aclasta] a biphosphonate that works by inhibiting osteoclast-mediated bone resorption thereby slowing the breakdown of bone to reduce the risk of fracrures. As of

August 14th 2009, there have been 139 post marketing reports of renal impairment following the use of Zoledronic Acid infusion worldwide. Many of these occur in patients with pre existing medical conditions or risk factors [elderly, renal impairment and or concurrent dehydration] or on NSAIDS or other concurrent exposure to other nephrotoxic agents. There have been rare cases requiring dialysis and fatal outcome have been reported in patients with pre existing renal impairment and concomitant risk factors [Health Science Authority, Singapore. Adverse Drug Reaction News. August 2010, Vol12, No 2. Pg2].

In a patient with renal impairment it is necessary to adjust the dose or the dosing interval of certain drugs which are excreted by the kidneys. Drugs which are excreted by the kidneys are water soluble. Lipophilic drugs are metabolised in the liver into water soluble metabolites before excretion by the kidneys. Apart from the excretion of the drug itself, one has also to consider the elimination of metabolites which may still possess significant pharmacological properties like cyclosporin A and its toxic metabolites.

In clinical practice, one generally administers an initial dose and the maintenance doses are reduced according to the degree of renal failure using various formulae based on the weight of the patient and the level of the serum creatinine.

For example: If one wants to prescribe gentamicin to a male patient weighing 60 kg with a serum creatinine of 3.2 mg/dl:

The loading dose would be 1 mg/kg BW which would be 60 mg of gentamicin.

The dosing interval in hours would be: Serum creatinine multiplied by a factor of 7, i.e. $3.2 \times 7 = 22.4$ hours or once a day dosing interval. The next dosing interval would depend on the next day's serum creatinine level. One could increase the dose and prolong the dosing interval or reduce the dose and shorten the dosing interval.

For amikacin, a factor of 9 is used in the calculation.

The above calculation at best is still a very crude approximation as too many assumptions have been made.

The dose and frequency for patients on hemodialysis [HD], peritoneal dialysis [PD] and continuous renal replacement therapy [CRRT] also has to be varied, e.g.

Gentamicin, for treating UTI, dose is 1mg/kg given post HD, every 48 hours for a PD patient and 24 to 48 hours for a CRRT patient.

For Tobramycin for UTI, also 1 mg/kg given post HD, every 48 hours for a PD patient and 24 to 48 hours for a CRRT patient.

For Amikacin, dose is 7.5 mg/kg given post HD, every 48 hours for a PD patient and 24 to 48 hours for a CRRT patient.

Serum peak concentration [for efficacy] and troughs [for toxicity] must be monitored. Obtain levels with the 4th dose after initiation of therapy or after dose adjustment. It is important to obtain serum concentrations earlier [with the 3rd dose] in patients with low CrCl [<50 ml/min]. Recheck only trough levels every 5 to 7 days to ensure levels remain low. A trough level must be obtained within 30 mins of a dose and a peak level at least 30 mins only after the end of an infusion. In patients with severe dysfunction, random levels taken around the time the subsequent dose is due should be obtained to determine the appropriate dosing interval. In hemodialysis patients, check a level prior to the next scheduled dialysis. In both patient groups, redose when level [troughs] falls to <2 mcg/ml for gentamicin/tobramycin and <10 mcg/ml for amikacin.

When prescribing we use a loading dose equivalent to that used in a patient with normal renal function to ensure that therapeutic drug concentration is rapidly achieved. Next the subsequent drug dose is determined. This dose is a fraction of the normal drug dose [Df] and is derived from the formula: Df = t1/2 normal divided by t1/2 renal failure. t1/2 is the elimination half life of a drug in a patient with normal renal function, and t1/2 renal failure is the elimination half life of the drug in a patient with renal failure. If we want to maintain the normal dose interval in a patient with renal failure, the amount of each dose is derived from the formula: Dose in renal impairment + normal dose × df. This dose is given in the same dose interval as for patients with normal renal function. This method is used for drugs with a narrow therapeutic range and a short plasma half life.

Another method of prescribing is to give the same dose as a patient with normal renal function but at a longer dose interval. This is useful for drugs with a broad therapeutic range and a long plasma half life. The formula used is as follows: Dose interval = Normal dose × interval divided by Df.

In patients with renal failure on dialysis and CRRT, the antibiotic dosages and the dose interval would also vary depending on the moiety of dialysis used. Intermittent HD [IHD] removes drugs by diffusion across the dialysis membrane. Drugs less than 500 daltons and are less than 90% protein bound are more easily removed. This will also vary with the use of high flux membranes with patients on high flux dialysis. A patient on daily dialysis may be underdosed and a patient on slow efficiency dialysis may also require a larger dose compared to someone on IHD.

For patients on CAPD, drugs are less efficiently removed compared to IHD. Here also drugs that are of smaller MW and less protein bound are more readily removed. Ideally for better concentration the drugs should be given intraperitoneally. As PD patients still have residual renal function, this is another factor to be considered.

For CRRT, the amount of drug removed depends on the membrane used, the rate of blood flow, whether dialysate is used and the MW of the drug itself. The volume of drug distribution is an important factor, just as the binding of the drug to protein. If a drug is about 80% protein bound, it is not readily removed by convection or diffusion during CRRT.

THE EFFECTS OF DRUGS ON THE KIDNEYS

I. Renal Haemodynamic Changes

1. NSAID or non-steroidal anti-inflammatory agents like indomethacin, naprosyn and mefenamic acid decrease GFR. They inhibit the synthesis of prostaglandins since they are

prostaglandin synthetase inhibitors and prostaglandins are important in maintaining vasodilation and promotion of renal blood flow.

2. ACEI and ARBs like enalapril and losartan can cause renal failure because they antagonise the angiotensin II receptors at the efferent arterioles of glomeruli, and thereby decrease intraglomerular BP resulting in lowered GFR.

3. Cyclosporin A can cause severe tubulo-interstitial injury as well as inhibition of prostaglandin synthesis resulting in renal failure. (See chapter on Renal Transplantation.) Cyclosporin A also causes increased platelet aggregation and predisposes to thrombosis of renal blood vessels.

II. Direct Tubular Toxicity

1. Lithium carbonate is toxic to the distal tubules and causes nephrogenic diabetes insipidus.

2. Amphotericin B produces tubular damage with renal impairment. It also causes Distal or Type I RTA.

3. Outdated tetracyclines cause Fanconi's syndrome (Type II RTA). Tetracycline too causes a hypercatabolic state with marked elevation of blood urea in patients with renal impairment.

4. Analgesics like aspirin, even paracetamol in high doses and NSAID cause papillary necrosis of the kidneys (analgesic nephropathy). The newer NSAIDS like vioxx and celebrax too have been known to cause not only renal impairment but also acute renal failure in some patients.

5. Aminoglycosides damage predominantly the proximal tubules.

Characteristically they produce non-oliguric acute renal failure. This occurs more commonly in the elderly, especially when they are dehydrated or given diuretics. Combination with cephaloridine further aggravates the nephrotoxicity. The second and third generation cephalosporins do not have a synergistic nephrotoxic effect with the aminoglycosides.

III. Blockage of Renal Tubules

1. Sulphonamides can cause crystalluria because of poor solubility especially in an acidic urine. It is therefore important to alkalinise the urine of patients who are prescribed sulphonamides.
2. Methotrexate in high dose can cause acute tubular necrosis due to its precipitation in the renal tubules.
3. Methoxyflurane causes oxaluria with intratubular precipitation of calcium oxalate crystals, giving rise to renal failure.
4. Triamterene (see chapter on Diuretics) can cause crystals and casts to form in the tubules, giving rise to triamterene stones.

IV. Immunologically Mediated Damage

1. Sulphonamides, bactrium, allopurinol, methicillin, even ampicillin can all cause an acute allergic interstitial nephritis associated with Steven Johnson's syndrome. See chapter on Renal Tubular Disorders.
2. Penicillamine produces a membranous glomerulonephritis resulting in the nephrotic syndrome.
3. Rifampicin can give rise to an immune complex glomerulonephritis and methicillin can cause a rapidly progressive glomerulonephritis due to formation of anti-glomerular basement membrane antibodies (anti-GBM antibodies).

V. Injury Related to Changes in Electrolytes

1. Diuretics can cause hypokalaemia inducing vacuolar degeneration of the tubules with nephrogenic diabetes insipidus.

2. Vitamin D therapy can induce hypercalcaemia predisposing to intrarenal calcification and tubular damage with renal impairment.

PRACTICE POINTS

1. In any patient with renal impairment it is always useful to take a drug history, especially with regard to the use of analgesics both from the point of analgesic nephropathy as well as NSAID related renal failure. Remember that ACE inhibitors and ARBs prescribed for hypertension or proteinuria can also cause renal impairment.
2. In a patient with rash and renal impairment, think of acute allergic interstitial nephritis. Enquire about the use of allopurinol, bactrium and other antibiotics given by other doctors. Check for eosinophilia and eosinophils in the urine.
3. Remember aminoglycosides as a very common cause of renal impairment when dealing with a patient who has sepsis and renal failure. Check the levels of aminoglycosides in the serum.
4. Withdrawal of the offending agent, e.g. ACE inhibitor or ARB will result in an improvement of renal function.
5. Sometimes a renal biopsy may have to be performed to confirm or exclude acute interstitial nephritis.

DRUGS WHICH REQUIRE CAUTION AND ALTERATION OF DOSAGE IN RENAL FAILURE

A 1. Antibiotics

- Aminoglycosides: Marked decrease in dose required. Monitor drug levels.
- Cephalosporins: Avoid cephaloridine which is very nephrotoxic. The newer generation may require some alteration of dosage.

- Ciprofloxacin: Adjust dose when large doses are used.
- Nitrofurantoin: Avoid in renal failure since it causes very painful neuropathy. Like nalidixic acid it is also useless in renal failure as both are not concentrated in the kidneys in renal failure to be of any use.
- Penicillin: Adjust dose only when large doses are used.
- Tetracycline: Avoid in renal failure because of catabolic effect. Doxycycline can be used.
- Acyclovir, Ganciclovir: Reduce dose; can cause mild renal impairment. In patients with renal failure or on hemodialysis always use reduced doses as these patients can develop acute brain toxicity with confusion, seizures and coma. Acyclovir, valaciclovir and valganciclovir accumulate in renal failure, resulting in CSF levels of both parent compound and metabolite resulting in neuropsychiatric side effects.
- Amphotericin B: Slight reduction in dose. Usually causes renal impairment even in patients with normal renal function. Nowadays the use of fluconazole or nizoral and other newer oral anti fungal agents have often obviated the need for amphotericin.
- Bactrium or Septrin (combination of sulphonamide and trimethoprim): Adjust dose in renal failure.
- Ethambutol: Reduce dose.
- 5-fluorocytosine: Marked decrease in dose.
- Isoniazid: Reduce in advanced renal failure.
- Para-amino-salicylic acid: Avoid in renal failure.
- Streptomycin: Marked reduction of dose.

A 2. Anti-Convulsants and Sedatives

- Phenobarb: Reduce dose in advanced renal failure.
- Phenytoin: Reduce dose in advanced renal failure. The absorption of phenytoin is slow. Its protein binding is decreased and volume distribution increased in renal failure. Look out for nystagmus as a sign of toxicity. Seizures may also occur.

Diazepams and chlordiazepoxide and phenothiazines can all cause prolonged sedation and care has to be exercised when prescribing these to patients with renal impairment.

Lithium carbonate has been used for depression. Dose reduction and plasma lithium level monitoring is required when prescribing for those with renal impairment. Hemodialysis can be used to remove overdose of lithium.

A 3. Anticoagulants and Anti-Platelet Agents

* Warfarin, heparin and dipyridamole: May be useful to reduce dose as patients with renal failure have a tendency to bleed. These agents should be withdrawn when serum creatinine exceeds 400 micro M/L as patients will require surgery for creation of arteriovascular fistulae for dialysis access. For all patients on warfarin, it has to be stopped 10 days to 2 weeks before surgery and commenced 10 days to 2 weeks post operatively. The combination of clopidogrel and aspirin has been associated with haemorrhagic complications in hemodialysis patients given these agents to prevent thrombosis of AV fistulae. The use of LMW heparins has resulted in excessive anticoagulation in patients with GFR <50%. It may be safer to half the dosage of LMW heparin if one has to use it in patients with renal impairment who need it for thromboprophylaxis.

A 4. Antineoplastic agents

* Cisplatin
  Primary site of nephrotoxicity is at distal tubular and collecting ducts.

  Use with moderate hydration (3 litres per day) and mannitol or frusemide diuresis to reduce nephrotoxicity.

  Do not exceed $120 \, mg/M^2$ body surface area as it causes irreversible toxicity.

- Nephrotoxicity due to these agents can be manifest as acute renal failure, chronic renal failure or specific tubular dysfunction.

C. Cardiac Drugs

- Digoxin: Marked reduction in dose.
  Be careful when using antiarrhythmic drugs because toxicity may occur. Monitor the ECG and look out for prolonged QT interval or widening of QRS complex.

D. Diuretics

In patients with renal impairment, the use of diuretics may cause dehydration and cause them to lose more renal function. Also, potassium sparing diuretics may cause severe hyperkalaemia which could be lethal.

- Frusemide and other loop diuretics: Require large doses to be effective.
  Burinex more effective (1 mg ≡ 40 mg of Frusemide). Beware of dehydration and aggravation of renal failure.
- Spironolactone: Avoid in renal failure as it is a potassium sparing diuretic.
- Thiazides: Not effective in renal failure. Thiazides lose their efficacy when GFR falls below 30 ml/min.

H 1. H 2 Antagonists

- Cimetidine, ranitidine: Reduce dose; ranitidine is preferred. Nowadays with the use of famotidine and omeprazole, cimetidine is less often prescribed for renal patients.

H 2. Hypolipidaemic Drugs

- Eicosapentanoic acid: Caution, reduce dose because of bleeding tendency in uraemics.
- Gemfibrozil: Caution, reduce dose in renal failure.
       Simvastation, Pravastatin: In severe renal failure, reduce dose.
- Never combine Gemfibrozil and statin as this will cause myoglobinuria with renal failure.

H 3. Hypotensive Drugs

- ACE inhibitors and ARBs: Reduce dose in renal failure, monitor renal function and serum potassium. *ACE inhibitor and ARBs are used to reduce intra-glomerular hypertension in patients with glomerular hyperfiltration. Withdraw when serum creatinine exceeds 400 micro M/L as danger of hyperkalaemia increased.
- Beta blockers: Reduce dose as metabolites are active (Atenolol).

I. Immunosuppressive Drugs

- Azathioprine: Reduce dose.
- Cyclophosphamide: Reduce dose.
- Cyclosporin A: Reduce dose, monitor levels.

N. Non-Steroidal Anti-Inflammatory Drugs (NSAID), Analgesics

Prostaglandins [PG] are important in maintaining vasodilation and renal autoregulation. NSAIDS are prostanglandin synthetase inhibitors and prevent production of PG in the kidney leading to deleterious vasoconstriction and renal failure. NSAIDS also cause hyperkalaemia and fluid retention in renal patients. Recently, NSAIDS have also been associated with cardiac deaths in those on long term usage. Antithrombotic effect of aspirin is also neutralized by NSAIDS.

- Aspirin, indocid, ponstan, naproxen, ketoprofen, diclofenac, sulindac, vioxx, celebrex (celecoxib, cycloxygenese-L-inhibitors): Try to avoid as they can cause or worsen renal failure.
  Codeine or Gingerol (Zinax) may be useful substitutes as analgesics. Gingerol is mild and slow acting.
  The accumulation of active metabolites of morphine and meperidine may cause prolonged sedation. Prolonged narcosis is seen with patients on codeine and dihydrocodeine and these durgs should be prescribed with caution in patients with renal impairment.

O. Oral Hypoglycaemics

- Avoid long acting oral hypoglycemics like Chlorpropamide, Glibenclamide in renal failure. Use short acting ones like Tolbutamide and Diamicron (Gliclazide) and short to intermediate acting ones like Minidiab (Glipizide). Both Glicazide and Glipizide must be used with caution as they can cause hypoglycaemia, Glicazide is preferable to Glipizide. Another alternative is to use Rosiglitazone which is a Thiazolidinedione which increases sensitivity of peripheral tissue to insulin action. Rosiglitazone does not require dose reduction in renal failure but should still be used with caution because of hypoglycemia as renal failure progresses.
- Metformin: Avoid in renal failure as there is risk of lactic acidosis. Avoid in patients with diabetic nephropathy. The

kidneys excrete metformin and the risk of metformin accumulation and lactic acidosis increases with age and is a problem in the elderly with renal impairment.

Renal Transplant: Drugs to avoid

- Allopurinol: Avoid in a transplant patient on Azathioprine. It interferes with metabolism of Azathioprine through purine pathway as it is a xanthine oxidase inhibitor, thus potentiating effect of Azathioprine and causing bone marrow suppression.
- Erythromycin: Caution in transplant patient on Cyclosporine A. Avoid if possible. Will cause CyA toxicity as it interferes with liver enzyme (Cytochrome P 450) which metabolises CyA. Check CyA levels and reduce dose of CyA.

Table 27.1 is a compilation of many of the common drugs used in patients with all forms of kidney diseases through the various stages of chronic kidney disease from CKD 1 to 5. For CKD 1 and 2, in most instances there is no necessity to modify the dose of the drug or increase the time interval for the next dose so as to reduce the total amount of drug given to the patient over a certain time frame in order to avoid drug toxicity both for the kidney as well as for the patient as a whole. Patients on hemodialysis, peritoneal dialysis and CRRT would also require modification of the dose or duration interval between drug dosing. In the table "100" means 100% of the standard dose. "50" means 50% of the standard dose and "25" means 25% of the standard dose. "Inj" means Injection through intravenous, intramuscular or subcutaneous route. Otherwise the presumed route of drug administration will be "Oral". "Precaution" means one should be cautious with the use of the drug and should advise the patient about possible complications e.g. when prescribing oral hypoglycemics to patients with diabetic nephropathy with renal impairment as there is a danger of the patient developing hypoglycaemia if the dose of

Table 27.1   List of Drugs which may Need Modification in Patients with Chronic Kidney Disease

DRUG	CKD 1,2 GFR >60ml SeCreat <150	CKD 3,4 GFR 60–15 ml/min SeCreat 150–300	CKD 5 GFR <15 ml/min Se Creat>300 μ mol/l	Hemodialysis	CAPD	CRRT
Acarbose	100% dose	100% dose	100% dose	no	no	no
Acyclovir	5 mg/kg 8hrly	5 mg/kg 12 hrly	5 mg/kg 24 hrly	5 mg/kg 24hrly	5 mg/kg 24 hrly	5 mg/kg 12 hrly
Allopurinol	200	100	100	100	100	100
Amiloride	100	50	no	no	no	no
Amikacin	100% 12 hrly Inj	75% 12 hrly Inj	50% 24 hrly Inj	5 mg/kg post HD	15 mg/kg EOD	15 mg/kg OM
Amytriptylline	100	100	100	100	100	100
Amiodarone	100	100	100	100	100	100
Amlodipine	100	100	100	100	100	100
Amoxycillin	100	100	50	50	50	100
Amphotericin	Inj 24 hrly	Inj 24 hrly	Inj 36 hrly	Inj 36 hrly	Inj 36 hrly	Inj 24 hrly
Ampicillin	Inj 6 hrly	Inj 8 hrly	inj 12 hrly	inj 12 hrly	Inj 12 hrly	inj 8 hrly
Aspirin	precaution	precaution	precaution	precaution	precaution	precaution
Atenolol	100	100	50	50	50	100
Azathioprine	100	75	50	50	50	75
Azithromycin	100	100	100	100	100	100
Aztreonam	100	75	50	50	50	75
Benzafibrate	75	50	no	72 hrly	72 hrly	50%
Captopril	100	75	50	50	50	75
Ceftazadine	1gm BD	1 gm OM	1 gm OM	1 gm post HD	1gm OM	1 gm OM
Ceftibuten	400mg OM	200 mg OM	200 mg OM	400 mg post HD	200 mg OM	200 mg OM

(Continued)

Table 27.1   *(Continued)*

Ceftriazone	100	100	100 post HD	100	100
Chlorpropamide	precaution	no	no	no	no
Cilazapril	75	50	50 post HD	50	75
Cimetidine	100	50	50	50	50
Ciprofloxacin	100	50	50	50	50
Cisplastin	75	50	50	50	75
Clavulinic Acid	100	75	75	75	100
Clindamycin	100	100	100	100	100
Codeine	100	100	100	100	100
Colchicine	100	100	100	100	100
Cyclophosphamide	50	50	no	no	no
Cyclosporine A	50 precaution	50 precaution	precaution	precaution	precaution
Dapsone	100	50	50	50	100
Diazepam	100	100	100	100	100
Diazoxide	100	100	100	100	100
Diclofenac	100	100	100	100	100
Digoxin	50	25	25	25	50
Diltiazem	100	100	100	100	100
Eicosapentanoic Acid	75	50	no	no	no
Erythromycin	100	75	75	75	100
Ethambutol	24 hrly Inj	36 hrly Inj	48 hrly Inj	48 hrly Inj	36 hrly Inj
Flucytosine	12 hrly Inj	12 hrly Inf	24 hrly Inj	24 hrly Inj	12 hrly Inj

(Continued)

Table 27.1 (*Continued*)

Foscarnet	25 mg/kg 8 hrly	15 mg/kg 8 hrly	10 mg/kg 8 hrly	no	no	no
Fosinopril	100	100	75	75	75	100
Frusemide	100	100	100	100	100	100
Gabapentin	400 mg 8 hrly	300 mg 12 hrly	300 mg 24 hrly	no	no	no
Ganciclovir	Inj 2.5 mg/kg 12 hrly	Inj 2.5 mg/kg 24 hrly	Inj 1.25 mg/kg 24 hrly	Inj 1.25 mg/kg 24 hrly	Inj 1.25 mg/kg 24 hrly	Inj 2.5 mg/kg 24 hrly
Gemfibrozil	100	100	100	100	100	100
Gentamicin	Inj 100% 12 hrly	Inj 75% 12 hrly	Inj 50% 24 hrly	Inj 50% Post HD	Inj 50% 24 hrly	Inj 50% 24 hrly
Glicazide	100% OM	precaution	precaution	precaution	precaution	precaution
Gingerol	100%	100	100	100	100	100
Glipizide	100	100	no	no	no	no
Glitazone	100	100	100 precaution	100 precaution	100 precaution	100 precaution
Griseofulvin	100	100	100	100	100	100
Guanethidine	Inj 24 hrly	Inj 24 hrly	Ing 36 hrly	no	no	no
Haloperidol	100	100	100	100	100	100
Heparin	100	100	100	100	100	100
Hydrallazine	100	100	100	100	100	100
Ibuprofen	100	100	100	100	100	100
Indapamide	100	100	100	100	100	100
Indomethacin	100	100	100	100	100	100
Isoniazid	100	100	75	75	75	100
Isosorbide	100	100	100	100	100	100

(*Continued*)

Table 27.1   *(Continued)*

Drug						
Isradipine	100	100	100	100	100	100
Itraconazole	100	100	100	100	100	100
Kanamycin	Inj 100% 12 hrly	Inj 75% 12 hrly	Inj 50% 24 hrly	Inj 50% 24 hrly	Inj 50% 24 hrly	Inj 50% 12 hrly
Ketoconazole	100	100	100	100	100	100
Ketorolac	100	75	50	50	50	75
Labetalol	100	100	100	100	100	100
Lamivudine	150 mg BD	100 mg BD	50 mg BD			
Levodopa	100	100	100	100	100	100
Levofloxacin	100	100	50	50	50	100
Lidocaine	100	100	100	100	100	100
Lincomycin	Inj 100% 8 hrly	Inj 100% 12 hrly	Inj 75% 12 hrly	Inj 75% 12 hrly	Inj 75% 12 hrly	Inj 100% 12 hrly
Linezolid	100	100	100	100	100	100
Lisinopril	100	100	75	50	50	75
Lithium Carbonate	100	75	50	50	50	75
Low Mol Wt Heparin	100	75	50	50	50	75
Mefenamic Acid	100	100	50	50	50	75
Melphalan	100	75	50	50	50	75
Meropenem	Inj 100% 6 hrly	Inj 100% 12 hrly	Inj 100% 24 hrly	Inj 100% 24 hrly	Inj 100% 24 hrly	Inj 100% 12 hrly

(Continued)

Table 27.1   (*Continued*)

Metformin	50 precaution	no	no	no	no
Methicillin	Inj 100% 6 hrly	Inj 100% 8 hrly	Inj 100% 12 hrly	Inj 100% 12 hrly	Inj 100% 8 hrly
Methotrexate	100	50	no	no	no
Methyldopa	100% 8 hrly	100% 12 hrly	100% 12 hrly	100% 12 hrly	100% 12 hrly
Methylprednisolone	100	100	100	100	100
Metochlorpropamide	100	75	50	50	75
Miconazole	100	100	100	100	100
Midazolam	100	75	50	50	75
Minoxidil	100	100	100	100	100
Morphine	100	75	50	50	75
Moxalactum	Inj 100% 8 hrly	Inj 100% 12 hrly	Inj 100% 24 hrly	Inj 100% 24 hrly	Inj 100% 12 hrly
Mycophenolate Mofetil	100	75	50	50	50
N Acetyl Cysteine	100	100	75	75	100
Nalidixic Acid	100	no	no	no	no
Neostigmine	100	50	25	25	50
Nicardipine	100	100	100	100	100
Nicotinic Acid	100	50	25	25	50
Nifedipine	100	100	100	100	100
Nitrofurantoin	no	no	no	no	no
Nitroglycerine	100	100	100	100	100

(*Continued*)

Table 27.1 *(Continued)*

Nitroprusside	100	100	100	100	100
Norfloxacin	100	50	50	50	75
Nortryptylline	100	100	100	100	100
Omeprazole	100	100	100	100	100
Ondansetron	100	100	100	100	100
Paclitaxel	100	100	100	100	100
Pancuronium	100	no	no	no	no
Paroxetine	100	50	50	50	75
ParaAmino Salicylate	100	50	50	50	75
Penicillamine	100	no	no	no	no
Pentamidine	Inj 100% 24 hrly	Inj 100% 48 hrly	Inj 100% 48 hrly	Inj 100% 48 hrly	Inj 100% 36 hrly
Pentobarbital	100	75	50	50	75
Pentoxyfylline	100	100	100	100	100
Perindropil	100	50	50	50	75
Phenobarbital	Inj 100% 8 hrly	Inj 100% 16 hrly	Inj 100% 16 hrly	Inj 100% 16 hrly	Inj 100% 12 hrly
Phenytoin	100	100	100	100	100
Pioglitazone	100	100 precaution	100 precaution	100 precaution	100 precaution
Piperacillin	Inj 100% 6 hrly	Inj 100% 8 hrly	Inj 100% 8 hrly	inj 100% 8 hrly	Inj 100% 6 hrly
Piroxicam	100	75	75	75	75

(Continued)

Table 27.1   (*Continued*)

Drug					
Prazosin	100	100	100	100	100
Primaquin	100	100	100	100	100
Probenecid	100	75	50	no	no
Procainamide	Inj 100% 4 hrly	Inj 100% 6–12 hrly	no	no	no
Promethazine	100	100	100	100	100
Propranolol	100	100	100	100	100
Propylthiouracil	100	75	50	50	75
Pyrazinamide	100	100	100	100	100
Pyridostigmine	50	33	25	25	33
Quinidine	100	100	100	100	100
Quinine	Inj 100% 8 hrly	Inj 100% 12 hrly	Inj 100% 24 hrly	Inj 100% 24 hrly	Inj 100% 12 hrly
Ramipril	100	75	50	50	75
Ranitidine	100	100	50	50	75
Ribavarine	100	100	50	50	75
Rituximab	100 precaution	100 precaution	100 precaution	100 precaution	100 precaution
Rosiglitazone	100 precaution	100 precaution	100 precaution	100 precaution	100 precaution
Simvastatin	100	100	10 to 20 mg OM	10 to 20mgON	10 to 20 mg ON
Spironolactone	100 precaution	100 precaution	no	no	no
Streptokinase	100	100	100	100	100
Streptozotocin	75	75	50	50	75
Sutenafil	100	100	100	100	100
Sulbactum	100	75	50	50	75

(*Continued*)

Table 27.1   (Continued)

Drug						
Sulphamethoxazole	100			50	50	50
Sulphinpyrazone	100			50	75	50
Sulindac	100			50	50	50
Tacrolimus	100			100	100	100
Tamiflu	100			50	50	50
Tamoxifen	100			100	100	100
Terazosin	100			100	100	100
Terbutaline	100			no	no	no
Tetracycline	100			50	50	50
Thiazide	100			no	no	no
Ticarcillin	100			75	50	75
Ticlopidine	100			100	100	100
Tolbutamide	100			100 precaution	100 precaution	100 precaution
Tramadol	100			75	50	75
Tranexamic acid	100			50	25	50
Triamterene	100			no	no	no
Trimethoprim	100			50	50	50
Valganciclovir	100			100 precaution	100 precaution	100 precaution
Vancomycin	100	500 mg 12 hrly	500 mg 24 hrly	500 mg post HD	500 mg thrice weekly	500 mg 48 hrly
Verapamil	100			100	100	100
Vincristine	100			100	100	100
Warfarin	100			100 precaution	100 precaution	100 precaution
Zidovudine	100			50	50	75

medication for diabetes is not reduced as renal failure progresses. This is why such patients should only be prescribed short acting oral hypoglycemics. "No" means that particular drug should be avoided.

Recent Changes in Vancomycin use in renal failure

Vancomycin is a key antibiotic for the treatment of serious gram positive infections. In the dialysis patient, infection is the next common cause of death after cardiovascular causes. The annual risk for bacteremia in HD patients ranges from 7.6% to 14.4% and 60–100% of these episodes are caused by staphylococcal species, esp Staph aureus. Vancomycin has served as the cornerstone antibiotic for years. Recently two evolutions in vancomycin usage have occurred. First is a progressive creep in minimal inhibitory concentration (MIC) for vancomycin in Staph aureus and this has dictated the use of higher therapeutic targets. Second, this means that the higher dose recommendations will result in more nephrotoxicity for vulnerable patients. The higher trough levels and longer duration of therapy will put more patients at risk. Most available normograms for vancomycin dosing in renal have much lower trough levels than the newer recommended trough levels of 15–20 μg/ml.

In patients undergoing high flux hemodialysis, 42% did not achieve the minimum target of 15 μg/ml when a 1000 mg loading dose followed by 500 mg doses after each HD session was administered. Target trough levels may be more readily obtained when a total body weight based loading dose of 20–25 mg/Kg was used instead of a fixed dose of 1000 mg. One additional shortcoming of such algorithms is that residual renal function is not taken into consideration.

The proposed vancomycin trough level targeted at 15–20 μg/ml engenders the risk of nephrotoxicity in CKD patients. Fortunately new drugs are now available for treatment of serious gram positive infections like lipopeptide daptomycin, the oxazolidin linezolid

broad spectrum cephalosporines with good activity against
ceftobiprole and ceftaroline are also in the pipeline. Ho'
drugs are to be positioned for use in CKD patients howeve
not clear [Vandecasteele SJ *et al.* Recent changes in vanc
use in renal failure. Kidney Int 2010, 77:760–764].

REFERENCES

1. MIMS Annual. Full Prescribing Information. Singapore 20(
2. DIMS Singapore 110th Edition, 2009.
3. British National Formulary, British Medical Association an
   Pharmaceutical Society of Great Britain, 2009.
4. Sanford Guide to Antimicrobial Therapy, Jay P Sanford M
   Edition, 2008.
5. Health Science Authority, Singapore. Adverse Drug Reactio
   August 2010, Vol12, No 2. Pg2.
6. Watanabe A *et al.* Targetted prevention of renal accumula
   toxicity of gentamicin by aminoglycoside binding receptor
   nists. *J Control Release*, 2004, **95**(3):423–433.
7. Vandecasteele SJ *et al.* Recent changes in vancomycin use
   failure. *Kidney Int* 2010, **77**:760–764.

CHAPTER 28

Acute Kidney Injury (Acute Renal Failure)

DEFINITION

In the context of Acute Renal Failure (ARF), several im
changes have been introduced. The term "renal" has no
changed to "kidney" and the term "failure" changed to "
so as to encompass the whole spectrum of renal failure ba
data showing that a small change in serum creatinine inf
the outcome. The term Acute Kidney Injury (AKI) ha
replaced ARF.

Acute renal failure [ARF] is a sudden temporary and
"reversible" failure of the kidneys to excrete waste prod
metabolism. The first sign is oliguria, usually defined a
volume less than 400 ml per day. In addition to tradit
described oliguric acute renal failure, there is non-oliguri
renal failure which is also transient and reversible where th
output is about a litre or more. Here there is less morbid
mortality compared to oliguric renal failure. Non-oliguri
failure is often caused by nephrotoxic antibiotics (in partic
aminoglycosides) and anaesthetics.

In recent years, the term Acute Kidney Injury [AKI] ha
introduced to replace the time honoured term of Acute
Failure. Basically, for all intents and purposes and in
practice, both terms can be used interchangeably. It has be
that Acute Kidney Injury is more embracing as it descri
sorts of conditions and situations of protean manifestatio
presentations where there is a decline of renal function, ba
GFR or eGFR, over any length of time varying from h

433

weeks associated with an increase in blood urea and serum creatinine representing retention of nitrogenous waste products. Acute Kidney Injury therefore consists of varying causes and mechanisms of variable duration and severity for the initiation phase, maintenance phase and recovery phase.

In contrast, it has been felt that the term Acute Renal Failure is rather limited and has a narrower focus defining any condition where there is a sudden and acute cessation of renal function with decreased urine output associated with abnormal renal function expressed as raised serum creatinine and blood urea representing retention of nitrogenous waste products of protein metabolism.

In clinical practice, the traditional classification of Acute Renal Failure [ARF] into pre renal Renal or intrinsic parenchymal causes and post renal or obstructive Acute Renal Failure still holds for patients with Acute Kidney Injury [AKI]. Hence the new terms used are Pre Renal AKI, Intrinsic AKI and Post Renal AKI. Similarly oliguric and non oliguric Acute Renal Failure is also still relevant for Acute Kidney Injury. In terms of diagnosis and management of patients, it is also the same for Acute Renal Failure [ARF] and Acute Kidney Injury [AKI]. The term Acute Tubular Necrosis [ATN] still applies to AKI and refers to a histological diagnosis as opposed to vasomotor nephropathy.

In a recent consensus conference sponsored by the Acute Dialysis Quality Improvement Initiative (ADQI), a new definition of ARF has been proposed which is now gaining acceptability [Bellamo R, Kellum J and Ronco C. Acute Renal Failure: time for consensus. Intensive Medicine. 2001, 27:1685–1688]. Due to the very broad spectrum of changes involved in AKI, a diagnostic classification scheme has been developed. This scheme is referred to by the acronym of RIFLE. There are three levels of Kidney Dysfunction, namely: 1. **R**isk of kidney dysfunction, 2. **I**njury to the kidney and 3. **F**ailure of kidney function. The scheme also includes two outcome categories: 4. **L**oss of renal function and 5. **E**nd stage kidney disease.

Criteria for RIFLE based on GFR and Urine Output:

1. R for Renal dysfunction is described as an increased in serum creatinine of 1.5 times of patient's previous serum creatinine which must be within normal [male up to $110\,\mu$mol/l and female up to $85\,\mu$mol/l] or GFR decrease >25% OR decrease in Urine Output 0.5 ml/kg/hr for 6 hours, the more severe of the two is selected 2.

2. I for Injury, increase in serum creatinine of twice, GFR decrease >50% OR Urine Output <0.5 ml/kg/hr for 12 hours.

3. F for Failure, increase in serum creatinine three times or GFR decrease >75% or serum creatinine ≥4 mg/dl [$350\,\mu$mol/l] OR Urine Output <0.3 ml/kg/hr or anuria for 12 hours.

4. L for Loss, persistent ARF+ complete loss of kidney function >4 weeks.

5. E for ESKD, End Stage Kidney Disease or End Stage Renal Failure >3 months.

Note: When the criteria is based on serum creatinine the subscript$_c$ is added, e.g.

RIFLE- F_c and if based on Urine Output, it is subscript $_o$. A worse RIFLE criteria score is associated with a worse APACHE II score with higher mortality at both 1 and 6 months.

Timely recognition of the syndrome is of the essence so that the correct diagnosis and management can be instituted. In general, the severity of the decline of GFR correlates with the onset of oliguria. However, in practice, many patients with severe renal failure are still nonoliguric. In AKI there is also poor correlation between the serum creatinine and the GFR. A serum creatinine based AKI diagnosis may bias one to an earlier diagnosis of a muscular patient in contrast to someone who is less muscular or malnourished elderly patient. The short Clearance Creatinine Test [2 to 4 hour CCT] may overestimate the GFR at low levels of renal function due to relatively high proportion of tubular secretion of creatinine. Obviously there is a need for more appropriate markers of renal function.

DIAGNOSTIC APPROACH AND INVESTIGATION

In the history one should always enquire about recent surgery, trauma, hypertension, drugs and previous renal diseases.

In the physical examination pay attention to the state of hydration of the patient whether he is dehydrated or in fluid overload (presence of oedema, jugular venous pressure (JVP), postural hypotension), external genitalia, palpation of the kidneys, urinary bladder, rectal and vaginal examination.

Establish whether patient is in "pre-renal" (hypovolaemia), "renal", or "post-renal" (urinary obstruction) failure.

Exclude Obstruction (Post Renal Failure)

In the history, enquire about renal calculi, prostatic symptoms, recent surgery, trauma to pelvis and cancer.

On examination look for a full urinary bladder or full and tender loin. An ultrasound of the kidneys, CT scan, MRI or cystoscopy and retrograde pyelogram may be necessary.

Once obstruction has been excluded, decide whether patient has "prerenal failure" (hypotension, dehydration, hypovolaemia, hypoperfusion) or "intrinsic renal failure" due to an intrinsic renal cause (acute tubular necrosis or vasomotor nephropathy).

INVESTIGATIONS

1. In "pre-renal failure" (hypovolaemia), the urine microscopy is normal but in vasomotor nephropathy (acute tubular necrosis) the urine contains some protein, tubular cells and casts.
2. If RBC casts are present in the urine the patient is likely to have glomerulonephritis as the cause of renal failure rather than vasomotor nephropathy or acute tubular necrosis.
3. If total urinary protein exceeds 2 gm, the diagnosis favours a chronic nephritis rather than vasomotor nephropathy.
4. Eosinophils in the urine should alert one to the possibility of allergic interstitial nephritis.

5. If the patient has total or absolute anuria and obstruction has been excluded, then a diagnosis of occlusion of the renal arteries has to be considered.
6. As and when appropriate, one may have to request for an ultrasound examination of the kidneys, a CT scan, MRI or renal arteriogram.

A high dose intravenous pyelogram may reveal the following:

1. Small smooth shrunken kidneys which would suggest chronic glomerulonephritis.
2. Small scarred kidneys which may suggest pyelonephritis (reflux nephropathy), diabetic nephropathy, analgesic nephropathy or even renal artery stenosis.
3. Total absence of the nephrogram phase would suggest arterial occlusion or a severe proliferative glomerulonephritis.
4. Early dense persisting nephrogram may favour vasomotor nephropathy or acute suppurative pyelonephritis.
5. A slowly developing dense nephrogram suggests acute glomerulonephritis.
6. A faintly persistent nephrogram suggests a chronic glomerulonephritis.

*High dose IVP is not done nowadays because of contrast media induced nephrotoxicity and also the newer imaging techniques like CT scan, MRI and Doppler ultrasonography have superceded the clinical usefulness of high dose IVP.

INTRINSIC RENAL FAILURE [INTRINSIC ACUTE KIDNEY INJURY]

The following are some of the possibilities:

1. Vasomotor nephropathy (VMN) or acute tubular necrosis (ATN)
2. Glomerulonephritis, vasculitis

3. Acute interstitial nephritis, drugs
4. Renal vascular thrombosis
5. Acute exacerbation of chronic glomerulonephritis

1. Vasomotor Nephropathy or Acute Tubular Necrosis

The term vasomotor nephropathy is now preferred to the traditional term acute tubular necrosis as it has now been shown that patients with ATN or VMN have vasoconstriction of the afferent arteriole. In many cases diagnosed clinically as acute tubular necrosis, the renal biopsies often show normal histology except for some mild vacuolar degeneration even though patients behave like classical ATN clinically.

Recognise the precipitating causes like shock, haemorrhage, dehydration, septicaemia and leptospirosis. There should be absence of evidence suggesting preexisting acute or chronic renal disease, allergic interstitial nephritis or vascular occlusion.

2. Glomerulonephritis, Vasculitis

Most patients in this category would give a history suggesting acute glomerulonephritis or a systemic illness like systemic lupus erythematosus.

If the urine microscopy demonstrates RBC casts, glomerulonephritis as a cause of renal failure is likely.

A total urinary proteinuria exceeding 2 gm suggests glomerulonephritis.

Low serum complement would indicate glomerulonephritis or SLE. A high ESR, positive LE cell, positive ANF, positive anti-DNA, positive ANCA would suggest a diagnosis of SLE or vasculitis.

Renal biopsy may show post infectious glomerulonephritis, crescenteric glomerulonephritis, lupus nephritis, polyarteritis nodosa.

3. Interstitial Nephritis, Drugs

Acute allergic interstitial nephritis presents with fever, rash, eosinophilia and eosinophils in the urine or eosinophiluria. A renal biopsy readily confirms the diagnosis through the presence of widespread tubulo-interstitial nephritis with plentiful cellular infiltrates including eosinophils. This condition should be treated with low dose [not more than 30 mg/day] prednisolone to prevent interstitial scarring and promote rapid healing and reversal of the allergic phenomenon. Methicillin, sulphonamides and allopurinol have all been implicated.

Contrast media used in radiology, antibiotics (gentamicin, amikacin, cephalosporin, streptomycin), and diuretics (thiazides) may also be responsible.

In Singapore, leptospirosis is a common cause of acute interstitial nephritis causing acute renal failure. The serum erythrocyte lysis (SEL) test should always be performed in any patient presenting with systemic infection and renal failure. Nowadays the SEL test have been replaced by newer serological tests.

Other causes of interstitial nephritis are toxins from bee stings and other insects, and venoms from snake bites.

4. Renal Vascular (Arterial Thrombosis, Embolism)

While taking a history, enquire regarding possibility of subacute bacteria endocarditis and mural thrombi. Loin pain and hypertension associated with oligo-anuria may suggest renal infarction.

Absent nephrogram on intravenous pyelogram or a renal radioisotope scan or a renal arteriogram showing no blood flow would indicate renal vascular obstruction.

Renal artery thrombosis may follow trauma or it could result from atherosclerosis. The patient would require urgent endarterectomy.

5. Acute Exacerbation of Chronic Renal Disease

The patient may reveal a history of previous symptoms of renal impairment, hypertension or urinary tract infection.

Urine microscopy may show RBC, casts, or protein. The total urinary protein usually ranges from 1 to 2 gm/day in these cases. A renal biopsy would confirm the diagnosis of preexisting glomerulonephritis.

In patients with "acute on chronic" renal failure, the acute elements causing acute renal failure may be dehydration, sepsis, uncontrolled hypertension, obstruction and nephrotoxic antibiotics as well as contrast agents and NSAIDS. When considering obstruction one should exclude obstruction to the urological tract as well as thrombosis of renal veins and arteries.

Tables 28.1 and 28.2 show the causes of acute renal failure in Singapore.

Table 28.3 shows the causes of AKI with dehydration as the commonest cause but with Sepsis as the next common cause followed by Drugs and Glomerulonephritis. In the older system as shown in Tables 28.1 and 28.2, using ARF rather than AKI, mild degrees of ARF which are more readily reversed

Table 28.1   Causes of Acute Renal Failure in Singapore (1976–1982)

		No. of Cases	%
1.	Infection	28	30%
2.	Glomerulonephritis	9	10%
3.	Renal Stone	6	7%
4.	Drugs	7	8%
5.	Poisoning	12	13%
6.	Pregnancy Related	8	8%
7.	Hepato-renal Failure	6	7%
8.	Post Surgery	9	10%
9.	Cancer	4	4%
10.	Others	3	3%
	TOTAL	92	100%

+Table 28.2 Causes of Acute Renal Failure in Singapore (1985–1989)

	Causes	No. of Patients	No. of Death
1.	Septicaemia	23	12
2.	Glomerulonephritis	3	1
3.	Hepatorenal Syndrome	1	1
4.	Drugs	2	0
5.	Poisoning	2	1
6.	Malignancy	1	1
7.	Renal stone	2	1
8.	Ruptured Viscus	2	2
9.	Trauma	4	2
10.	Miscellaneous*	8	4
	TOTAL	48	25 (52%)

* Acute Myocardial Infarction, Pancreatitis, Rhabdomyolysis, Hornet sting.
+ Courtesy of S S Wei.

Table 28.3 Causes of Acute Kidney Injury (AKI) at Singapore General Hospital

		No. of Cases	%
1.	Dehydration	59	34%
2.	Sepsis	47	27%
3.	Drugs	18	10%
4.	Glomerulonephritis	18	10%
5.	Hypotension	15	9%
6.	Obstruction	6	3%
7.	Others (Hepatorenal Syndrome, Pre-Eclampsia)	10	6%
	TOTAL	173	100%

This table shows the number of cases of AKI seen at the Singapore General Hospital from June 2009 to May 2010. By courtesy of Dr Elizabeth Oei.

like those due to dehydration and drugs may not have been captured under the definition of ARF. Hence the present term AKI is all encompassing and has a wider spectrum which would account for the large number of cases with AKI compared to those with ARF.

CLINICAL COURSE OF ACUTE RENAL FAILURE [ACUTE KIDNEY INJURY]

I. Onset Phase

Often the problem is one of diagnosis at onset rather than problem of immediate treatment. At this stage the patient has few symptoms or signs of renal failure other than oliguria. There is mild elevation of blood urea and serum creatinine and deteriorating electrolyte disturbance.

II. Oliguric Phase

In the majority of patients, there is often fluid overload with hyponatraemia associated with ankle oedema and pulmonary oedema. A routine chest X-ray should be performed in all patients.

If the patient has hyponatraemia it is important to exclude depletional hyponatraemia due to dehydration or gastrointestinal loss due to vomiting.

Hyperkalaemia is often due to oliguria, release of K^+ from cells as a result of trauma, haemolysis, catabolism, infection or acidosis. Symptoms of hyperkalaemia may manifest as paresthesia, weakness of muscles and cardiac arrhythmias.

Acidosis occurs because the damaged kidneys cannot excrete H^+, hence the Kussmaul's respiration.

Acute Uraemic Syndrome

The acute uraemic syndrome is due to uraemic toxins affecting the cardiovascular, gastrointestinal, central nervous and the haematological systems.

Cardiovascular system: Patients may present with hypertension, arrhythmias, congestive heart failure and pericardititis.

Gastrointestinal: Anorexia, nausea, vomiting, diarrhoea, gastrointestinal bleeding (gastric erosion, colitis, oesophagitis) and pancreatitis.

Central nervous system: Confusion, twitching, asterixis and fits due to uraemic encephalopathy may be present.

Haemopoietic system: The anaemia of renal failure is a normochromic, normocytic anaemia. It is caused by decreased erythropoietin. Sometimes, depending on the cause of renal failure, haemolysis or blood loss may contribute to the anaemia. Platelet function may be abnormal. This takes the form of decreased platelet adhesiveness and decreased platelet aggregation.

The patient with renal failure is also prone to pneumonia, urinary infections, skin infections and decreased wound healing as he has decreased phagocytosis and immune paralysis due to the depression of the immune system by the uraemic environment.

III. Diuretic Phase

Restoration of renal function is heralded by the diuretic phase. The onset of this phase is unpredictable and may occur anytime from 24 hours to even 2 months. It is related to the removal of excess water and salt as well as to impaired renal concentration. The danger to the patient at this stage is excess loss of water, dehydration and hypokalaemia. During this time patients experience a sense of well-being. There is loss of nausea and the appetite returns.

MANAGEMENT OF ACUTE RENAL FAILURE [ACUTE KIDNEY INJURY]

I. Oliguric Phase

At this stage one strives to keep the patient alive until his kidneys undergo a cure. It is important to monitor the electrolytes as well as the blood urea and serum creatinine daily. Maintain an intake and output chart. When the patient is oliguric his fluid intake should not exceed 500 ml/day unless he is dehydrated. Usually, patients tend to be overloaded as they are not passing into the urine the amount of water they have been drinking.

Serum potassium especially has to be monitored from the daily electrolyte profile. Hyperkalaemia (serum K^+ > 6 mEq/l) should be treated. An injection of 10 units of soluble insulin together with 50 ml of 50% dextrose is given in a bolus dose or in a drip infusion over half to 1 hour. If the patient can take orally, commence Resonium A 15 gm 8 hourly. If the patient cannot take orally, commence Resonium retention enema 30 gm 8-hourly. Also administer I.V. calcium gluconate or chloride 10 ml slowly to combat the effects of hyperkalaemia on the heart. Repeat serum K^+ four hours later and if serum K^+ proves difficult to control, dialysis may be required or a second bolus of insulin and dextrose may be given.

The caloric intake of the patient must be adequate to prevent catabolism of the body proteins. Anaemia is corrected by transfusion of packed red blood cells. Hypertension and heart failure should be treated. Infections should be treated with the correct antibiotics. The choice of antibiotics and the dosage is important. The use of aminoglycosides should be monitored by drug levels (gentamicin or amikacin levels).

If necessary the patient should be dialysed. The patient should be dialysed when serum creatinine is about 400 micro mol/L (sometimes even earlier). Other indications for dialysis are uraemic symptoms, pericarditis, hyperkalaemia, severe acidosis, pulmonary oedema or a hypercatabolic state. In patients with unstable BP, continuous renal replacement therapy (CRRT) like hemofiltration or hemodiafiltration is performed.

II. Diuretic Phase

The hazard at this stage is excessive loss of fluid, Na^+ and K^+. The high urea content in blood induces an osmotic diuresis. In addition, a defect in tubular concentration due to ATN is another cause for the diuretic phase. Sometimes efforts to keep up with the diuresis may perpetuate it.

One should maintain a strict intake and output chart. Check urine volume, serum urea, creatinine and electrolytes. Fluids and K+ should be replaced accordingly.

III. Post Diuretic Phase

The urine output of the patient slowly normalises as the renal blood flow and GFR gradually increase. Tubular functions like concentration and dilution may take a longer time to recover.

Continuous Renal Replacement Therapies (CRRT)

Continuous Renal Replacement Therapy or CRRT is the modality of renal replacement therapy used in patients with acute renal failure [acute kidney injury] as it does not result in intermittent drop of the patients' BP as in the case of Intermittent Hemodialysis (IHD) which is the modality used for patients on the chronic or regular hemoldialysis programme. The advantage of CRRT in the patient with acute renal failure apart from pre-serving whatever renal function the patient may still have as the kidneys start to recover from the acute insult is that it can remove large volumes of fluid and solute in the patient with acute renal failure with little drop in BP compared to conventional or IHD. With the introduction of the double lumen venous catheters, CRRT options are now usually continuous venovenous modalities (CVVH) or Continuous Venovenous Hemofiltration. In the 1970's, CRRT used to be arterial based, i.e. CAVH or Continuous Arterial Venous Hemofiltration, a technique first described by Kramer where the blood flow and filtration were determined by blood pressure. This has the advantage of not causing a drop in BP. But it was not as efficient when large volumes of ultrafiltra-tion was required for metabolic control. Also, CAVH requires a large bore femoral artery catheter which has its complications. Hence the use of CVVH nowadays.

CRRT modalities are used for fluid and metabolic control and involves high volumes of ultrafiltrate and require replacement fluid, dialysate or both. CVVH requires an extracorporeal circuit, a double lumen catheter which is hooked to an extracorporeal system with a blood pump, a high efficiency or high flux dialysis membrane and replacement fluid. The ultrafiltrate is produced by pure convection unlike hemodialysis which depends on osmosis and diffusion. The patient requires replacement fluid which is titrated with his volume status and metabolic and electrolyte status.

CVVHD or Continuous Venovenous Hemodialysis requires an extracorporeal circuit with a double lumen venous catheter hooked to an extracorporeal system with a blood pump, high efficiency or high flux dialysis membrane and dialysis fluid. The dialysate runs countercurrent to the blood pathway. Both convection and diffusion are involved with this form of CRRT. CVVHDF or Continuous Venovenous Hemodiafiltration consists of an extracorporeal circuit with a double lumen venous catheter hooked to an extracorporeal system with a blood pump, high efficiency or high flux dialysis membrane plus both replacement fluid and dialysate. This combination is used to increase clearance in the patient with hypercatabolic acute renal failure. Others use this modality to simplify citrate delivery for anticoagulation.

In the old days, in the 1970's, leptospirosis was very common in Singapore and patients often present with hypercatabolic acute renal failure and they require long hours of daily hemodialysis. Such patients can now be well maintained using CVVHDF. Previously, we sometimes had to resort to CAVH alternating with IHD or CAVHDF which is Continuous Arterial Veno Hemodialfiltration [1].

Slow low efficiency daily dialysis or SLEDD can be used for patients with low BP and this gentle form of dialysis allows easier adjustment of volume control and solute clearance compared to IHD. It approaches the benefits of CRRT and is useful for both acute as well as chronic renal failure with low BP or those with low left ventricular ejection fraction with less stable cardiac status.

In Slow continuous ultrafiltration or SCUF the extracorporeal circuit has a blood system which is hooked inline with a high efficiency or high flux membrane. As blood passes through the membrane, plasma water and solutes pass through the membrane to allow formation of an ultrafiltrate, which is then discarded. In this modality, there is no need for replacement fluid or dialysate as this is a convective modality. The ultrafiltrate is therefore limited and is useful for patients with residual renal function and not too severe oliguria. This is useful for the patient with acute renal failure whose serum creatinine is not too high about 350 to 400 micromol/l and not too oliguric.

PROGNOSIS

Recovery depends on the nature of the underlying disease, i.e. the cause of renal failure. 50% of hospital acquired acute renal failure [acute kidney injury or AKI] are multifactorial. Patients with trauma, infection and shock do worse. A healthy young patient does better than an old patient. The crude mortality rate among those patients with intrinsic AKI remains about 50% and has been so over the past three decades.

Efficient management is also important in determining prognosis. The mortality rate is about 15% for obstetric cases and 30% in toxic related AKI. Patients with sepsis have mortality rate of 60% to 90%. For simple acute renal failure patients, with no other illness, outside ICU, mortality rate is 7–23%. Mortality in ICU patients is 50–80%, average about 37%. Survival depends on severity of underlying illness and number of failed organs, that is, co-morbid illness [2].

20% of all deaths are due to infections and in 60%, infections are contributory factors. Factors indicating poorer prognosis are male sex, elderly patients, oliguric patients [urine output <400 ml/day, rise in serum creatinine of greater than 3 mg/dl, presence of multiorgan failure [3].

REFERENCES

1. Raghavan M *et al.* Acute Kidney Injury in non-severe pneumonia is associated with an increased immune response and lower survival. *Kidney Int* 2010, **77**:527–535.
2. Tolwani AJ *et al.* Simplified citrate anticoagulation for continuous renal replacement therapy. *Kidney International*, 2001, **60**:370–374.
3. Star RA. Treatment of Acute Renal Failure. *Kidney International*, 1998, **54**:1817–1831.
4. Kellum JA *et al.* Patients are dying of acute renal failure. *Critical Care Medicine*, 2002, **30**:2156–2157.
5. Muntner P *et al.* Acute Kidney Injury in sepsis: Questions answered but others remain. *Kidney Int* 2010, **77**:485–487.
6. Schrier RW. ARF, AKI or ATN? *Kidney Int, Editorial, Nature Reviews Nephrology*, 2010, **6**:125.

CHAPTER 29
Chronic Renal Failure

DEFINITION

Chronic renal failure is the gradual onset of an "irreversible" and persistent impairment of both glomerular and tubular functions which is so severe that the kidneys are no longer able to maintain the normal internal environment. This definition includes mild asymptomatic functional impairment, sometimes called chronic renal impairment.

AETIOLOGY

1. **Primary glomerular disease:** Acute glomerular disease including rapidly progressive glomerulonephritis. Chronic glomerulonephritis is the second commonest cause of ESRF in Singapore.
2. **Primary tubular disease:** Chronic hypercalcaemia, chronic hypokalaemia, heavy metal poisoning like lead and cadmium.
3. **Vascular disease:** Ischaemia of the kidneys due to congenital or acquired renal artery stenosis; accelerated or malignant hypertension, hypertensive nephrosclerosis.
4. **Infection:** Chronic atrophic pyelonephritis (reflux nephropathy), tuberculosis.
5. **Obstruction:** Renal stones, retroperitoneal fibrosis, prostatomegaly, urethral strictures and tumours.
6. **Vasculitis:** Systemic lupus erythematosus, polyarteritis nodosa, Henoch — Schonlein nephritis, scleroderma, Wegener's granulomatosis. In Systemic Vasculitis, anti-neutrophilic cytoplasmic

449

antibody (ANCA) is usually positive, while it is usually negative in SLE.

7. **Metabolic renal disease:** Diabetes mellitus (commonest cause of ESRF in Singapore), amyloidosis, analgesic nephropathy, gout, primary hyperparathyroidism and **milk** alkali syndrome.

8. **Congenital abnormality:** Hypoplastic kidneys, reflux nephropathy, medullary cystic disease, polycystic kidneys.

With a population of 4.8 million people in 2008 in Singapore, about 700 patients or 146 per million population, would be in end stage renal failure. As of 2010, the population is 5.08 million.

Table 29.1 lists the causes of chronic renal failure in Singapore.

CLINICAL PRESENTATION

Central Nervous System

One of the most subtle changes in uraemia is a neuro-behavioural change. It may take the form of a personality defect. The patient tends to speak in short sentences. He has a short attention span and performs mental arithmetic poorly. Later he becomes disorientated and then develops delirium, fits and lapses into a

Table 29.1   Causes of chronic renal failure in Singapore. About 700 new ESRF patients are seen every year

		%
1.	Diabetic Nephropathy	54%
2.	Chronic Glomerulonephritis	25%
3.	Hypertensive Nephrosclerosis	9%
4.	Polycystic Kidney	3%
5.	Vasculitis	2%
6.	Kidney Stones	1%
7.	Chronic Pyelonephritis	1%
8.	Causes Unknown	5%
	TOTAL	100%

coma. The electroencephalogram shows slow waves indicative of a metabolic encephalopathy. Physical examination would reveal asterixis.

The peripheral nervous system is also involved and neuropathy may take the form of the restless leg syndrome, burning feet syndrome or even foot drop due to paralysis.

The urinary bladder may show a large residual volume due to an autonomic neuropathy.

Myopathy may be an added feature of the uraemic syndrome.

Patients are also prone to cerebrovascular accidents in the form of cerebral thrombosis, embolism or haemorrhage as they have accelerated atherogenesis.

Ophthalmic Changes

Acute visual loss due to cortical blindness may be a manifestation of uraemia.

Patients may have calcium deposits in the cornea due to metastatic calcification causing a red eye syndrome or "conjunctivitis".

There may be amino acid deposits in the lateral aspects of the cornea giving rise to wedge-shaped "penguinculae".

Examination of the fundi may show changes of a hypertensive fundus. One may see papilloedema due to accelerated or malignant hypertension. The finding of a macular star in the fundus should alert one to the possibility of chronic renal failure.

Gastrointestinal

Nausea and vomiting are the classical features of the uraemic syndrome. This is due to the decomposition of urea to ammonia by gastrointestinal flora which causes irritation of the gastrointestinal tract. Acute gastric erosions may cause haematemesis and melaena. Gastrointestinal bleeding may also be due to uraemic colitis which may cause diarrhoea or lower intestinal bleeding.

Other gastrointestinal manifestations of uraemia include hiccups, parotitis and sometimes pancreatitis.

Dermatological

Uraemic itch is commonly due to the dry and scaly skin in uraemic patients because of atrophy of the sweat glands causing decreased sweating. Other causes of the uraemic itch include hypercalcaemia resulting from tertiary hyperparathyroidism, and peripheral neuropathy. Uraemic frost is seldom seen nowadays. This is the result of precipitation of uraemic crystals in the skin. Improved standard of hygiene and nursing care may account for the rarity of uraemic frost.

The brown nail arc is another cutaneous feature. This is due to deposits of lipochrome and urochrome in the outer edges of the nails.

Due to severe itch patients tend to scratch their skin and platelet dysfunction and capillary fragility in these patients would contribute to easy bruising seen together with the scratch marks on the skin.

The skin of the uraemic patient is also prone to bacterial, viral and fungal infections as they have decreased cell mediated immune function.

Cardiovascular System

Congestive cardiac failure may be due to severe anaemia or severe hypertension or a combination of uncontrolled hypertension with fluid overload.

Uraemic pericarditis may be a cause of chest pain. When the pain disappears it may mean that the patient has now developed pericardial effusion. The development of pericardial tamponade is always a potential danger in anyone with an effusion. This is especially so in patients who are on regular haemodialysis where heparin is routinely used. Such patients may require pericardial tapping when there is a moderate pericardial effusion.

Uncontrolled hypertension may give rise to acute left ventricular failure with paroxysmal nocturnal dyspnoea due to acute pulmonary oedema. Severe fluid overload per se is another cause of pulmonary oedema. This is contributed to by increased capillary permeability and the chest X-ray occasionally shows the classical appearance of batwings, sometimes termed uraemic lung due to pulmonary oedema.

Haematological System

The anaemia of chronic renal failure is a normochromic normocytic anaemia. This is due to decreased erythropoietin production because of uraemia. Patients may sometimes have folate deficiency as evidenced by hypersegmented polymorphonuclear leukocytes. The red blood cells in a uraemic environment have a shortened lifespan because of the uraemic toxin. The bleeding tendency associated with renal failure is the result of impaired platelet function in the form of decreased platelet adhesion and aggregation.

Respiratory System

A deep sighing respiration due to severe metabolic acidosis called Kussmaul's breathing is often seen in the patient with uraemia. Pulmonary oedema is another cause of severe dyspnoea and a chest X-ray may show the typical batwing appearance over both lung fields.

Patients with uraemia are also prone to pneumonia because of decreased resistance to infection as they have impaired cell mediated immunity as well as decreased phagocytosis in the leukocyte.

Renal Osteodystrophy

This is another term for renal bone disease which in clinical practice usually implies a combination of osteomalacia and secondary hyperparathyroidism. It is the result of impaired calcium and vitamin D metabolism. In renal failure the renal tubules are unable to convert 25-dihydroxycholecalciferol to 1,25-dihydroxycholecalciferol. This leads to decreased absorption of calcium from the bowels which in turn stimulates the parathyroid gland to secrete more parathormone. The stimulated parathyroid gland undergoes hypertrophy giving rise to secondary hyperparathyroidism where the patient has low serum calcium and high serum phosphate, and increased serum alkaline phosphatase levels. Persistent hypercalcaemia is a feature of tertiary hyperparathyroidism when the glands have become autonomous.

If the skeleton can respond to excess parathormone the patient has osteitis fibrosa cystica and if the calcium phosphate product exceeds 55 (in mg) or 4.4 (in S.I. units), metastatic or ectopic calcification results. The patient then has calcium deposited in the cornea of the eyes and presents with the red eye syndrome or he may have band keratopathy. Metastatic calcification may also involve the joints and soft tissues of the body including various organs. Deposition in the skin causes severe pruritus while deposition in the blood vessels can make subsequent renal transplant very difficult technically.

If the skeleton cannot respond to excess parathormone then osteomalacia or adult rickets is the result.

The patient with renal osteodystrophy may present with a waddling gait or he may walk with a limp and complain of bone pain or chest pain because of fracture of the ribs. Pain in the hip may be the result of fracture of the neck of the femur.

MANAGEMENT

Search for reversible treatable chronic diseases of the kidney and treat them as this may arrest or slow down the progression of renal deterioration. In this respect, infections like renal tuberculosis and chronic pyelonephritis (reflux nephropathy) are noteworthy. The course of analgesic nephropathy can also be arrested if the patient can be made to stop the abuse of analgesics. Hypercalcaemic nephropathy, hypokalaemic nephropathy and renal disease due to drugs and chemicals should also be identified and treated. Finally, obstructive uropathy due to stones and enlarged prostate can be treated.

Look for reversible factors adversely affecting the course of irreversible renal disease, among which are causes such as urinary and any other forms of sepsis that could cause renal impairment. Dehydration or salt depletion, evident by the presence of postural hypotension, loss of tissue turgor, decreased JVP, low serum sodium and chloride can also be easily identified and treated. Hypokalaemia and heart failure are also reversible causes of renal impairment. Uncontrolled or accelerated hypertension from whatever cause also needs to be treated aggressively. Finally, nephrotoxic agents, in particular the aminoglycosides, cephalosporins, bactrium, tetracycline, allopurinol, NSAID and many others should be thought of in a patient with renal failure. Drugs and antibiotics can give rise to renal impairment either because of a direct nephrotoxic effect or due to a hypersensitivity reaction giving rise sometimes to unsuspected interstitial nephritis.

Always exclude Dehydration, Sepsis, uncontrolled Hypertension, Obstruction (to urological tract or renal vessels — thrombosis of veins or arteries) and Drugs including nephrotoxic antibiotics and NSAIDS.

Dietary Treatment and Supplements

It has been long established that protein reduction can slow the rate of GFR decline in CKD patients. A vegetable diet has less protein and phosphates and could be advantageous provided the patient has an adequate intake of high biologic protein to prevent malnutrition. A dietician's help with food exchange would be advisable in the formulation of the diet. We would advise that patients take a 0.8 gm/Kg BW protein diet as opposed to a 0.6 gm/Kg BW protein diet as the latter diet may result in malnutrition. Vegetarian diet would also improve lipid abnormality. A high intake of polyunsaturated fat would reduce the risk of coronary artery disease [CAD] whereas a diet consisting high trans fat and unsaturated fatty acids would increase the risk of CAD. Consumming trans fat would raise LDL cholesterol and lower HDL cholesterol and would be deleterious. Most patients with CKD would be prescribed statins to treat lipid abnormalities which would be present in more than 80% of patients with CKD. Uncontrolled lipid abnormalities like uncontrolled BP would lead to a more rapid decline in the GFR. In addition to the use of statins, patients with CKD 4 to 5 should also be on Renalvite or Renal Vitamin which consists of water soluble B vitamins like thiamine, riboflavine, B6 and B12 as well as folic acid and Vitamin C. Folic acid must be sufficient for erythropoietin [EPO] to be effective. This is because folic acid found in fruit and vegatables may be destroyed by cooking. Iron is given as a supplement in the form of iron fumarate or gluconate. The fumarate form causes less constipation. Vitamin C in a dose of 50 mg is useful as an antioxidant and is also included in Renalvite. The fat soluble vitamins like Vitamin A and E are not recommended. Vitamin A impairs bone remodelling and the value of Vitamin E is doubtful in the CKD patient. Zinc has been reported to boost lymphocyte counts and may be of value as a trace element but aluminium must be avoided as it reduces the efficacy of EPO.

Causal Role of Uric Acid in Cardiovascular and Kidney Disease

Recent studies have raised the contributory role of Uric Acid in Cardiovascular and renal disease [Nakagawa T *et al.* Kidney Int 2006, 69:1722–1725]. Hyperuricemia can cause a fall in nitric oxide and activate the renin angiotensin system in the first phase of injury and in the second phase it mediates microvascular renal disease which resembles the renal arteriolosclerosis of hypertension. Uric acid is an independent predictor of hypertension. Among new onset hypertensives, about 90% have elevated serum uric acid [Feig DI *et al.* Kidney Int 2003, 42:247–252]. Uric acid is also associated with the metabolic syndrome. Ingestion of fructose is strongly associated with the development of the metabolic syndrome. Fructose is the only sugar that causes a rise in uric acid. It has been hypothesised that a rise in uric acid could have a role in the development of insulin resistance through a **urate induced inhibition of endothelial nitric oxide**. Lowering of uric acid improved most of the features of the metabolic syndrome in fructose fed rats [Nakagawa T *et al.* Nat Clin Pract Nephrol 2005, 1:80–86]. Hyperuricemia in experimental studies can cause the development of albuminuria, microvascular disease, glomerulosclerosis and tubulointerstitial fibrosis [Nakagawa T *et al.* Am J Nephrol 2003, 23:2–7]. Uric acid also has a contributory role in preeclampsia [Kang DH *et al.* J Hypertens 2004, 94:932–935].

In general, as renal failure progresses, with decreased creatinine clearance there is also associated decreased urate clearance, hence the increased serum uric seen in patients with raised serum creatinine with renal failure. The fractional clearance of uric acid clearance in fact rises markedly when the GFR is below 15 ml/min and the ratio of urate excreted to GFR increases about fivefold because there is increased tubular urate secretion and reduced reabsorption [Danovitch GM *et al.* Clinical Science, 1972, 43:331–341]. The steady state excretion of uric acid falls from 300 mg to 100 mg a day as renal failure progresses. In clinical practice one seldom sees serum uric levels exceeding 10 mg/dl in CKD patients. This is because blood urea itself dissolves the uric acid. In addition, patients with CKD also tend to eat less protein and this contributes to less urate production. Also the degradation of uric acid is increased as more bacteria flourish in the bowels of patients with CKD. A pathogenic role for uric acid has been established in relation to production and progression of vascular disease [Johnson RJ *et al.* J Amer Soc Nephrol 2005, 16:1909–1919]. High serum uric acid is also associated with salt sensitive hypertension which means that a high serum uric acid level would further cause renal deterioration. Some have advocated the use of low dose allopurinol but there is no basis for this. In fact patients with CKD are more prone to allopurinol hypersensitivity and development of Steven Johnson's syndrome. What is important to note is that as renal failure progresses there will be some CKD patients who would be prone to more frequent attacks of gout. For this group of patients they should be treated with colchicine and a small dose of allopurinol of 100 mg a day could be used possibly with a smaller test dose of 50 mg to ensure there is no allopurinol sensitivity which could lead to allergic interstitial nephritis induced by allopurinol hypersensitivity. One should avoid the use of NSAID wherever possible. If the attacks are too severe and painful and associated with renal deterioration, one would have to administer steroids with the help of a Rheumatology colleaque to abort and reduce the frequency and severity of the gouty attacks which would be causing a rapid decrease of residual GFR or even precipitating acute on chronic AKI with a need for dialysis in the less fortunate patient.

A high protein diet can reduce GFR by 0.15 ml/min/year for every 10 gm increase protein in the diet for patients with GFR between 56 to 79 ml/min. Conversely a low protein diet where protein intake is reduced by 0.2 gm/Kg BW/day could slow the decline in GFR by 1.15 ml/min/year based on the MDRD study [Levey AS, Adler S, Caggiula AW *et al.* Amer J Kidney Disease, 1996, 27:652–663]. There are some who argue that patients should receive a trial of protein restriction before initiating dialysis, particularly if the mode of dialysis is hemodialysis which does not preserve the residual renal function unlike peritoneal dialysis. This is because during HD there are intermittent drops of BP which would erode whatever residual GFR the patient may still have on initiating HD. In addition there are psychological impacts of life on dialysis and the mortality on dialysis is 10 times during that of the predialysis period [Division of Kidney UAHDNN:USRDS 2002 Annual Data Report: Atlas of ESRD in the United States. Bethesda, NIH 2003].

Low Protein Diet

It is important to remember when instituting a protein restricted diet in a uremic patient that there must be adequate intake of essential amino acids or their ketoanalogues. The intake of these carbon skeletons is to ensure that protein metabolism is not impaired. A protein restricted diet that does not contain sufficient high quality amino acids may be detrimental. Di Landro in a study of 44 patients on a 3 year diet of 0.6 gm/Kg BW protein compared to another group of 46 patients on 0.3 gm/Kg BW plus a supplement of essential amino acids and their ketoanalogues found that progression of renal disease in the group with the ketoacid analogues was slower based on the reciprocals of the serum creatinine [Di Landro *et al.* Contrib Nephrol 1990, 81:201–207].

Restriction of dietary protein relieves symptoms of uraemia like nausea and vomiting but imposition of an unpalatable diet is not an easy task and may sometimes be considered unkind. The first problem is to get the patient to take the low protein diet. The second is to persuade him to continue it.

Traditionally it has been taught that low protein diet will not prevent the progression of underlying renal disease, and often there is a decrease in the level of blood urea but serum creatinine remains the same or worsens. The diet serves to prevent the accumulation of potentially toxic metabolites and relieves symptoms of uraemia but nutrition suffers eventually.

The aim of imposing a low protein diet in a patient with renal failure therefore is to cause a decrease in the metabolic end proteins of nitrogen metabolism which accumulates in his body.

20 gm Protein Diet

The 20 gm protein diet contains only 3 gm of nitrogen which is the smallest quantity of nitrogen required to maintain nitrogen balance in most uraemics, though in most patients it often leads to malnourishment.

Giovanetti and Giordano introduced essential amino acids into the 20 gm low protein diet which was supplemented with higher calories. They obtained much better results as evident by a more dramatic lowering of blood urea, and in a substantial number of their patients there was also improvement or stabilisation of serum creatinine levels. Nowadays a 20 gm protein diet is not prescribed as it is considered a starvation diet.

0.8gm/kg Body Weight (BW) Protein Diet

Most individuals require at least 35 gm (0.5 gm/kg BW) of protein in order to maintain nitrogen balance reasonably well. At the Singapore General Hospital, a low protein diet usually means a 0.8 gm/kg BW protein diet. Therefore a 50 kg weight patient would require a 40 gm protein diet and a 60 kg weight patient a 50 gm protein diet. It is important to stress that patients on low protein diet require not only high biological protein with essential amino acids but also high calorie carbohydrate and fat.

Excellent nutritional care may minimise complications such as malaise, nausea, vomiting, haemorrhage, anaemia, osteodystrophy, neuropathy, infections, and psychological problems.

Glomerular Hyperfiltration and Relevance of Low Protein Diet (0.8 gm/kg BW)

Nowadays most nephrologists believe that in today's setting, protein restriction should be commenced when the serum creatinine is above normal (>110 micro mol/L for males and >85 micro Mol/L for females) or eGFR <60 ml/min as it is thought that early protein restriction in patients with mild renal impairment may decrease the damage due to glomerular hyperfiltration. Protein restriction is not necessary once serum creatinine is above

400 micro mol/L. Patients should have a normal protein diet at this stage. Otherwise the patient may have malnutrition by the time he needs dialysis.

Keto Acid Analogues

Keto and hydroxy analogues of the amino acids have been much popularised. These agents are transaminated in the liver by non-essential amino acids to the corresponding essential amino acids which are then used for protein synthesis. 20 gm high biological value protein diets supplemented with keto acid analogues in patients with creatinine clearance of less than 15 ml/min have resulted in slowing and even temporarily reversing the progression of chronic renal failure. Compliance may be a problem in these patients as it involves a Giovanetti type high biological value diet together with keto acid analogue supplements. The practical role of these agents may be restricted to patients for whom dialysis is not readily available.

Role of Nutritional Therapy (NT) and Quality of Life in Kidney Disease

Reference: Kalantar-Zadeh K [Amer J Kid Disease, 2001, Nephrol Dial Transpl 2004].

1. There is a high risk of death in CKD patients in the USA. Dialysis accounts for 46% of deaths, worse than that of many cancers. The 10 year survival is only 15% for HD patients. Protein Energy Malnutrition (PEM) and underweight causes more deaths than being overweight and obese. Correction of PEM with gain in dry weight will lower the mortality rate (MR) in these patients.
2. Characteristics of patients with Protein Energy Wasting (PEW) are: BMI <20 kg/m^2 (24%), Muscle mass <90% (62%), Serum

Albumin <35 g/l (20%), Serum Transthyretin or Prealbumin <300 mg/l (36%), nPNA <1 g/Kg (35%).

3. Serum creatinine of dialysis patients is another index. Those with very low serum creatinine as opposed to those with high serum creatinine are the ones with a high relative rate (RR) for death. Their RR is 3.8 versus 0.3 for those with high serum creatinine despite dialysis. So under nutrition kills faster than high cholesterol or obesity.

4. Dr Kalantar would ask his patients routinely "How is your appetite today?". Those with a good appetite would have a lower MR compared to those with a poor appetite.

5. The KDOQI guidelines recommended protein intake of 1.0 to 1.2 gm/Kg BW/Day with an energy intake of 35 kcal/Kg BW/day for those <60 years and 30 kcal/Kg BW/day for those >60 years. Yet more than 50% of HD patients receive nPCR or nPNA <1.0 gm/Kg/day. Those with higher protein intake >1.4 gm/Kg BW/day have lower RR of death compared to those with <1.2 gm/Kg BW/day.

6. Too rigid or strict restriction of Phosphorus (P) in the diet may also outweigh the benefit. The P intake in the diet depends on the protein intake.

7. Serum Albumin is a strong, robust and linear predictor of survival. Patients with serum albumin <3 gm/l have a higher hazard ratio of death compared to those with serum albumin 4.2 gm/l. So if the patients's serum albumin is falling it is a poor prognostic index compared to one where it is rising. The same refers to the serum prealbumin.

8. The TIBC is another predictor. Malnourished HD patients have a low TIBC. It is a marker of the nutritional status of the patient. Low TIBC equates with high MR. Low serum albumin is a poor prognostic marker for both HD and PD patients.

9. Nutritional Therapy and Nutrition Support:

   (i) Oral therapy: patients should be allowed to have their meals on dialysis. Those who eat during dialysis do better. For the CKD patient his oral nutritional needs are important. Those who cannot feed themselves should have tube feeding.

(ii) Parenteral therapy: IDPN (intra-dialytic parenteral nutrition) or TPN (total parenteral nutrition). Those who cannot feed orally or thro' the tube should have IDPN or TPN.

(iii) Pharmacologic support: appetite stimulant, anti depressants, anti inflammatory, anabolic and/or muscle enhancing.

(iv) It is a good practice for the patient to have 1 can of Nepro during HD.

10. Nutritional Objectives: 1.2 gm protein/Kg BW /Day and 30 to 35 kcal/Kg/day

11. As eGFR falls, the serum Albumin will also fall. Therefore, patients with low eGFR usually tend to have low serum albumin [Koppler *et al.* Kidney Int 2000, 75:1688–1703].

12. CKD stages and PEM/PEW. For those patients with CKD stage 1 to 4, 24% to 48% would have PEW and for those in stage 5, up to 75% have PEW. PEW is therefore uremic malnutrition [Fouque, Kalantar, Koppler *et al.* Kidney Int 2008, 73:391–398].

13. Among 1,220 US veterans with non dialysis dependent CKD, those with low serum albumin (as low as <2.5 g/l) have high hazard ratio for death compared to those with higher serum albumin (as high as >5.4 g/l). 29% of them have serum albumin <3.5 g/l, 55% have <3.8 g/l and 74% have <4.0 g/l [Kovesdy *et al.* Amer J Clin Nutrition, 2009].

14. Vandana Menon [Menon V *et al.* Amer J Kid Disease, 2009, 53:208–217] in a study of 229 non diabetic stage 1 to 4 CKD patients who were given either a low protein diet of 0.58 gm/Kg BW protein diet/day versus those given a very low protein diet of 0.28 gm/Kg BW protein diet/day plus supplements with keto acid analogs of essential amino acids, **those on a very low protein diet did not delay progression of kidney failure and appeared to have increased risk of death.** There is a grave risk of putting patients on a very low protein diet as they would develop PEW which is associated

with **hypoalbuminemia of <3.8 gm/l,** worsening quality of life, increased infection rates and hospitalisation rates and increased mortality rates [Kovesdy *et al*. Amer J Clin Nutrition, 2009]. Oral protein supplements will decrease these risks. All CKD patients from stage 1 to 4 should have oral supplements like Suplena plus ketoanalogs.

15. **Conclusion**:

    (i) Periodic Nutrition Assessment and Dietary Counselling is important. Assess dry weight and check lab data like serum albumin.
    (ii) Indication for nutrition intervention if serum albumin <4.0 g/l. Start oral supplements.
    (iii) Assess patients on a monthly basis. Those who improve, continue treatment with oral supplements. Those who do not improve, increase the quantity of oral supplements. If necessary use tube feeding or IDPN if serum albumin <3 g/l.
    (iv) Use adjunctive pharmacology if needs be: appetite stimulant, anti depressant, anti inflammatory, anabolic or muscle enhancing therapy.

16. **Summary and Conclusion**:

    (i) Measurement of Nutrition Status correlate strongly (rather than conventional risk factors) with CKD mortality.
    (ii) A change in Nutritional Status may be a particularly sensitive as an indicator of clinical outcome.
    (iii) Serum albumin is the strongest predictor of survival in dialysis patients. Serum prealbumin can be as sensitive or even more.
    (iv) A nutritional intervention that can increase serum albumin by as little as 0.3 g/l may have an impact of improving survival of CKD patients.
    (v) Oral nutritional intervention can oppose or even reverse catabolic/sarcopenic effects of HD leading to a lasting anabolic effect even after the end of a dialysis session.

(vi) The oral nutritional intervention may improve outcome and survival of CKD patients.

(vii) Consider oral nutritional supplements with pill intake (to replace fluid intake).

The above is a transcript of a power point presentation by Dr Kalantar when he delivered the Plenary Lecture during the Singapore Society of Nephrology (SSN) Annual Meeting on 18th Sept 2010. This is reproduced by kind courtesy of Dr Kalantar through the auspices of the SSN.

Maintaining Internal Environment

In the management of patients with chronic renal failure one should try to maintain the internal environment as near normal as possible.

Prevent dehydration and salt depletion as well as fluid overload. Examine the patient and monitor the neck veins, tissue turgor and tongue. Check the blood pressure for postural hypotension and the serum electrolytes. The patient may require salt supplement. In cases of severe acidosis where the plasma bicarbonate is less than 15 mEq/1, one may have to administer sodium bicarbonate infusions or oral sodium bicarbonate.

Hyperkalaemia

Treat hyperkalaemia with insulin and dextrose and at the same time start the patient on Resonium A.

Anaemia and Erythropoeitin

1. If the patient is anaemic with Hb of 7 gm and less, or if he has symptoms due to anaemia he should be transfused with packed red blood cells. However if the patient has been on

regular follow-up by a nephrologist, he should be given injections of Erythropoeitin [EPO] when Hb is less than 10 gm together with iron supplements. EPO is usually given in a weekly dose of 4,000 units per week together with iron supplements. Sufficient iron must be present in the body in order to form Hb. A patient deficient in iron will not have a rise in Hb despite EPO injections.

2. Several forms of rHuEPO [Human recombinant EPO] are available. These are EPO alpha and beta produced through recombination of the human EPO gene. The half life of EPO alpha is between 4 and 12 hours when given intravenously [IV] and prolonged to 25 hours if given subcutaneously [SC]. The beta EPO has a slightly larger volume of distribution and 20% longer elimination half life after IV route and delayed SC absorption when compared to the alpha form. Clinical efficacy is comparable in both. In the late 1990s Darbepoeitin [DPO] alpha was introduced into the market. This is a hyperglycosylated rHuEPO analog which was described as a novel erythropoeisis stimulating protein. It has a very long half life compared to EPO [25.3 versus 8.5 hours] and clinically is as efficacious as EPO alpha and beta. The initial dose is 0.45 to 0.75 U/kg and can be given weekly or fortnightly initially and later maintained once every 2 or 3 or even up to 4 weekly [MacDouggal JC *et al.* Nephrol Dial Transpl 2003, 18:576–581]. The dose in our local formulary is 20 mg or 40 mg and patients can be maintained at 40 mg once every 2 to 3 weeks, in some even monthly. This is convenient and equally efficacious for many patients instead of the weekly injections of EPO. Patients with CKD not yet on dialysis or on PD can have EPO or DPO by SC route and those on HD can have the IV route during dialysis.

3. Recently, another new pegylated form of Continuous Erythropoietin Receptor Stimulator [CERA] has been introduced and this can be given monthly and in terms of convenience should be as good as DPO.

4. Patients with CKD should start EPO or DPO when the Hb is less than 10 mg/l and once they reach a level of 12 gm or more it should be maintained at that level. There is no necessity to go up to 13 gm/l as a higher Hb level may cause complications. The complications include hypertension, seizures, impaired solute clearance with dangerous accumulation of serum K resulting in hyperkalaemia despite dialysis. There is also a tendency for strokes and thrombosis of vascular access [AVF].

5. Failure to respond to EPO include iron deficiency, secondary hyperparathyroidism, aluminium toxicity, haemoglobinopathies, haemolytic anemia, folic and B12 deficiency, infections, underlying cancers. All these causes should be seen to. For a patient who has well maintained Hb on EPO, if there is a severe decline in Hb of a few grams in a short period, one of the commonest causes of anemia is blood loss due to gastrointestinal bleeding. We should investigate with a gastroscopy followed by a colonoscopy if necessary. If no gastric ulcers are detected other causes of blood loss should be considered including undetected malignancy.

6. Anti rHuEPO antibodies.
    From 1898 to 1998 there was an unusual complication arising from the use of EPO. It was a pure red cell aplasia [PRCA]. Those patients affected produced antibodies that neutralised rHuEPO and inhibited erythroid colony formation from the bone marrow. Subsequently it was discovered that the cause was due to leachates from uncoated rubber syringe stoppers in the EPO delivery package that induced the antibodies which caused PRCA [Boven K *et al.* Kidney Int 2005, 67:2346–2353]. This problem has since been solved and should not recur.

7. In a recent report by Patel [Patel NM *et al.* Vit D deficiency and anemia in early CKD. Kidney Int 2010, 77:715–720], in a study of 1661 patients with CKD it was found that the mean Hb concentration significantly decreased with decreasing tertiles of 25 Vit D and 1,25 Vit D. These trends remain significant

after adjusting for age, gender, ethnicity, eGFR, diabetes and PTH. Patients with a significant dual deficiency of 25 D and 1,25 D had a 5.4 fold prevalence of anemia compared with those replete for both. This study is consistent with previous studies showing that Vit D supplement with calcitriol and ergocalciferol increased the sensitivity of erythropoietin as evidenced by the requirement for less erythropoeisis stimulating agents [ESA] [Saab G *et al*. Prevalence of vit D deficiency and the safety and effectiveness of monthly ergocalciferol in HD patients. Nephron Clin Pract 2007, 105:c132–c138].

8. TREAT. The trial to reduce cardiovascular events with Aranesp therapy, a large trial involving 4038 patients with diabetes and CKD with anemia, 2,012 patients were assigned to receive darbepoeitin alpha to achieve a Hb of 13 gm/l, the rest of the patients were assigned placebo with rescue darbepoeitin when Hb was less than 9 gm/l. The primary end points were composite outcome of death or CV event (nonfatal MI, CHF, stroke or in hospital IHD) and of death or ESRD. The use of darbepoeitin in these patients not undergoing dialysis did not reduce the risk of either of the 2 primary composite outcomes and was associated with an increased risk of stroke. In another trial, the CHOIR or Correction of Hb and outcomes in renal insufficiency trial, involving 222 patients over 16 months, there was a higher risk of CV events in the group assigned to a target Hb of 13.5 gm versus the group with 11.3 gm [Marc De Broe. A trial of darbepoeitin alfa in type 2 diabetes and CKD. Kidney Int 2010, 77:382].

REFERENCES

1. MacDouggal JC *et al*. Correction of anemia with Darbepoeitin in patients with CKD receiving dialysis. *Nephrol Dial Transpl* 2003, **18**:576–581.

2. Boven K *et al.* The increased incidence of pure red cell aplasia with an Eprex formulation in uncoated rubber syringes. *Kidney Int* 2005, **67**:2346–2353.
3. Patel NM *et al.* Vit D deficiency and anemia in early CKD. *Kidney Int* 2010, **77**:715–720.
4. Saab G *et al.* Prevalence of vit D deficiency and the safety and effectiveness of monthly ergocalciferol in HD patients. *Nephron Clin Pract* 2007, **105**:c132–c138.
5. Marc De Broe. A trial of darbepoeitin alfa in type 2 diabetes and CKD. *Kidney Int* 2010, **77**:382.

Iron Therapy

1. Many patients are given Iron [Fe] supplement together with EPO, because if the patients are deficient in Fe the EPO would not be able to increase the manufacture of Hb in the patients. Fe is often given as 200 mg twice daily of Ferrous Fumarate or Gluconate. Fe sulphate causes more constipation compared to the other 2 preparations. Some patients find oral Fe difficult to take and have GI side effects like dyspepsia, bloating and constipation.
2. Compliance of patients is therefore a problem with oral Fe. Also taking oral Fe with Phosphate binders will interfere with Fe absorption. Fe should be taken 1 hour apart from phosphate binders. Because of these 2 factors, some patients on EPO may not respond due to inadequate Fe intake.
3. Intravenous Fe is preferable to oral Fe due to poor efficacy of oral Fe. They come in the form of Fe dextran, Fe sucrose and Ferric gluconate. Giving IV Fe instead of oral Fe will improve the rate as well as response of patients to EPO. The requirement for EPO can also be reduced by about 40% when patients are given IV Fe instead of oral Fe. There is cost savings as well as efficacy.
4. Fe sucrose is preferable to Fe dextran as there is the risk of anaphylaxis with Fe dextran [about 0.6%]. Intravenous Fe sucrose is given as 1000 mg either as 2 separate infusions of 500 mg or 5 infusions of 200 mg over 14 days. Patients once

stabilised can be monitored every 3 months for adequacy of Fe. Another strategy is to give the patient small weekly doses of Fe sucrose to maintain Fe stores. Patients with CKD and on PD can be treated with oral Fe as they do not lose blood regularly like the HD patient during dialysis.

5. The Fe status of the patients can be monitored using Fe and TIBC or total iron binding capacity. Serum Ferritin is also a useful index to measure storage of Fe and reflect Fe deficiency when when the concentration is less than 100 ng/ml. Transferrin saturation often gives false positives of Fe deficiency due to poor specificity. Serum Ferritin may also be too sensitive. We may therefore obtain discordant results of Fe deficiency as expressed by Transferrin saturation and Fe overload as expressed by Serum Ferritin. Inflammation can also give such results. So we should also rely on clinical judgement when interpreting lab results. A useful test is the percentage of hypochromic RBCs [PHR] as a measure of Fe stores. If the PHR is more than 6% it is likely that the patient has Fe deficiency. This test is about 90% accurate [Cullen P *et al.* Nephrol Dial Transpl 1999, 14:659–665].

6. For patients with CKD not on dialysis or those on PD, the KDOQI guidelines for Serum Ferritin is >100 ng/ml and for those on HD it is >200 ng/ml [NKF KDOQI guidelines and clinical practice recommendations for anemia in CKD. Amer J Kidney Disease, 2006, 47S:S1–S146].

Phosphate Binders

High phosphate is now considered an independent risk factor for a more rapid decline in renal function and a higher mortality from myocardial infarction during the pre dialysis phase. Plasma phosphate within the normal range is of vital importance in the pre dialysis patients. Among a group of 6730 CKD patients, 3490 patients had serum phosphate measured during the previous 18 months. After adjustment, serum phosphate levels >3.5 mg/dl

(>1.13 mmol/L) were associated with a significantly increased risk of death. Mortality rate increased linearly with each subsequent 0.5 mg/dl (0.16 mmol/L) increased risk of death [JASN 2005, 16: 520 to 528]. In another study in North America, it was shown that patients on hemodialysis who had high serum phosphate above 6.5 mg/dl (2.1 mmol/L) had a 27% higher risk of death than those whose phosphate levels were between 2.4 and 6.5 mg/dl (0.8 to 2.1 mmmol/L [Block GA *et al.*, Association of serum phosphorus and calcium x phosphate product with mortality risk in chronic hemodialysis patients: a national study. Amer J Kidney Disease, 1998, 31:607–617]. Subsequent analyses showed that an excess risk of death was associated with both high and low levels probably indicating malnutrition. The increased risk of cardiovascular mortality is probably related to accelerated progression of vascular calcification.

Calcium carbonate and phosphate binders should be used whenever the serum phosphate exceeds 1.45 mmol/L or 4.5 mg/dl. Good control of the serum phosphate will cause an increase in serum calcium and also decrease the incidence of metastatic calcification. Patients are usually prescribed calcium carbonate or calcium acetate as phosphate binders. The calcium present will also supplement low calcium levels due to renal bone disease [secondary renal osteodystrophy]. Apart from calcium carbonate and calcium acetate which are the usual drugs used there are newer agents like sevelamer, an ion exchange resin first released as sevelamar hydrochloride. A meta-analysis of 5 randomised trials involving 2429 patients however showed no significant difference between patients treated with sevelamer and calcium based agents [Tonelli M *et al.*, Systemic review of the clinical efficacy and safety of sevelamer in dialysis patients. Kidney Int 2007, 72:1140–1137]. However, among the elderly, 2 prospective outcome studies showed significant survival benefit in incident dialysis patients and in elderly prevalent patients [Suki WN. Response to "Lack of mortality benefit with sevelamer", letter in Kidney Int 2008, 73:1093–1094]. Short term clinical trials have shown it to be effective for controlling serum phosphate with lower episodes of hypercalcemia. Total doses averaging 5 to 6 gms were sufficient to maintain phosphate levels at 5.8 to 6 mg/dL or 1.6 to 2 mM among HD patients [Chertow GM *et al.* Nephrol Dial Transpl 1999, 14:2709–2714].

Lanthanum carbonate is a non aluminium, non calcium phosphate–binding agent. At present there have been no adequately powered trials to examine the clinical effect of lanthanum. None of the trials so far have shown significant differences between lanthanum carbonate and calcium based agents with respect to bone fractures, quality of life and cardiovascular complications [Tonelli M *et al.*, Oral phosphate binders in patients with kidney failure. New Engl J Med 2010, 362:1312–1324]. The capacity of this agent to bind phosphorus is greater than that of Ca acetate, Ca carbonate or Sevelamar. Several clinical trials of Lanthanum carbonate with doses as high as 3000 mg per day have documented its efficacy in patients on dialysis, both HD and PD patients [Baaj A *et al.* Nephrol Dial Transpl 2005, 20:775–782], [Hutchison AJ *et al.* Nephron Clin Prac 2005, 100:c8–c19].

Calcium, Vitamin D Supplements

Calcium supplements are usually given early as many patients have low calcium when GFR is less than 30 ml/min. It is given as calcium carbonate or calcium acetate. Calcium supplements are contraindicated in the presence of severe hyperphosphataemia. The use of the new synthetic vitamin D analogues will depend on the type and degree of renal osteodystrophy. Patients should probably start calcitriol [Rocaltrol] or 1-∝-di(OH)-D_3 as soon as the serum alkaline phosphatase starts to rise. Some prescribe this earlier, two or three times a week instead of daily. However, with the introduction of the KDOQI Clinical Practice Guidelines for Renal Bone Disease in CKD and the availability of new Vitamin D Sterols and Calcimimetic agents much more can now be done to help treat renal bone disease inpatients with CKD.

Recommended values from KDOQI guidelines:

CKD	eGFR range [ml/min]	Phosphorus [mg/dL]	Calcium [mg/dL]	Ca X P	Intact PTH [pg/ml]
3	30–59	2.7–4.6	8.4–10.2		35–70
4	15–29	2.7–4.6	8.4–10.2		70–110
5	<15, dialysis	3.5–5.5	8.4–9.5	55	150–300

For SI units

CKD	eGFR range [ml/min]	Phosphorus [mmol/dL]	Calcium [mmol/dL]	Ca X P	Intact PTH [pmol/L]
3	30–59	0.87–1.48	2.10–2.55		3.85–7.7
4	15–29	0.87–1.48	2.10–2.55		7.7–12.1
5	<15, dialysis	1.13–1.77	2.10–2.38	4.4	16.5–33.0

Treatment for patients with CKD 3 and 4, not yet requiring dialysis

Treatment with Vit D is recommended to lower plasma PTH levels in stages 3 and 4 when levels exceed 70 pg/ml and 110 pg/ml respectively. Vit D [calcitriol] is useful as it will lower plasma PTH levels, enhance intestinal calcium absorption to raise calcium levels and correct hypocalcemia. Standard dose used is 0.25μg/day or every other day and adjusting upward to correct hypocalcemia or lower PTH levels. Watch out for hypercalcemia and hyperphosphatemia and adjust dose accordingly. For patients with symptoms like bone pain or muscle weakness these can improve as the level of PTH decreases. Caution in patients when they develop hypercalcemia as this can cause deterioration of residual renal function. Newer analogs of Vit D like doxercalciferol and paricalcitriol as oral preparations are now available. They are less potent than calcitriol in causing calcium and phosphate absorption from the intestine and less likely therefore to cause hypercalcemia. Hence they would offer more favourable safety profile to patients in CKD 3 and 4.

Treatment for patients on hemodialysis or peritoneal dialysis, CKD 5

For these patients thrice weekly or daily doses of calcitriol range from 0.125 to 1 μg/day is often used. Watch out for hypercalcemia and hyperphosphatemia and adjust dose accordingly. Thrice weekly or twice weekly doses will reduce incidence of hypercalcemia and hyperphosphatemia. Newer analogs of Vit D like docercalciferol, paricalcitol, maxacitol are available as parenteral preparations which are given during hemodialysis to treat secondary hyperparathyroidism [SHPT]. Studies have shown that intravenous calcitriol given thrice weekly [dose 0.5 to 2.25 μg] can lower plasma PTH levels after 2 weeks [Slatopolsky E *et al.*, Marked suppression of secondary hyperparathyroidism by administration of 1, 25 dihydroxycholeciferol in uremic patients. J Clin Invest 1984, 74:2136–2143]. However, there are no long term data beyond 2 years and the impact on bone mass and the need for surgical parathyroidectomy are still unknown. Also there is always the problem of hypercalcemia and hyperphosphatemia which limit the safety of these agents with long term usage. **Long term outcome seems to suggest higher cardiac morbidity and mortality** due to vascular calcification. Because of such concerns parenteral calcitriol have been replaced by the newer Vit D analogs like doxercalciferol and paricalcitriol.

Doxercalciferol and paricalcitriol have been shown to lower plasma PTH levels in short term and long term studies of patients with secondary hyperparathyroidism [SHPT] [Maung HM *et al.* Efficacy and side effects of intermittent and oral docercalciferol (1-hydroxyvitamin D^2) in dialysis patients with secondary hyperparathyroidism; a sequential comparison. Am J Kidney Dis 2001:532–543.] [Lindberg J *et al.* A long term multicenter study of the efficacy and safety of paricalcitriol in end stage renal disease. Clin Nephrol 2001, 56:315–323].

Persistent hypercalcemia and hyperphosphatemia occurred less with paricalcitriol than with calcitriol. However, there are no long term outcome studies regarding bone mass and skeletal fracture rates. Treatment with intermittent oral doses of doxercalciferol [dose range 2.5 to 10 µg thrice weekly] lowers plasma PTH levels in hemodialysis patients with SHPT. Values decrease by 60% after 16 weeks. Occasional hypercalcemia and hyperphosphatemia resolve after 3 to 7 days after temporarily withholding treatment [Tan AU *et al.* Effective suppression of parathyroid hormone by 1 alpha-hydroxy vitamin D in hemodialysis patients with moderate to severe secondary hyperparathyroidism. Kidney Int 1997, 51:317–323]. Present evidence would suggest that it may be safer to have patients on long term paricalcitriol or doxercalciferol rather than calcitriol as there is less cardiac morbidity and mortality due to vascular calcification. But the prohibitive cost of these newer Vit D analogs are a limiting factor as many patients would not be able to afford. In the meanwhile judicious use of the usual Vit D analogues like calcitriol and 1 alpha dihydroxy choleciferol would have to suffice for most patients with frequent monitoring of serum calcium, phosphate and PTH levels.

Calcimimetic agents

These are small organic molecules that function as allosteric activators of the CaSR, the molecular mechanism that mediates calcium regulated PTH secretion by parathyroid cells [Nemeth EF *et al.* Calcimimetics with potent and selective activity on the parathyroid calcium receptor. Proc Natl Acad Sci USA, 1998, 95:4040–4045]. Calcimimetics bind to the membrane spanning portion of the CaSR and lower the threshold for receptor activation for calcium ions [Hammerland LG *et al.* Allosteric activation of the calcium receptor expressed in Xenopus laevis ooocytes by NPS 467 or NPS 568. Mol Pharmacol, 1998, 53:1083–1088]. They inhibit PTH secretion and lower PTH levels. This action is different from that of Vit D and therefore provides another pathway for lowering PTH levels in patients with secondary hyperparathyroidism in dialysis patients. In patients on dialysis, phosphate control is a problem as the amount of phosphate removed by dialysis is inadequate compared to the amount of dietary phosphate ingested. This is especially so among dialysis patients who ingest a high protein diet where the phosphate component is significantly more. High phosphate levels precludes the use of Vit D to control the high PTH levels due to the danger of vascular and soft tissue calcification. Use of large doses of calcium acetate or calcium carbonate to control high phosphate levels may also lead to hypercalcemia which in turn also precludes the use of Vit D to control the high PTH levels. With this scenario, calcimimetics like cinacelcet can lower plasma PTH levels without aggravating phosphate retention or raising serum calcium. Use of cinacelcet may in fact lower both calcium and phosphate levels. Also, even in the presence of high calcium and phosphate levels, cinacelcet can be given to lower plasma PTH. Sustained lowering of PTH levels can be achieved up to 3 years. There have been reports that cinacelcet therapy may also reduce the need for parathyroidec-tomy in dialysis patients and the risk of fractures have also been reduced [Cunningham J *et al*. Effects of calcimimetic cinacelcet HCl on cardiovascular disease, fracture and health related quality of life in secondary hyperparathyroidism. Kidney Int 2005, 68:1793–1800]. Serum calcium in some patients on cinacelcet may be low [7.5 to 8.0 mg/dL] and they may require Vit D and calcium acetate or carbonate or increase in calcium concentration in the dialysate.

Some additional notes on Phosphate and Calcium binding agents

Phosphate retention in dialysis patients is a problem because the usual dialysis regime does not remove phosphate adequately. Hence we have to resort to the use of phosphate binders which are not without problems. Alternative regimes of hemodialysis like daily dialysis and nocturnal hemodialysis is another strategy for phosphate removal as patients on these regimes have more markedly cumulative weekly removal of phosphate [Musci I *et al*. Control of serum phosphorus without any phosphate binders in patients treated with nocturnal hemodialysis. Kidney Int 2000,

35:1226–1237. For patients with CKD 3 and 4, phosphate removal is still adequate and there is not much cause for concern. It must be stressed that phosphate control is important as hyperphosphatemia contributes to vascular calcification with increased cardiovascular mortality. KDOQI guidelines for CKD 3 and 4 is to maintain serum phosphorus levels at normal levels and for CKD stage 5 values of 3.5 to 5.5 mg/dL are acceptable. If aluminium hydroxide gel were to be resorted to for phosphate control we should use for only short term, not more than 3 months and in as low a dose as possible. Plasma aluminium levels have to be monitored for aluminium toxicity.

Calcium acetate and carbonate are still commonly used as phosphate binders but not calcium citrate because citrate enhances intestinal aluminium absorption. The use of large doses of calcium in the form of phosphate binders may lead to undesirable vascular and soft tissue calcification. It should not exceed a total of 2000 mg calcium for both dietary and medicated calcium. One solution then is to prescribe sevelamer and lanthanum carbonate which are both calcium free phosphate binders. Sevelamar binds to phosphorus in the bowel thereby reducing its absorption. Sevelamar is effective in reducing serum phosphate levels without causing hypercalcemia and is as effective as calcium acetate. In a dose of 5 to 6 gm a day sevelamar can maintain serum phosphorus between 5.8 to 6 mg/dL or 1.8 to 2 μM in hemodialysis patients with secondary hyperparathyroidism. One useful effect of sevelamer is that it also reduces total cholesterol and LDL cholesterol and increases HDL cholesterol. For patients on sevelamar, the coronary and aortic vascular calcification did not change among patients on sevelamar in contrast to those on calcium acetate or carbonate. Both the hydrochloride and carbonate forms of sevelamar exert actions of bone modelling and skeletal anabolism and inhibition of vascular calcification. However, in patients with ESRF on hemodialysis, the hydrochloride component may worsen acidosis and adversely affect bone metabolism and contribute to renal bone disease. Acidosis has been associated with malnutrition and inflammation and decreased survival in hemodialysis patients. Sevelamer carbonate may be preferable in this respect as the carbonate may combat renal acidosis. Compared to the hydrochloride which may worsen acidosis [Delmez J *et al.* A randomised, double-blind, crossover design of sevelamar hydrochloride and carbonate in patients on hemodialysis. Clin Nephrol 2007, 68:386–391].

Lanthanum carbonate is another potent phosphate binder. It binds phosphorus in vitro like aluminium hydroxide and is in fact more powerful than calcium acetate and carbonate as well as sevelamer. Doses of up to 3000 mg a day have been used with great efficacy in controlling serum phosphate levels among dialysis patients. Safety and efficacy data have been obtained up to 3 years [D'Haese PC *et al.* A multicenter study on the effects of lanthanum carbonate on renal bone disease in dialysis patients. Kidney Int Supple 2003, 85:S73–S78].

Phosphate Control in Patients with CKD 3 and 4

1. For those with raised serum phosphate levels they should be treated with calcium acetate or carbonate [phosphate binders]. If serum PTH levels are raised, they should be prescribed dietary phosphate restriction in addition to phosphate binders. Generally, patients with eGFR >30 ml/min should not have phosphate retention.
2. For those with hypocalcemia, small doses of Vit D [calcitriol] can be prescribed as this will enhance calcium absorption from the bowels and also lower plasma PTH levels. It is also safe to give such patients with secondary parathyroidism smaller doses of oral doxecalciferol or paricalcitriol. They will lower PTH levels without changing calcium and phosphate levels. There is also evidence that unlike calcitriol, the newer Vit D analogs like doxercalciferol and paricalcitriol will not cause vascular calcification, but their cost is prohibitive. It may be useful to screen patients for Vit D deficiency.

3. Calcimimetic agents like cinacelcet can be used in patients with CKD 3 and 4 with secondary hyperparathyroidism [not on dialysis yet]. Their serum phosphate levels usually remain unchanged during cinacelcet therapy but the serum calcium levels may be low and this may limit the doses required to control secondary hyperparathyroidism. For the moment, further studies are required to determine safety and efficacy of cinacelcet in this group of patients.

Phosphate Control in Patients with CKD stage 5

1. It is mandatory to control high serum phosphorus levels in dialysis patients as elevated phosphate levels are associated with a high cardiovascular morbidity and mortality rate. Dietary phosphate restriction goes hand in hand with phosphate binding medications. The total dose of oral calcium should not exceed 1500 mg/day, otherwise the risk of vascular and soft tissue calcification will be increased. In this respect the use of sevelamer and lanthanum would be preferable but their cost is prohibitive. In some patients on these calcium free phosphate binders, the dietary intake of calcium may not be adequate, in which case they may need a combination with a small dose of calcium acetate or carbonate.

2. The level of serum PTH has to be monitored whilst the patients are on phosphate binders and if PTH levels are high, the next step would be to use Vit D sterols or calcimimetic drugs which would lower PTH levels. At this point most patients are prescribed calcitriol or 1 alpha dihydro-choleciferol as the cost of these are much more affordable to patients. The newer Vit D analogs like paricalcitriol and doxercholecalciferol would be preferable as patients treated with these newer drugs do not develop vascular and soft tissue calcification compared to the older Vit D analogs, but the prohibitive cost of these newer agents is a major factor influencing the choice of these agents.

Paricalcitriol is usually given thrice weekly and it is very effective, causing the high PTH levels to decrease steadily over a few months to reach an acceptable target range of between 150 to 300 pg/ml.

3. One caution with the use of Vit D analogs and paricalcitriol is that while the level of PTH decreases, the level of serum calcium may increase causing hypercalcemia or phosphate increases causing hyperphosphatemia, so all these levels need monitoring. If this happens, then the Vit D sterols or paricalcitriol would have to be temporarily withheld. Serum calcium levels should not exceed 9.5 to 10 mg/dL or 2.4 to 2.5 mmol/dL and serum phosphate not exceed 5.5 mg/dL or 1.8 mmol/dL as mortality will increase with these values.

4. One alternative for patients who repeatedly have high serum calcium with Vit D treatment is to convert to the use of calcimimetic like cinacelcet which tends to cause hypocalcemia. Cinacelcet lowers plasma PTH levels as well as serum calcium and serum phosphate during therapy and so would be useful for patients with secondary hyperparathyroidism with high serum calcium and serum phosphate. Cinacelcet can also be used when the serum calcium and phosphate are normal or high, whereas Vit D would be more useful for those patients who have low serum calcium. Cinacelcet is available as an oral preparation. Do not exceed a dose of more than 30 mg initially as it may lower serum calcium dramatically. Over a period of 12 weeks or so with incremental doses of cinacelcet, the plasma PTH will decrease. Expect also a decrease of serum calcium especially during the early few weeks of treatment. Serum phosphate levels will also decrease steadily. If serum calcium falls too much and the dose of cinacelcet cannot be increased further to reduce plasma PTH levels to the target level, then add Vit D which will help to decrease plasma PTH as well as increase the serum calcium level. Hence titrating both the doses of Vit D and cinacelcet may allow one to have adequate control of plasma PTH as well as serum calcium and phosphate levels in the patients.

5. A final word on dialysate calcium levels. A low dialysate calcium will stimulate PTH secretion and cause parathyroid hyperplasia. So do not keep the dialysate concentration of calcium below 2.5 mEq/L or 1.25 mmol/L.

Calcium Phosphorus Product

The assumption that ectopic calcification will occur when a particular threshold of calcium phosphorus product is exceeded has no scientific basis. It is no longer considered a sound assumption. However, it is imperative that we keep the calcium, phosphorus and serum PTH levels of our patients within the limits of the recommended guidelines bearing in mind the potential pitfalls with regards to calcium phosphate binders and use of Vit D analogs.

Although ectopic calcification can occur anywhere, the focus should be on vascular calcification which is the most common site and most likely to affect patient outcomes.

Although the KDOQI guideline that the Ca X P product should not exceed 55 mg^2/dl^2 or 4.4 in SI units this is not considered evidenced based since there is no data to support this [O'Neill WC. The fallacy of the calcium-phosphorus product. Kidney Int 2007, 72:792–796].

Blood Pressure Control

Judicious control of blood pressure is important as it may retard the progression of chronic renal failure. Calcium channel blockers form the mainstay of treatment together with beta blockers. Alpha terazoxin, an alpha blocker is a useful addition for patients whose BP is difficult to control. Though thiazides are no longer of use as diuretics when the GFR is less than 30 ml/min, they are still useful as vasodilators. Frusemide is the diuretic of choice.

For patients with renal failure with serum creatinine less than 400 micro M/L, ACE inhibitor or Angiotensin Receptor Antagonist

(ATRA) can be used to reduce intra-glomerular hypertension due to Glomerular Hyperfiltration. Monitor serum potassium and renal function.

Once serum creatinine exceeds 400 micro M/L, ACE inhibitor or ATRA is withdrawn as the danger of hyperkalaemia is increased with worsening renal failure.

Vitamins

Multivitamin and iron supplements are usually prescribed.

Investigations

During radiological investigations, the patient with CKD stage 3 and 4 should not be dehydrated. Beware of contrast induced nephropathy which may push the patient into CKD stage 5. In the case of a patient with CKD stage 3 and 4 with cardiac problem who may need a coronary angiogram, use the smallest dose of contrast and do not dehydrate the patient. Warn the patient that despite the reduced contrast load he or she may still end up with CKD stage 5 requiring dialysis. However, in most cases patients have not much choice but to proceed with the angiogram which is necessary as part of the cardiac management with a view to angioplasty or coronary artery bypass surgery [CABG]. If the heart problem is not solved the patient may die. As for the kidney patient with ESRF there is always the option for a renal transplant or dialysis. Blood taking in the forearm must be avoided as it may be difficult to create arteriovenous fistulae later if the forearm veins are traumatised or thrombosed. Similarly, BP measurement should not be performed on the arm with an AV fistula.

Sympathy

Remember that the patient is human and you must be too. Show an interest in him. Ask about the food he eats. Enquire about his appetite, his fluid allowance, his sleeping pattern and even his sex life. Listen to his feelings and his fears. Be aware of depression and suicidal tendencies. Some patients go through a phase of "denial" before they can "accept" their illness. They suffer from "reactive depression" and may require psychiatric counselling.

RECENT ADVANCES: Renoprotective Effects of Vitamin D Analogs

1. The activities of 1, 25 $(OH)_2 D_3$ are mediated by the Vitamin D receptor (VDR), a member of the nuclear receptor super family. VDR is expressed in all tissues of the body. The noncalcemic activities of Vit D include regulation of the RAS and the nuclear factor $(NF)_k B$ pathway. The current Vit D analogs include paricalcitriol, docercalciferol and 22-oxacalcitriol. **These analogs suppress PTH activity** but has less calcemic effects than calcitriol.

2. These newer Vit D analogs have renoprotective activity which include inhibition of renal fibrosis, reduce renal inflammation and suppress proteinuria. Interstitial fibrosis is the hallmark of disease progression and its prominent feature is increased deposition of extra cellular matrix (ECM). **Paricalcitriol can suppress ECM production by suppressing the profibrotic TGF pathway**. In rats with 5/6 nephrectomy, paricalcitriol also suppressed the activation of the local RAS in the kidney leading to reduction in BP and proteinuria.

3. In the USA, 7.8% of the population have diabetes and diabetes is the cause of ESRF in 44% of patients and is the leading cause of CKD. High glucose activates the RAS and the $(NF)_k B$ pathway in the kidney. Recently, VDR has been found to have a renoprotective role against the development of Diabetic nephropathy (Diab Nx).

4. The current usage of ACEI, ARBs for Diab Nx though useful in reduction of proteinuria does not halt the epidemic of

CKD. This is because these agents give rise to a compensatory increase in renin synthesis caused by the disruption of the feedback inhibition loop by the inhibitors themselves. Renin build up in the plasma and interstitial space stimulates the conversion of Ang I to Ang II. Ang II accumuation eventually limits the efficacy of RAS inhibition and explains why the current RAS inhibitors are only suboptimal clinically. Zhang *et al.* [Zhang *et al.* Renoprotective effect of the role of Vit D receptor in diabetic nephropathy. Kidney Int 2008, 73:163–171] treating diabetic rats with paricalcitriol and losartan ameliorated kidney injury, restored Glomerular filtration, reduced Glomerular sclerosis accompanied by suppression of ECM proteins, pro fibritic and pro inflammatory cytokines like TGF-β, MCP-1 and VEGF with reversal of decline of slit diaphragm proteins.

5. The antiproteinuria effect of Vit D analogs was reported by Agarwal *et al.* [Agarwal R *et al.* Anti proteinuria effect of paricalcitriol in CKD. Kidney Int 2005, 68:2823–2828]. Here despite treatment with ACEI and ARB, the effect of paricalcitriol was still obvious. The study indicated that the Vit D analog has synergistic effects with ACEI/ARB in reducing proteinuria.

6. Alborzi [Aborzi P *et al.* Paricalcitriol reduces abbuminuria and inflammation in CKD: a randomised double blind pilot trial. Hypertension, 2008, 52:249–255] in a recent study of 24 patients with CKD 2 to 3, reported that paricalcitriol treatment for a month significantly reduced proteinuria and inflammation status in the treated subjects independent of its effects on hemodynamics and PTH suppression.

7. **Vit D analogs protect the kidney by targeting 2 major P/W, the local RAS and the (NF)$_k$ B pathway.** Hyperglycemia, renal insufficiency and Vit D deficiency can activate the local RAS leading to production of Ang II. Ang II causes vasoconstriction and oxidative stress, induces cell proliferation, inflammation and fibrosis. The other P/W, the (NF)$_k$ B

pathway is a master regulator of immune response and is involved in the regulation of inflammatory cytokines and chemokines like MCP-1, PAI-1 and TNFα which are involved in development of kidney disease. 1, 25 $(OH)_2 D_3$ and Vit D analogs like paricalcitriol can inhibit renin expression as well as suppress $(NF)_k B$ activation.

8. There is growing evidence for the renoprotective role of Vit D and its analogs [Li YC. Renoprotective effects of Vit D analogs. Kidney Int 2010, 78:134–139]. We need to introduce such new therapeutics in order to stem the growing tide of patients afflicted by CKD progression to ESRF every year.

What is current guideline for use of Vit D in patients with CKD and those on renal replacement therapy?

1. In a recent review by Anca Gal-Moscovici [Gal-Moscovici A *et al*. Use of Vit D in CKD patients. Kidney Int 2010, 78: 146–151] it has been stated that administration of VDRa, be recommended for those undergoing renal replacement therapy only for treatment for hyperparathyroidism. It has been suggested that Vit D therapy should be stopped or not initiated when phosphate concentrations are >5.5 mg/dl or 1.8 mmol/l, when PTH concentrations are <150 μg/ml, or when the calcium phosphate product >55 mg^2/dl^2. For SI units the Ca x P product is 4.4, the equivalent of 55 of the traditional mg/dL unit. There is no comment on the use of Vit D to correct the deficiency of Vit D in these patients.

2. In patients with CKD 3 and 4 it is recommended to correct 25 Vit D deficiency when hyperparathyroidism is present with the use of ergocalciferol or cholecalciferol. Only if hyperparathyroidism persists, it is recommended to use a VDRa for treatment.

Vit D nomenclature

Term	Sterol		Comment
Vitamin D	Cholecalciferol	D_3	
	Ergocalciferol	D_2	
25 Vit D	Calcidol (25(OH) D3)	D_3	
	Ercalcidol (25(OH) D2)	D_2	
VDRa	Calcitriol (1,25(OH)2D3	D_3, **natural** hormone	
	Alphacalcidol (1(OH) D3)	D_3, synthetic prohormone[a]	
	Doxercalciferol (1(OH) D2)	D_2, synthetic prohormone	
	Paricalcitriol (19nor, 1,25 (OH)2D2)	D_2, synthetic **analog**	
	Maxacalcitriol (22oxa, 1,25 (OH)2D3)	D_3, synthetic **analog**	

Abbrev: VDRa = Vitamin D receptor agonist; 25 Vit D = 25 hydroxy D.

[a]Prohormone = requires 25 hydroxylation by the liver to become an active analog.

Above Table (Modified from Anca Gal-Moscovici (Refer to above article in Kidney International).

Alternative nomenclature

[With Courtesy and Modified from Kalantar-Zadeh K *et al.* Kidney bone disease and mortality in CKD: revisiting the role of vitamin D, calcimetics, alkaline phosphatase and minerals. Kidney Int 2010,78S:S10–S21]

Nutritional Vit D (ergocalciferol and cholecalciferol)
Vit D receptor **activators** (calcitriol*, alphacalcidiol, doxercalciferol)
Vit D **mimetics** (paricalcitriol, maxacalcitriol)
Calcimimetics (calcicinet)
Recombinant PTH (teriparatide)

Receptor activator of nuclear factor — $_k$ B ligand modulators (denosumab).

* calcitriol is also referred to as **active** Vit D

3. In most patients with CKD, calcium and phosphate disorders are not evident till CKD stage 4, hence the high risk of Cardiovascular disease in this group cannot be attributed solely to calcium and phosphate disorders. But the level of calcitriol concentrations in CKD stage 2 is already at the lower limit of normal and by stage 3 and 4 the levels are even lower [Levin A *et al.* Prevalence of abnormal serum vitamin D, PTH, calcium and phosphorus in patients with CKD: results of the study to evaluate early kidney disease. Kidney Int 2007, 71:31–38]. Therefore, just like patients undergoing dialysis, such patients will also run the risk of increased cardiovascular disease with increased morbidity and mortality. Why is calcitriol low in these patients? This is the result of decreased renal mass.

5. In a recent study by Coyne [Coyne D *et al.* Paricalcitriol capsule for the treatment of secondary hyperparathyroidism in stages 3 and 4 CKD. Amer J Kidney Disease, 2006, 47:263–276] of 220 patients, PTH concentrations fell significantly (42%) and this was associated with a significant decrease in bone specific alkaline phosphatase compared with placebo subjects.

6. **In conclusion**, Vit D deficiency develops very early in CKD and with the evidence showing that VDRa can lower morbidity and mortality in these patients we need to think carefully about how we can offer our patients better protection. Based on current guidelines, all CKD patients should be treated with ergocalciferol or cholecalciferol to correct Vit D deficiency. However, for those patients with raised plasma PTH levels, VDRa therapy should be considered [Gal-Moscovici A *et al.* Use of Vit D in CKD patients. Kidney Int 2010, 78:146–151].

7. How should we do it based on knowledge we have today? It is my belief that for CKD 1,2 and 3A there is no need for Vit D therapy as they have enough kidney function to produce adequate natural Vit D, given the evidence that the conventional Vit D like calcitriol actually increases the vascular calcification in these patients, hence explaining the higher CVS mortality in these patients. For those who are in CKD 3B and 4 they should be on oral paricalcitriol if they can afford. Otherwise we may have to prescribe the usual calcitriol that we now use. Those in CKD 5 on dialysis with high plasma PTH should have paricalcitriol by injection [higher dose required] if they can afford it. Calcimetics like cinacelcet could be considered for high calcium, high phosphate, high Ca X Phosphate product or raised plasma PTH, whichever is more affordable, paricalcitriol versus cinacelcet. **Paricalcitriol is marketed as Zemplar and cinacelcet is marketed as Regpara locally.**

New Insight into Phosphorus Metabolism in CKD

1. In today's terms, once a diagnosis of CKD is made the prognosis is dismal as there is a high risk of death from cardiovascular Disease (CVD). So far neither the quality of dialysis or therapeutic intervention has made a significant impact. The ray of hope could lie with the discovery of **fibroblast growth factor 23(FGF23)** as a means of providing early diagnosis of a **perturbation in Phosphorus Metabolism** at an **early subclinical state** thus providing an **opportunity for early therapy** before the ravages of CVD have set in.

2. As stated earlier hyperphosphatemia is an independent risk factor for CVD and mortality for patients on dialysis. The present KDOQI guidelines recommended that for patients with **CKD 4 and 5**, the serum P levels should be between **2.7 to 4.6 mg/dl (0.87 to 1.48 mmol/l)** and for those **on dialysis** it should be between **3.5 to 5.5 mg/dl (1.13 to 1.78** mmol/l).

However, this has not been satisfactory as the high CVD death rate in these patients have not been abated. In fact, the reported risk estimate for death in one of the pre dialysis CKD studies was **23% per 1 mg/dl (0.3 mmol/l)** increase in se P level, yet **50% of patients had levels within the range of 2.5 to 3.5 mg/dl (0.80 to 1.13 mmol/l)** [Kestenbaum B *et al.* J Am Soc Nephrol 2005, 16:520–528]. The hazard ratio for kidney disease progression was reported to be 1.07 for every 0.3 mg/dl (0.1 mmol/l) increase in serum P level. To compound the problem, the diurnal variation for serum P is up to 1 mg/dl (0.3 mmol/l).

3. Sensitive biomarkers are urgently needed for screening, early diagnosis and initiation of therapy for disordered P metabolism. **Fibroblast growth factor 23 (FGF23) is a key regulator of P and Vit D metabolism.** It is a 251 amino acid protein secreted by osteocytes in adults and by other tissues during development. FGF 23 binding to FGF receptor 1c-klotho complex **induces phosphaturia by decreasing P reabsorption in the proximal tubule**. This in turn inhibits conversion of 25 hydroxy Vit D (25D) to 1,25 dihydroxy Vit D. FGF23 regulates P and 1,25D homeostasis in health.

4. **FGF23 is elevated in patients with CKD** as a compensatory response to maintain normophosphatemia. **Low rates of hyperphosphatemia, yet markedly increased levels of FGF23 are found in pre dialysis patients.** As increased FGF23 levels are found in early CKD patients long before hyperphosphatemia, **increased FGF23 may be a more sensitive biomarker of disordered P metabolism than concommittant se P levels. Increased FGF23 levels at initiation of dialysis has been associated with increased mortality** during the 1st year of dialysis. **This result was independent of serum P levels**. There was an association with ascending quartiles of FGF23 and linear increase in mortality. The **highest FGF23 quartile was nearly 600% increased risk of death**, which was marked greater than the **parallel analysis for serum P showing only 20% increase for mortality**.

5. The increased mortality of high levels of FGF23 may seem at odds with survival benefit of active Vit D therapy [Teng M *et al*. Survival of patients undergoing HD with paricalcitriol or calcitriol therapy. New Eng J Med 2003, 349:446–456]. It is possible that the effect of FGF23 excess on mortality can be modified by treatment with active Vit D. Patients who die despite active Vit D therapy could be those with the highest baseline FGF 23 levels. There is likely a **therapeutic window for active Vit D therapy whereby too high a dose could be harmful by raising FGF23 excessively**, while lower doses might promote less elevation of FGF23 while garnering the beneficial effects of Vit D.

6. **FGF23 is associated with CVD**. FGF23 bears a strong relationship to vascular disease and **LVH. It is related to impaired vascular reactivity and arterial stiffness** and is also associated with significant increased **risk of severe coronary arterial calcification**. FGF23 is therefore a marker of coronary and vascular disease.

7. **FGF23 and Kidney Disease Progression.** During a median follow up period of 53 months, **FGF23 levels >35 pg/ml was associated with more rapid progression of CKD**, independent of age, gender and baseline eGFR, Proteinuria and serum levels of calcium, phosphorus and PTH levels. **FGF23 is a marker of CKD progression long before there is any increase of serum P**.

8. So far, no studies assessed have shown that phosphate binders are associated with decreased mortality on dialysis, until a recent study from Isakova [Isakova T *et al*. Am J Kid Dis 2009, 20:388–396]. However, recently Nagano and Others [Nagano N *et al*. Effect of manipulating serum P with phosphate binders on circulating PTH and FGF23 in renal failure rats. Kidney Int 2006, 69:531–537] have shown that **P binders lower FGF23 in animals, healthy humans and dialysis patients** [Burnett SM *et al*. J Bone Mineral Res 2006, 21:1187–1196].

9. CKD stage 3 and 4 occurs in millions of patients. Yet 90% of them have normal serum P levels despite markedly elevated FGF23 levels. Only about 30% of CKD 4 patients and 20% of CKD 3 patients are on phosphate binders.

10. The authors of this review article which I have summarised have proposed a placebo controlled randomised trial of phosphate binders in patients with CKD stage 3b and 4. Eligible patients should have serum P of <4.6 mg/dl without previous phosphate binder treatment and an FGF23 of a certain level to be determined. Those who develop hypophosphatemia would reduce or discontinue the use of phosphate binders. A trial of 1000 patients in each arm for 2 years would provide 90% power with a 2 sided alpha of 0.05 to detect 20% reduction in mortality in the treatment group assuming an incidence density of 10 deaths per 100 patient years in the placebo group, equivalent to median survival of 5 years. From the authors internal data, they have found 69% of patients with CKD stage 3b and 4 had C terminal FGF23 levels >100 RU/ml and 46% had levels >150 RU/ml respectively. The trial is hoped to show sustained FGF23 level reduction in the target group.

Reference: Isakova T *et al.* A blueprint for randomised trials targetting phosphorus metabolism in CKD. *Kidney Int* 2009, **76**:705–716.

Summary of FGF23 by courtesy of Dr Robert Guiberteau

1. FGF23 provides an assay for identifying genetic disorders affecting minerals.
2. It is an exciting tool for unraveling new physiologic pathways.
3. It is the most sensitive marker of early phosphate retention and is possibly the new target for phosphate binder titration in therapy.
4. It is a most promising marker for morbidity and mortality.

Dr Guiberteau also delivered a lecture at the Singapore Society of Nephrology Annual Meeting on 18th Sept 2010.

REFERENCES

1. Bellizzi V *et al.* Very low protein diet supplemented with ketoacid analogs improves blood pressure control in chronic kidney disease. *Kidney Int* 2007, **71**:245–251.
2. Altmann P *et al.* Cognitive function in Stage 5 CKD patients on hemodialysis: No adverse effects of lanthanum carbonate compared with standard phosphate binder therapy. *Kidney Int* 2007, **71**:252–259.
3. Suresh Matthew *et al.* Reversal of Adynamic Bone Disorder and Decreased Vascular Calcification in CKD by Sevelamer Carbonate Therapy. *J amer Soc Nephrol* 2007, **18**:122–130.
4. Delmex J *et al.* A randomised, double blind, cross over design study of sevelamer hydrochloride and sevelamar carbonate in patients on hemodialysis. *Clin Nephrol* 2007, **68**:386–391.
5. Tonelli M *et al.* Oral phosphate binders in patients with kidney failure. *New Engl J Med* 2010, **362**:1312–1324.
6. Brancaccio D *et al.* Lanthanum carbonate: time to abandon prejudices? *Kidney Int* 2007, **71**:190-192.
7. O'Neill WC. The fallacy of the calcium-phosphorus product. *Kidney Int* 2007, **72**:792–796.
8. Li YC. Renoprotective effects of Vit D analogs. *Kidney Int* 2010, **78**:134–139.
9. Agarwal R *et al.* Anti Proteinuria effect of paricalcitriol in CKD. *Kidney Int* 2005, **68**:2823–2828.
10. Zhang *et al.* Renoprotective effect of the role of Vit D receptor in diabetic nephropathy. *Kidney Int* 2008, **73**:163–171.
11. Verstuyf A *et al.* Vit D: A pleiotropic hormone. *Kidney Int* 2010, **78**:140–145.
12. Gal-Moscovici A *et al.* Use of Vit D in CKD patients. *Kidney Int* 2010, **78**:146–151.
13. Kalantar-Zadeh K *et al.* Kidney bone disease and mortality in CKD: Revisiting the role of vitamin D, calcimetics, alkaline phosphatase and minerals. *Kidney Int* 2010,**78**S:S10–S21.
14. Isakova T *et al.* A blueprint for randomised trials targeting phosphorus metabolism in CKD. *Kidney Int* 2009, **76**:705–716.

CHAPTER 30

Hemodialysis

A patient should be considered for dialysis or transplantation as soon as it is clear that he or she has chronic renal failure, usually when serum creatinine is about 400 micro mol/L. Remember to screen patients for Hepatitis B, C and HIV infection so that precautions can be taken in positive patients.

Dialysis is usually started when the serum creatinine is about 600 to 700 micro mol/L though occasionally it is indicated on symptomatic grounds at an earlier stage. The aim should be to start dialysis before complications of uraemia occur (pericarditis, nausea and vomiting), so that it should be possible for a patient to continue full-time employment.

SELECTION

Acceptance policies vary considerably in different countries. Some countries accept any patient while many others, because of financial restrictions, select patients based on age, medical, economic and other factors.

CENTRE DLALYSIS

Centre dialysis in the Singapore General Hospital is usually required for the initiation of dialysis and for a short period after transplantation. Patients on dialysis in stand alone dialysis centres run by the Voluntary Welfare Organisations [VWO] like the National Kidney Foundation, the Kidney Dialysis Foundation or People's Dialysis Centre or Private dialysis patients with complications such as hypertension, vascular access difficulties and severe infections also need to be dialysed at the Centre whilst their problems are sorted out during the in hospital stay. Such complications require a high staff-patient ratio with one nurse attending to 3 patients [1:3] in contrast to the stand alone VWO centres with a staff-patient ratio of about 1 to 10. In centre hospital dialysis also provide more sophisticated and more complicated forms of dialysis unlike the usual conventional intermittent standard dialysis of 4 hour dialysis provided by stand alone VWO and other private centres. The non standard dialysis are also more costly and labour intensive requiring more specialised doctors and nurses and patients can dialysis at prices subsidised by the government.

HOME DIALYSIS

This is the best option for the patient on dialysis. The patient can dialyse himself after office hours at his own convenience with the aid of his spouse or partner. Employers are happier and such patients are more productive compared to those on centre or self dependency dialysis. In Singapore the set-up for home dialysis which includes the dialysis machine and water treatment unit (reverse osmosis or deioniser) cost about S$60,000 to S$90,000, with a monthly maintenance expenditure for disposables like dialysers, blood-lines and dialysate which together cost about S$1,800 monthly expenditure. It is obvious therefore that not many can afford to dialyse at home. For those who can afford more, the private nephrologist can provide a dialysis nurse with the dialysis machine and other set up to perform the dialysis in the comfort of the patient's home. The cost can vary from S$500 upwards a session. Some of the richer patients can have daily short hour dialysis [2 hours plus] compared to the conventional thrice weekly schedule of 4 hours a session. Alternatively, some patients can opt for nocturnal daily dialysis at an even higher cost. For those patients on daily dialysis they have better serum phosphate control as the cumulative dialysis time is more. They are also those who can afford the use of the more costly newer Vit D analog like paracalcitriol and more expensive calcium free phosphate binders like lanthanum carbonate or sevelamer carbonate.

The Cost of Starting and Maintaining a Large Home Hemodialysis Program

Home hemodialysis (HHD) improves some measurable biological and quality of life parameters over conventional in-center dialysis. This is a report from Komenda [Komenda P *et al*. British Columbia Provincial Renal Agency, Vancouver, Canada], article published in Kidney International [Komenda P *et al*. Kidney Int 2010, 77:1039–1045]. It covered 122 patients of which 113 were still in the programme at study end. The majority performed nocturnal home HD in this 2 year retrospective study. All training periods, both in-center and in-home dialysis, medications, hospitalisations and deaths were captured. Comparative data from provincial database and pricing models were used for costing purposes. The total comprehensive costs per patient — incorporating startup, home and in-center dialysis, medications, home remodelling and consumables was $59,179 for years 2004–2005 and 48,648 for 2005–2006. This study described a valid comprehensive funding model delineating cost estimates of starting and maintaining a large home based HD programme.

The HHD patients were on the whole younger, have less diabetes and likely to have less CVD. Starting cost for programme cost $510,000 including training the first cohort of 53 patients. Each patient started on HD cost about $11,665. Estimate of programme cost per patient for 2004–2005 was $18,830. Startup cost for patients who started in 2005–2006 was $17,306 per patient. At end of 2005–2006, it cost 1.95 million $ to deliver 65.58 patient years of HHD to 113 patients. Maintenance dialysis cost per patient was $40,349 per patient in 2004–2005 and $31,342 per patient in 2005–2006.

This model found significantly magnified savings when quality adjusted life years were taken into account ($129,845/ quality-adjusted life years for in-center HD versus $71,443/ quality-adjusted life years for nocturnal HD).

REFERENCE

Komenda P *et al.* British Columbia Provincial Renal Agency, Vancouver, Canada. The cost of starting and maintaining a large home hemodialysis program. Kidney International *Kidney Int* 2010, **77**:1039–1045.

SELF DEPENDENCY DIALYSIS CENTRES

These centres are developed in most countries to provide a more convenient dialysis location for patients who cannot dialyse at home. To keep costs down, emphasis is placed on self dialysis with a low staff-patient ratio. This policy also retains the advantages of home dialysis in placing the responsibility for care on the patient himself, with a consequent better survival and rehabilitation rate. However, nowadays in Singapore, many patients opt for Assisted Dialysis in the various centres which include those run by the National Kidney Foundation (NKF), the Kidney Dialysis Foundation (KDF) or the Peoples Dialysis Centre (PDC) or the other private dialysis centres where patients are dialysed by the staff in these centres without the need for a spouse or helper, though at a higher cost than the self dependency dialysis centres. Assisted dialysis frees the spouse or family member from turning up at the dialysis centre thrice weekly.

In a few cases, there may be difficulties related to access, or to cramps and hypotension on dialysis but for the majority it provides a reliable and effective form of renal replacement therapy. Haemodialysis is usually performed 3 times per week for 4 hours per session. With newer techniques (high efficiency dialysis) using special membranes and more sophisticated machines, and with AV fistulae with good blood flow rates, haemodialysis can now be shortened to only 3½ hours. Newer membranes which are more biocompatible have been introduced recently and will doubtless make their impact on the local scene.

When Should Dialysis be Initiated?

There have been some controversies in this regard. Most would initiate dialysis when the eGFR is between 8 to 12 ml/min, perhaps around 10 ml/min, certainly when it is about 5–6 ml/min. Recently there have been concerns that those who start too early die faster, perhaps due to loss of residual renal function with the drop in BP intermittently during HD. The rationale for early start was based on the ideas that residual renal function contributed to adequacy of dialysis, reduces intradialytic weight gain, associated with better nutritional status, lower EPO requirements and better outcome [Canaud B *et al.* Residual renal function: the delicate balance between benefits and risks. Nephrol Dial Transpl 2008, 21:411–418]. In the USA the percentage of patients starting dialysis at eGFR >10 ml/min more than doubled between 1996 and 2005 from 25% to 54%. In France it was stable at 30%. More recent studies showed decrease of survival with higher eGFRs at initiation [Sawhney S *et al.* Survival and dialysis initiation: comparing British Columbia and Scotland Registries. Nephrol Dial Transpl 2009, 24:3186–3192] despite comorbidities.

To resolve this controversy, Lasalle [Lasalle M *et al.* **Age and comorbidity** may explain the paradoxical association of an early dialysis start with poor survival. Kidney Int 2010, 77:700–707] measured mortality hazard ratios associated with the Modification of Diet in Renal Disease and eGFR at dialysis initiation for 11,685 patients from the French REIN Registry, with sequential adjustment for covariates.

The 15th deci-decile eGFR, including values around 10 ml/min was their reference point. The patients more likely to begin dialysis at a higher eGFR were older male patients, had diabetes, CVS diseases, low body mass index, and low serum albumin or were started with PD. During a median follow up of 21.9 months, 3,945 patients died. The 2 year crude survival decreased from 79 to 46% with increasing eGFR from less than 5 ml/min to over 20 ml/min. Each 5 ml/min eGFR increase was associated with a 40% increase in crude mortality risk. The authors concluded that **age and patients comorbidities were the strongest determinants for the decision to start dialysis** and this would explain most of the inverse association between eGFR and survival. Considering that early start of dialysis is costly and has major consequences in the personal life of the patient, strong evidence is required to justify an early start. As to whether starting at a higher eGFR affects overall quality of life and morbidity, further studies are required.

In my opinion, if the modality of dialysis results in a progressive decline of residual renal function, this should be the strongest deterrant to an early initiation of dialysis. Early HD will subject the patient to loss of residual renal function resulting from drop in BP sustained during IHD. Based on consensus, it is now believed by most that early dialysis i.e. eGFR >10 ml/min should be discouraged. To compound the problem, many of these early dialyses are performed via I/J catheters or permcatheters which also put patients at risk of sepsis and worse still if they develop septic emboli. Therefore, instead of hemodialysis catheter placement and immediate dialysis, every consideration should be given to placing a fistula, graft or PD catheter, and deferring initiation of dialysis until the access is usable.

Extended Daily Dialysis [EDD]

The standard dialysis for most patients are thrice weekly intermittent dialysis [IHD] for about 4 hours per session. Some patients may require more extensive dialysis or for some others who can afford more, and want to optimise their dialysis therapy, Extended Daily Dialysis is another option. This is also sometimes used for patients with Acute Kidney Injury with Acute Renal Failure. Using a conventional hemodialysis, dialysis is performed 6 to 7 times a week at a low blood flow rate of 100 to 200 ml/min compared to the usual blood flow rate of 300 to 400 ml/min. The dialysate flow rate is about 300 ml/min compared to the usual rate of 500 ml/min. Each treatment may last 6 to 8 hours. The advantage of EDD is better clearance of uremic toxins, better control of salt and water balance and including potassium intake compared to conventional thrice weekly dialysis where patients have to be very strict about salt, potassium and fluid intake. One very important advantage is better phosphate removal and this translates into less cardiac morbidity and mortality.

Slow Long Hemodialysis [SLHD]

This is another alternative to conventional intermittent thrice weekly dialysis [IHD] first introduced by Tassin. Slow long HD is also thrice weekly HD but the sessions last from 6 to 8 hours with blood flow rate of 200 to 250 ml/min. This has better benefits than IHD but not as good as EDD.

Short Daily Hemodialysis [SDHD]

This consists of 5 to 7 dialysis sessions weekly lasting 1.5 to 2.5 hours a session using high flux biocompatible membranes with blood flow rate of 400 ml/min and dialysate flow rate of 500 to 800 ml/min.

Nocturnal Hemodialysis [NHD]

This is performed 5 to 7 times a week like SDHD and each session lasts 6 to 8 hours using biocompatible membranes with blood flow rates of 200 to 300 ml/min and dialysate flow rates of 200 to 300 ml/min.

Single-pool KT/V values:

Conventional IHD — 1.2 to 1.8
Slow long HD — 1.6 to 1.8
Short Daily HD — 0.2 to 0.8
Nocturnal HD — 0.9 to 1.2

Advantages and Outcome of Various Dialysis Regimes

Slow Long HD

Dietary protein intake [DPI] is as high as 1.3 ± 0.42 gm/Kg/day and serum albumin is 4.2 ± 0.5 gm/dL compared to DPI of 1.0 ± 0.3 gm/Kg/day and serum albumin 3.8 ± 0.3 gm/dL for patients on IHD. Hence DPI and serum albumin reflecting nutritional status of patients on Slow long HD is superior to that of those on IHD. Good nutrition equates with longevity on HD as there is less CVD and CV deaths.

Short Daily HD

This therapy is also associated with improvement in protein catabolic rate [PCR] from 1.0 gm/Kg/day to 1.7 gm/Kg/day and serum albumin levels increased from 38.6 gm/dL to 40.8 gm/dL after 18 months on SDHD [Lindsay RM *et al.* Short Daily Hemodialysis. Adv Renal Replace Ther 2001, **8**(4):236–249].

Nocturnal HD

The dietary protein intake [DPI] and serum albumin of patients on Nocturnal HD [NHD] is superior to that of conventional thrice weekly Intermittent HD. One great advantage is that patients on NHD have much superior phosphate removal and less problems with renal bone disease. The serum phosphate of those on NHD fell from 6.0 mg/dL to 3.9 mg/dL. Patients were on a normal phosphate diet and they could do without the use of phosphate binders and in some patients, they even required addition of phosphate to the dialysate [Mucsi I *et al.* Control of serum phosphate without any phosphate binders in patients treated with nocturnal hemodialysis. Kidney Int 1998, **53**: 1399–1404].

Comparing Nocturnal HD with Short Daily HD

Here are two different dialysis regimes, Nocturnal HD requires 7 to 8 hours at a lower blood flow and dialysate rate whilst Short Daily HD requires shorter treatment duration of 1.5 to 2.5 hours at high blood flow rates. Nocturnal HD has better KT/V and better removal of high molecular weight toxins. The dry weight and protein catabolic rate of both modalities are much improved. The serum albumin is better with Daily Short HD but phosphate removal is better with Nocturnal HD. Nocturnal HD is more home based whilst Daily Short HD can be done at home or at the dialysis centre. These modalities are for patients who can afford better quality of dialysis and who can also afford the time for extended dialysis. But in terms of overall KT/V, Extended Daily HD [EDD] appears superior.

Quantification of Dialysis

The Kt/V is traditionally used to determine the adequacy of dialysis. However the curve relating dialysis dose and survival is J shaped. Therefore low dialysis dose is associated with high mortality and mortality declines with increased doses of dialysis. Kt/V being an index of LMW solute removal begs the question of whether LMW solute removal is the most important index in determining survival. Smaller individuals are more likely to have higher Kt/V than larger individuals because their urea volume or V is smaller. African Americans tend to have body mass greater than Whites and Black Americans survive better than White Americans [Frankenfield DL. Relationship between urea reduction ratio, demographic characteristics and body weight for patients in the 1996 National ESRD Core Indicators Project. Am J Kidney Dis 1999, 33:584–591]. A low body mass is an independent risk factor for death in dialysis patients [Collins AJ. Urea index and other predictors of hemodialysis patient survival. Amer J Kidney Dis 1994, 23:661–669]. V the urea volume may be an independent variable for survival. It is felt that various elements in the Kt/V equation may offset one another and the result is that if patient survival is assessed as a function of Kt, the J shaped curve would disappear and mortality would decline over the entire range of Kt. Mortality was lower in patients with larger body size and decreased as a function of the dose of dialysis delivered. There is a valid relationship between Kt/V and mortality, but patients' size has also to be taken into account as indices of body size is taken as a surrogate for nutritional status since we all know that a poor nutritional state predicts poorer survival.

Alternative to Kt/V

URR or the **Urea Removal Ratio** is the ratio of pre dialysis BUN minus post dialysis BUN divided by pre dialysis BUN. The URR depends on the changes of urea levels during hemodialysis. The URR is an index of survival also recognised by the KDOQI guidelines. URR cannot be used to assess adequacy of peritoneal dialysis as the urea of patients on peritoneal dialysis is in a steady state.

The SRI or solute removal index measures the amount of urea removed during dialysis rather than the fractional change as in URR. Urea removal can be considered as a surrogate for small molecular toxins.

For Daily Short HD and Nocturnal HD, at this time there is no agreed dose measures which are considered totally acceptable. An alternative is the standard Kt/V. This is a dose measure that combines treatment dose with treatment frequency and it also allows various intermittent therapies to be compared with continuous therapies [CRRT]. Standard Kt/V is defined as the continuous removal rate divided by the average peak concentration.

Standard Kt/V Urea: A Method of Calculation That Includes Effects of Fluid Removal and Residual Renal Function

Reference: Daugirdas JT *et al. Kidney Int* 2010, **77**:637–643.

In the above equation, K is the dialyzer clearance for urea, t is the treatment time, and V is the patient's volume of urea distribution. The new clearance is based on achieving equivalent average pre dialysis BUN concentrations, regardless of how many dialysis sessions are given per week. It was calculated as G/(mean pre-dialysis BUN) in which G is the patient's urea nitrogen generation rate. This is called "standard" clearance Kt/V, or std K and is expressed as weekly stdKt/V, in which t is the number of minutes in a week (10,080) and V is expressed in mls.

In addition, many patients have residual native kidney urea clearance (Kru). Kru exerts an effect to lower the pre dialysis BUN and contributes to stdKt/V. This equation therefore is more accurate and takes into consideration how U/F and Kru affect the calculation of stdKt/V. It has been found that this new equation predicted modelled stdKt/V with a high level of accuracy, even when substantial fluid removal and residual urea clearance were present.

Shorter time dialysis was associated with higher mortality among HD patients as reported by Brunelli SM comparing a cohort of 8,552 patients on thrice weekly in center HD. Those dialysed <4 hours a session had 42% increase in mortality [Brunelli SM *et al.* Kidney Int 2010, 77:630–636].

Medical Problems Still Present
in Patients on Dialysis

1. **Nutrition:** Malnutrition remains one of the major problems facing the patient on dialysis and is associated with
   great morbidity and mortality. Of utmost importance is the
   term protein calorie malnutrition as this would mean a host
   of factors which come into play, amongst which are inadequate intake of protein/calorie, metabolic acidosis, hormonal changes, nutrient losses during dialysis, dialysis
   induced hypercataboilsm. All these predispose to infection, incurring readmitted admissions to hospital with
   additional comorbidities and further exposure to other hospital acquired comorbidities resulting in the early demise
   in as much as up to 30% of patients during the first 2 years
   of hemodialysis. This is compounded by the loss of residual eGFR which also occurs during the first 2 years of
   starting hemodialysis which does not occur with peritoneal
   dialysis as there is no associated intermittent drop of BPs
   during peritoneal dialysis compared to intermittent
   hemodialysis.

   In order to prevent protein calorie malnutrition, various
   parameters must be assessed and monitored amongst which
   are the serum albumin which is the reflection of the visceral
   protein stores of the patient, serum creatinine, BUN. Some
   also measure transferrin, prealbumin and insulin like growth
   factor-1 [IGF-1]. The serum albumin is the most reliable. It
   is readily accessible and relates well to the patient's intake of
   protein in the diet. Others like BUN or urea are also reliable.
   BUN is the composite measure of protein intake, volume of
   distribution and renal and dialyzer clearance and urea is the
   metabolic end product of dietary protein intake. The recommended protein intake is 1.2 gm/Kg BW/day. 50% of the protein should be of high biologic value. Recommended daily
   energy intake is 35 kcal/Kg BW/day for those patients who
   are less than 60 years old and 30 kcal/Kg BW/day for those

60 years and over. Patients should be monitored and their intake assessed and topped up as when necessary. For those unable to feed, they may require enteral feeding or in the case of some even total parenteral nutrition. Trace elements are retained in renal failure and there is no necessity for supplementation except for selenium and zinc in those who are deficient. Selenium deficiency may be associated with cardiovascular disease as selenium is a co-factor in antioxidant enzyme function. Water soluble B vitamins and folic acid supplementation may be required. This is especially so for folic acid which is present in foods that patients have to avoid in order not to develop hyperkalaemia. Vit C prevents oxidative injury and aids iron metabolism. Fat soluble vitamins are adequate in hemodialysis patients except for Vit D. Avoid Vit A because of potential toxicity. Vit E may be useful in reducing cardiovascular complications in hemodialysis patients [Boaz M *et al.* Secondary prevention with antioxidants of cardiovascular diseases in end stage renal disease (SPACE): Randomised placebo controlled trial. Lancet, 2000, **356**(9237):1213–1216].

2. **Itch**, sometimes intense and generalised, is often still a problem for the patient on dialysis. A soothing aqueous cream and antihistamines may help. Some patients may respond to a course of ultraviolet therapy.

3. **Bone disease** is still a problem and this is often related to the number of years the patient has been on dialysis though most patients will have histological changes on bone biopsy. Some will have radiological changes of osteomalacia or hyperparathyroidism. Patients with renal bone disease will require control of serum calcium and phosphate with calcium carbonate or calcium acetate. Those who can afford can be prescribed lanthanum or sevelamer. Vitamin D analogues may also be required. Some patients may require partial parathyroidectomy if they do not respond to Vitamin D therapy. These are patients with elevated serum calcium and high serum alkaline phosphatase and high plasma PTH levels with

severe changes of osteodystrophy on skeletal survey. Patients should be on Vit D analog like 1,25-dihydroxycholecalciferol (calcitriol), 0.25 micro gm once daily on alternate days. Patients with normal liver function can be treated with 1-∝-(OH)-D_3 or alphacalcidol. The newer Vit D analogs like paricalcitriol or doxercholecalciferol can be prescribed for those who can afford.

What has been found to be disturbing is that recent studies have shown that indeed, life is all about affordability. In the USA, because dialysis is covered by Health Insurance, intravenous Vit D in the form of paricalcitriol has become the standard therapy in for profit dialysis centres. Here it has been found that mortality was higher for patients on calcitriol compared to paricalcitriol. Doxercalciferol, a second Vit D being used is also available. It has been found that mortality rates were identical in those on paricalcitriol and doxercalciferol 15.3 and 15.5) compared to those on calcitriol (19.6, $p < 0.001$) among a study population of 7,731 patients on HD in the USA. In all models, however, mortality was still higher for those on no Vit D compared to those on calcitriol [Tentori T *et al.* Kidney Int 2006, 70:1858–1865].

Paricalcitriol and doxercalciferol are a new class of drugs, the **Vit D receptor activators** which should be used in place of the older Vit D analogs like calcitriol (rocaltrol, 1α OH D3, etc.) as the older forms of Vit D are associated with increased vascular calcification with resulting increased CVS morbidity and mortality. Animals with renal failure treated with hypercalcemic doses of calcitriol and paricalcitriol showed an increase in systolic BP. However, diastolic BP was only raised significantly in animals treated with paricalcitriol, but not in those on calcitriol. Hence those on calcitriol had an increase in pulse pressure, likely caused by extensive calcification observed in arteries of animals treated with calcitriol which was not present in those treated with paricalcitriol [Cardus A *et al.* J Bone and Mineral Research, 2007, 22: 860–866].

Recent evidence from animal and human studies supports an association between Vit D Receptor Activators (e.g. Paricalcitriol) and reduced risk of cardiovascular deaths, irrespective of PTH levels. New pathways of Vit D regulation also have been discovered involving fibroblast growth factor-23 and klotho [Patel TV and Singh AK. Role of Vit D in CKD. Semin Nephrol 2009, 29:113–121]. Klotho gene is now associated with aging. It may be possible to prevent aging of kidneys by modulating the Klotho gene. See Chapter on Aging and the Kidney.

Historically, in the old days at SGH in the early 1970's, we saw patients with Osteomalacia that did not respond to Vitamin D therapy. We subsequently discovered that these patients had aluminium induced osteomalacia. This was the result of aluminium in tap water which was used in the dialysate which we manufactured locally in our pharmacy. One of the common causes of death was due to dialysis dementia, the result of aluminium toxicity in the brain. The aluminium came from the untreated tap water. At that time, people all over the world had not recognised the syndrome of Aluminium induced Dialysis Dementia and Aluminium induced osteomalacia due to aluminium in tap water used for the dialysate. Since the introduction of reverse osmosis and deionisers to treat our dialysate water, the incidence of dialysis dementia and aluminium induced osteomalacia has become a thing of the past.

4. **Anaemia:** Most patients on regular haemodialysis can tolerate Hb of 10 gm reasonably well. They are transfused if Hb drops below 8 gm or when they have symptoms of anaemia. The advent of human recombinant DNA Erythropoeitin has been a boon for patients with anaemia. Most patients are now on it, maintaining Hb level of around 12 gm or more. Patients should be on erythropoeitin even before they start dialysis [CKD stage 3 to 4] to keep Hb about 12 gm. Iron supplements have to be given too. The KDOQI target for Hb is 12 gm and recent reports have questioned the safety of

achieving high levels of Hb levels with erythropoeisis stimu-lating agents [ESA] [McFarlane PA *et al*. International trends in erythropoietin use and Hb levels in hemodialysis patients. Kidney Int 2010, 78:215–223].

Traditionally, **Erythropoeitin** [EPO] injections are given as Eprex or Recormon in a weekly dose of 4,000 units once or twice weekly. This is often given when the patient comes for dialysis. Recently with the introduction of newer forms of Erythropoeisis Stimulating Agent (ESA) like C.E.R.A. or Continuous Erythropoeitin Receptor Activator and Darbepoeitin Alpha [DPOA] a long acting EPO, patients now have the convenience of having the injections on a monthly basis instead of a weekly basis. CERA once every 4 weeks has been found to correct anemia in patients with CKD not on dialysis as well as those on dialysis and the safety and efficacy for both CERA and Darbopoeitin Alpha [DPOA] are comparable.

In a study by Roger SD (Cordatus Study) comparing 153 patients on CERA versus 154 on DPOA, the most common treatment related side effect was hypertension occurring in 4.7% of CERA group versus 9.7% in the DPOA group (p = 0.12). The incidence of side effects in the 2 groups was also comparable. The once monthly dosing interval (QAW) of CERA demonstrated successful correction of anemia in patients with CKD not on dialysis, with fewer patients exceeding 12 gm/l during the first 8 weeks of treatment compared to DPOA. The Hb of 12 gm/l was also maintained in both groups.

Reference: Boudville NC *et al*. Clin J Amer Soc Nephrol 2009, **4**:738–750.

In another study by Carrera F (Patronus Investigators) for 245 patients on CERA versus 245 patients on DPOA, all on intermittent HD given monthly IV injections of CERA and DPOA. Target Hb was 12 gm/l. The response rate was significantly higher in the CERA group, 64% compared to the DPOA group of 40% (p < 0.001) after 26 weeks. Between week 27 and the next 26 week period, Hb was unchanged for the CERA group but the Hb in the DPOA group decreased by 1.09 gm/l. The incidence of adverse events and serious side effects were similar in both groups with no deaths in both groups.

Reference: Levin NW *et al.* Lancet, 2007, **370**:1415–1421.

5. **Hypertension:** In most patients, hypertension is controlled by salt and water depletion by dialysis as well as diet and strict fluid control. About 30% to 40% of patients will still require antihypertensive medication. Control of salt and water related hypertension is important, as patients with left ventricular ejection fraction less than 50% have a high risk of dying from cardiac complication and are not candidates for renal transplant.

The Magnitude of the Problem

(i) **Management of BP in patients with CKD stage 5 on dialysis** is a great challenge. In such patients with CKD stage 5, BP is determined by a complex interplay of fluid volume and prescription of post dialysis target weight, sodium load, the RAS and sympathetic nervous system and other factors like the administration of erythropoeisis stimulating agents [ESA]. In a recent conference to improve global outcomes for BP in CKD stage 5 patients [Levine NW *et al.* **Blood pressure in CKD stage 5- report from a Kidney Disease: Improving Global Outcomes controversies conference**. Kidney Int 2010, 77:273–284]. The conference discussed (1) optimum BP in relation to end organ damage in dialysis patients, (2) pharmacological therapy for cardioprotection and to achieve BP targets (3) nonpharmacological therapy to achieve BP targets-focus on volume and salt control.

(ii)   In the past, severity of HPT was classified based on diastolic BP which was considered the best predictor of CKD risk, with increased pulse pressure as an independent CVD risk factor in addition to DBP. DBP generally increases from birth to the 5th decade followed by a decline starting at 50–60 years. The pulse pressure increases markedly in later life, and isolated SBP becomes the predominant form of HPT after 60 years.

(iii) However, in dialysis (Dx) patients, increased SBP and decreased DBP are both associated with CVD events. This is due to arterial stiffness. In addition, decreased SBP following previous HPT is associated with adverse outcomes. The pathophysiology of BP patterns in these patients are complex reflecting (1) cardiac function (2) arterial stiffness — large blood vessels (3) intensity of wave reflections — principally vasomotor tone of resistance arterioles. Added to this complexity are the effects of ultrafiltration (U/F) and variable plasma volume refilling rates frequently resulting in hypotensive episodes during dialysis. Relationship of low SBP with CVD is also complex, as low SBP in some patients may represent ideal control but in others it may indicate increase mortality.

(iv)   The relative merits of calcium channel blockers (CCB), ACEI, ARB, β adrenergic blockers alone and in combination with centrally acting sympatholytic agents are not satisfactorily established. Recent review suggest problem of aldosterone activation with blood vessel wall fibrosis with ACEI and ARB. There is also problem of hyperkalaemia with the use of these agents.

(v)   For patients with fluid overload, what they need is more U/F and longer dialysis time and more frequent dialysis in some patients.

(vi)   Recent finding that excess sodium is stored without osmotic activity at concentrations of 180–190 meq/l in the skin, bound to glucoaminoglycans could revolutionise our views of sodium balance. The skin sodium acts as a buffer to exogenous sodium and this sodium store can be released into the circulation giving rise to hypervolumia and oxidative stress. With aging and catabolism, among the old they may lose the capacity to store sodium in the skin.

(vii) Current thrice weekly HD of 3–4 hours is common in the US with no efforts to decrease the sodium exposure of patients. The sodium concentration of the dialysate is also higher than that in the patients' serum. This can lead to increased thirst, ECF expansion and weight gain. Also there is problem of habitual salt intake among patients. Saline is also used for "sodium profiling" or to maintain plasma volume during U/F.

(viii) The sequelae of all these long term hypervolumia, activation of RAS, hyperactivity of the Sympathetic Nervous System, obesity, sleep anoxia, chronic inflammation, oxidative stress are elevated arterial pressure, cardiac arrhythmias, increased myocardial demand and in concert with arterial HPT, reduced compliance of large arteries. In addition sodium exerts pro inflammatory and pro fibrotic effects with potential of aggravating kidney disease and CVD.

(ix) The attainment of normal body hydration or "dry weight" (DW) expressed in practice by recognition of and attainment of post dialysis weight is difficult without adequate means of measurement. This is not satisfactory and work is ongoing to address this issue.

(x) Overall, with the severity of CVD in dialysis patients, fluctuations of BP with each dialysis treatment, associated with inflammation and vasoactive substances, pro fibrotic factors, sympathetic excess, poor volume control and salt overload....the management of BP in the dialysis patient is a very difficult and complex problem. Guidelines are being worked out and will be addressed in clinical practice guidelines.

Addressing the Problems

(i)   How and when should BP be measured?
      Use pre and post dialysis BP.

(ii) What components of BP to measure?
      Use SBP and DBP, not mean arterial BP.

(iii) What BP level defines HPT in HD patients?
      SBP >139 mm Hg or DBP >89 mm Hg.

(iv) What are treatment goals for BP in HD patients?
      A self measured home SBP range between 120 and
      145 mm Hg.

(v)   What are special considerations for anti HPT agents in
      dialysis patients?
      Use of ACEI have generated much controversies. β Blockers
      have been suggested to be cardioprotective in HD patients.

(vi) Should vasoactive agents be used for their anti HPT
      effects or independent cardioprotective effects?
      Until more or better evidence, ACEI/ARB, β Blockers and
      CCB could be used as in general population.

(vii) Which anti HPT are recommended?
      Aliskiren was recently approved for treatment of HPT.
      Experience in CKD stage 5 is rather limited. Small trials
      have shown beneficial effect of a specific β Blocker,
      carvedilol on hard CV end points.

(viii) Regarding pharmacokinetics and timing of drug
      administration.
      Two long acting anti HPT drugs, atenolol and lisinopril
      recommended for thrice weekly given immediately after
      HD. Shown to have 44 hours sustained anti HPT effects.

(ix) What are nonpharmacological therapy to achieve BP
      targets? — focus on volume and salt control.
      Longer and or more frequent dialysis sessions allows the
      decrease in U/F rates and reduces risk of intradialytic com-
      plications. Hence alternative dialysis methods like short
      daily, long daily and long conventional HD improve LVH,
      sympathetic overactivity and or vascular reactivity and
      improve ejection fraction in patients with heart failure.

Conclusions

(i) HPT is an ubiquitous problem in HD patients with major implications for survival.

(ii) Evidence for superiority of self measured BP at home over pre HD BP measuring is impressive.

(iii) Modifying effect of cardiomyopathy in HPT patients resulting in decline in BP make it difficult without further cardiac investigation to distinguish patients with a satisfactory target BP from those with severe cardiac disease. Use of echocardiography is essential to understand problem.

(iv) In general, all anti HPT drugs can be used. However the concomitant cardioprotective effects of these drugs should be considered.

(v) The two major aspects differentiating managing of HPT in HD patients compared to general population are the extremes of ECF volume present in majority of HD patients who have lost their residual renal function and the nature of dialysis. Short intense removal of fluid and the impaired CV response in many patients to this result in intradialytic hypotension which is much dreaded by patients.

(vi) The role of combined sodium restriction together with the use of anti HPT drugs has not been clarified. However, since most patients are in positive salt balance and would benefit from sodium restriction, both inter- and intradialytically, this may be the best practice. Long or more frequent dialysis may solve this problem.

6. **Hepatitis:** An effective vaccine has now been developed and those at risk of Hepatitis B (patients, helpers, nurses and doctors) are now routinely immunised. Hepatitis C remains a problem. Patients with hepatitis B and C should be referred to a hepatologist and assessed and if necessary started on lamuvidine for those with Hepatitis B and those with Hepatitis C should have treatment with interferon and ribavarine. Otherwise, untreated the presence of hepatitis will pose a risk to these patients when they do get transplanted.

7. **Infections:** Apart from the above, patients on dialysis are still prone to **infections** like lung infections and septicaemia. Infection is the second leading cause of death in hemodialysis after cardiovascular causes accounting for about 20% mortality rate in the dialysis patients and 75% of these patients succumb to septicaemia. For the hemodialysis patient the septicaemia rate is 100 fold more than that of the general population and the major source of infection is often related to the infection of the dialysis catheters [internal jugular and permanent catheters]. These catheters are a constant risk of infection causing septicaemia with septic embolisation and septic shock in the already immunocompromised hemodialysis patient. One of the concerns is bacterial endocarditis and methicillin resistant staph aureus [MRSA] septicaemia. This is why patients should be encouraged to have an AV fistula created when the serum creatinine is about 400 mE/L so that vascular access is ready when the patient needs dialysis, thus obviating the need for insertion of internal jugular catheters which carry a high risk of infection. Apart from this, whenever a patient is being needled for hemodialysis he or she also runs the risk of contamination and subsequent infection due to repeated disruption of the dermal integrity during needling of the AV [Arteriovenous] fistulae. Dialysis patients are prone to viral infections including Hepatitis B and C. The incidence of pneumonia has also been high and about 50% are due to Streptococcus pneumoniae. It is therefore recommended that all dialysis patients should be immunised against Hepatitis B, influenzae including H1N1 as well as pneumococcal pneumonia.

8. As a result of accelerated atherogenesis, arteriosclerosis and hypertension, dialysis patients are prone to **myocardial infarction** and **cerebrovascular accidents**. Observational studies have suggested a link between higher serum phosphate, calcium and PTH levels and cardiovascular mortality. In a recent report based on an observational study by Block [Block GA *et al.* Cinacelcet hydrochloride treatment significantly

improves all-cause and cardiovascular survival in a large cohort of hemodialysis patients. [Kidney Int 2010, 78: 578–589]. Among 19,186 patients on HD in the USA, 5976 received cinacelcet over 26 months. Unadjusted and adjusted time dependent Cox proportional hazards modelling found that all-cause and and cardiovascular mortality were significantly lower for those treated with cinacelcet than those without cinacelcet. This observational study found a significant survival benefit associated with cinacelcet prescription in patients receiving i.v. vitamin D. Definite proof, however, of a survival advantage awaits the performance of randomised clinical trials.

PRINCIPLES INVOLVED IN HAEMODIALYSIS

Dialysis is a process which separates solutes dissolved in water across a semipermeable membrane.

In haemodialysis the patient's blood is let out of his body where it is treated with anticoagulant (heparin) to prevent it from clotting and passed over a semipermeable membrane in the dialyser (artificial kidney) through which exchange of solutes (dialysis) takes place. The exchange occurs across the membrane of the artificial kidney into a solution called the dialysate which has a composition similar to a solution of the body's salts but without any of the waste products.

By means of osmosis and diffusion the waste products of metabolism like urea, creatinine, and potassium which are at a higher concentration in the blood compartment of the artificial kidney pass across the membrane into the dialysate compartment since the latter has a lower concentration of these substances.

During the process of haemodialysis the blood from the patient flows continuously through the dialyser while fresh dialysate is passed through it on the other side of the membrane so that a high gradient of toxic substance is always present on the blood side. The blood returning to the patient after passing through the dialyser is almost devoid of toxic substances accumulated in renal failure.

HAEMOFILTRATION (CRRT)

Excess water from the patient's body is removed by means of haemofiltration using a special dialyzer. A pressure gradient is generated across the membrane using a pump which raises the pressure in the blood compartment, causing more water to be lost through the membrane and into the dialysis compartment.

Hemodiafiltration is a useful procedure for patients with unstable BP and fluid overload as we can remove excess fluid from the patient and dialyse the patient at the same time in spite of the low BP. Hemofiltration and Hemodiafitration are referred to as Continuous Renal Replacement Therapy (CRRT), ideal for patients with Acute Renal Failure in ICU setting as it does not cause intermittent drop in BP of patients as in the case of Intermittent Hemodialysis [IHD]. For the patient recovering from acute renal failure, this is important, as every bit of renal function left in the patient, or whatever renal function that can be salvaged in the patient, will determine the long term outcome and prognosis of the patient. Nowadays, most centres would put patients with acute renal failure on CRRT to preserve and protect renal function, rather than utilise IHD which will further jeopardise renal function.

Slow Low Efficiency Dialysis [SLED]: For patients with low BP, another form of hemodialysis known as SLED or slow low efficiency dialysis can also be used as it does not cause hypotension to occur in contrast to the usual conventional hemodialysis which causes intermittent hypotension in patients.

Vascular Access and How It is Made Possible

In order to get blood out of the patient repeatedly to pass through the artificial kidney machine and back into the body after it has been cleansed, a vascular access is necessary. Put simply, the access is a point of entry into the bloodstream so the patient can be connected to the machine.

The commonest form of access is the arteriovenous (AV) fistula usually done over the wrist or forearm. This involves a small operation to join the radial artery with a vein in the arm. The vein would increase in size and develop a thick wall after 3 to 6 weeks. It is then very easy to put a needle into this vein and connect the patient to the machine.

Nowadays for immediate access, an internal jugular catheter is inserted. It is a catheter which is inserted into the internal jugular vein by the side of the neck. This method of access is a temporary measure which provides immediate access for dialysis while the AV fistula which is usually done about the same time matures. The internal jugular catheter cannot be used beyond a few weeks as it tends to get blocked by clotted blood or the site of insertion gets infected. An alternative is the perm-catheter which lasts longer.

Most kidney doctors usually electively have an AV fistula created for the patient when his serum creatinine level is about 400 micro mol/L since it takes about 6 weeks to mature and be ready for needling. This will obviate the need for an internal jugular catheter. The patient is usually started on dialysis when the serum creatinine level is around 600 to 700 micro mol/L depending on whether he has symptoms or other complications of end stage kidney failure by then.

According to the KDOQI guidelines patients should be referred for surgery for construction of an AV fistula when the eGFR is <25 ml/min or serum creatinine >4 mg/dl (>352 micro mol/l). However, in a recent study [O'Hare AM *et al*. When to refer patients with CKD for vascular access: Should age be a consideration? Kidney Int 2007, 71:555–561] it was found that the ratio for unnecessary to necessary procedures after 2 years of follow up was 5:1 for patients aged 85 to 100 years but only 0.5:1 for those aged 18–44 years. Therefore for the very elderly patients we should have a more targeted approach directed at the minority that will begin dialysis within the desired time frame as suggested by O'Hare.

Types of Dialysers (Artificial Kidneys)

1. The hollow fibre dialyser: In this dialyser blood is passed through thousands of minute hollow fibres of membrane around which dialysate (dialysis solution) flows.

2. The flat plate dialyser: Here membranes are stacked together like a sandwich with spaces in between through which dialysate and blood flow in different compartments.

These dialysers though said to be disposable can in fact be reused for 3 to 6 times or more after washing and sterilising at the end of each use.

DIALYSATE

Dialysate is the fluid or solution used for dialysis. For haemodialysis the concentrated dialysate is mixed with 30 to 40 times its volume of water by means of a proportioning pump. The dialysate after mixing is warmed to body temperature and its composition checked by special meters as it passes into the dialysis machine before going into the dialyser.

The Tap Water Used for Haemodialysis

In Singapore, as in most centres, the water used for dialysis has to be treated by reverse osmosis or passed through deionisers to get rid of impurities in the water, especially aluminium. If accumulated in the body of patients with kidney failure, aluminium may cause a degenerative disease of the brain (dialysis dementia) whereby the patient behaves abnormally, has slurred speech, facial distortions, develops repeated convulsions and finally dies. The accumulated aluminium also results in aluminium bone disease which causes bone pain and fractures.

EQUIPMENT REQUIRED FOR HAEMODIALYSIS

The patient will require a haemodialysis machine with a built-in monitoring system and various sets of pumps; the dialyser or artificial kidney; lines for letting out and returning blood to the patient; dialysate or dialysis solution, water treatment unit (deionser or reverse osmosis) and vascular access for the patient (usually an AV fistula).

Functions of the Monitoring System in the Dialysis Machine

The monitoring system ensures a series of automatic checks such that the dialysis procedure is safe for the patient. It incorporates a system of alarms which will go off if a fault is detected.

The following checks are made by the monitoring system:

1. The dialyser is not leaking blood into the dialysate compartment. This can occur if there is a break in the dialyser membrane. The membranes are very thin (ranging from 5–40 microns depending on the type of membrane used). The diameter of the pores in the membrane ranges from 1–7 nano metres depending on the type of membrane used.
2. No bubbles are returning to the patient in the venous line as the entry of air into the vein can cause death through air embolism. A bubble trap is usually installed in the system and the presence of air would set off an alarm system.
3. The temperature of the dialysate must be the same as that of the normal body temperature. This is recorded by a temperature gauge.
4. The composition of the dialysate must be correct. This is checked by a conductivity meter.
5. The blood pressure on the arterial and venous lines must be appropriate.

THE EFFECT OF HAEMODIALYSIS ON THE PATIENT

For most patients haemodialysis remains the preferred form of dialysis. It provides a reliable and effective form of kidney

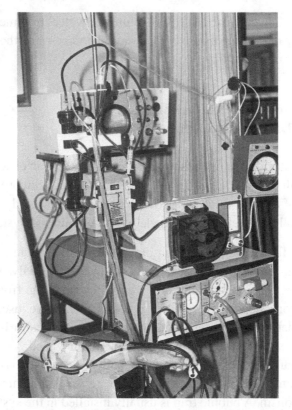

Fig. 30.1   A hemodialysis machine with built-in monitors

replacement therapy. Haemodialysis is usually performed 3 times per week for 4 hours per session.

Initially, most patients will find difficulty with life on haemodialysis. Some may feel unwell and washed out at the end of each dialysis. During dialysis they may have cramps, vomiting or hypotension. These effects are due to the changes occurring in the composition of his body fluids. However, most patients get over these effects after a few weeks. The majority of patients will have the feeling that they have been given a new lease of life. Gone are the symptoms of end stage renal failure, the worse being the nausea and vomiting, not to mention the shortness of breath, giddiness, tiredness and general malaise.

Food takes on a new taste and everything in their body seems to be working again.

DIETARY RESTRICTIONS FOR A PATIENT ON HAEMODIALYSIS

The patient still has to observe certain dietary restrictions very strictly. However, a patient on dialysis must have adequate protein intake of at least 1.2 gm/KgBW a day with 35 kcal/day to maintain a serum albumin of at least 38 gm/l, ideally of 42 gm/l. Otherwise he runs the risk of death due to Protein Energy Malnutrition (PEM). See section on Diet by Dr Kalantar in preceding Chapter.

He is allowed to take normal amounts of meat and carbohydrates but he must restrict potassium, salt and water in his diet. This is because he can still retain lethal amounts of potassium, salt and water in between dialysis. He must avoid all foodstuff containing potassium, some of these being fruits and vegetables. Fruits include preserved fruits such as jams and other preserves. Citrus fruits, especially oranges and grapes are worst. Our local specialty, the durian, has claimed many a life on dialysis, as it has particularly high potassium content. Patients who cannot resist its temptation and take a few seeds can meet with sudden death due to arrhythmias induced by severe hyperkalaemia. The only fruits patients can take as a concession are apples and pears, as their potassium content are much lower. However, these too have to be taken sparingly. Phosphate containing foodstuff too have to be reduced. We take meat and meat itself contains high amounts of phosphate. Hence serum phosphate levels will be raised in the patients. This is the reason why all patients will require phosphate binders. If patients do not have an adequate protein intake in the form of meat they risk having malnutrition and will succumb to infections which still remains an important cause of death for patients on dialysis.

Vegetables to be taken must be boiled and the water containing the extracted potassium poured away before the vegetable is eaten.

Patients on haemodialysis hardly pass more than about 200 to 300 ml of urine, some even less. Water sometimes accumulates very rapidly in between dialysis. This water is from the food and drinks ingested, as well as the result of the body's metabolic process. In fact, in most patients, accumulation of excess water in the body is due to failure in observing the rules regarding salt and water restriction. Despite being told to reduce their salt intake and restrict the total amount of fluid intake to not more than 500 ml a day, some patients could not help breaking these rules. The recalcitrant ones are those who die suddenly from pulmonary oedema, causing them to drown in their own fluids, which is a terrible way of dying.

Uncontrolled intake of salt and water in a dialysis patient will also cause the patient to develop very high blood pressure which can lead to heart failure, or the bursting of a blood vessel in the brain causing cerebral haemorrhage and death.

Patients in danger of death from fluid overload can have the fluid removed by ultrafiltration through the haemodialysis machine if they go to the hospital in time. This method of fluid removal however will cause severe cramps and unpleasant hypotension especially if more than 2 litres of fluid are removed. The result is that the patient feels terrible but hopefully more compliant the next time.

THE PSYCHOLOGICAL EFFECTS ON THE DIALYSIS PATIENT

For some patients, the thought of being on dialysis for the rest of their lives or until they can get a kidney transplant may mean the end of the world to them and some may even become suicidal. This is especially so in younger patients who find it more difficult to accept a rigid and restricted lifestyle. There is great stress on family members and in some cases, marriages break up and children who are already neglected by a parent's illness prior to the time of dialysis are finally left destitute when the family breaks up.

Many have decreased earnings and others may already have lost their jobs because of their illness. Many too would have to give up whatever social life they previously had as their leisure hours are now occupied by the thrice weekly dialysis. In those who are dependent on a helper, usually the spouse, he or she is also similarly tied down by the dialysis schedule. Added to all the above problems, males become impotent and females lose their libido, both of which are due to poisonous wastes retained in kidney failure affecting their sexual glands.

Some patients rebel against and refuse to accept the fact that they have kidney failure. Given time however, and support from the medical staff, most finally accept their fate and learn to come to terms with their illness. In fact, these very same patients are the ones who sometimes ironically turn out to be model patients and strict disciplinarians of the various impositions on their new lifestyle.

Most patients therefore do overcome the initial trauma, fears and resentment regarding their illness. They adapt very well and their courage has to be admired. They bear testimony to the belief that the human spirit is indefatigable and indomitable. On a cheerful note, they can also plan to travel abroad as many dialysis units overseas do accommodate visiting patients. For the dialysis patient, it is of utmost importance that he dialyses and maintains himself well in preparation for the day when he should be called up to receive a cadaver transplant. Our national policy is to encourage patients to opt for a living related donor transplant from one of the relatives. Ideally, if a patient can find a suitable donor, he or she should have a pre emptive renal transplant. This means that he or she can have a kidney transplant from a living donor when the serum creatinine is about 500 micro mol/l without the need of undergoing dialysis. It spares the patient the pain and inconvenience of undergoing thrice weekly dialysis. After the kidney transplant, all the patient has to do is to continue his or her renal transplant medicine to prevent kidney rejection. The quality of life with a kidney transplant is superior to one on dialysis.

HALLMARKS OF A WELL DIALYSED PATIENT

The patient who is well dialysed should:

- have a sense of well-being
- have well controlled blood pressure
- absence of heart failure, adequate left ventricular ejection fraction, more than 50%
- haemoglobin of more than 10 gm, about 12 gm. Here I must add that in a study, patients randomised to a HB level >13 gm had 34% higher risk of CHF, AMI, Stroke and death [See Ref 9 of this Chapter]
- adequate nutritional status with normal serum albumin and satisfactory dry weight
- absence of bone disease and neuropathy, well controlled serum phosphate, calcium and plasma PTH levels
- pre-dialysis serum creatinine less than 500 micro mol/L and Kt/V more than 1.8.

FUTURE PERSPECTIVE OF HEMODIALYSIS

Dialysis is a life saving procedure and today many patients are kept alive on hemodialysis. The ideal renal replacement is a kidney transplant. Peritoneal dialysis is an equally viable option compared to hemodialysis. Many more patients opt for hemodialysis as it is more convenient compared to peritoneal dialysis. Hence with a large hemodialysis market, today's state of the art hemodialysis has reached a stage where it has plateaued in the sense that every possible avenue has been explored to better the lives of patients on hemodialysis. The latest advance would be the hybrid dialyser which would combine the excretory function of the artificial kidney with that of bionic cells that can help regulate phosphate control and some other functions of the renal tubule which would then provide a more holistic approach to renal replacement approximating that of the live kidney. The ultimate question concerning the patient is whether hemodialysis as we have it today can offer improved mortality. Despite adequate doses of dialysis using high flux membranes, the overall mortality of patients have not increased significantly, suggesting that since the 1990's nothing revolutionary has appeared on the dialysis scene to extend mortality. This would suggest that we must look at alternatives to the present system if we are to answer the challenges of the genomic era with markedly improved life expectancy for the general population. We must address the issues of vascular access, membrane biocompatibility, delivery of adequate dialysis by individual prescription, phosphate removal and improvement of nutritional status. This means employing translational medicine to harness both glomerular and tubular functions of the kidney, removal of all possible forms of uremic toxins through both metabolic and hybrid cellular processes, in effect to create an artificial kidney transplant in the form of a hybrid bionic dialyser which will be a match for the cadaveric or living related donated kidney. Developers of the bionic artificial kidney will be competing with a team which are now engaged in clinical trails using stem cells and cloning to harness the functions of the renal glomerulus and tubules in terms of organogenesis without the problems of allogenecity and xenogenecity associated with heterotopic renal transplants. There is a bright glimmer of hope for the renal patient and this does not seem to be the mirage of the oasis we glimpse in the desert and as I see it, extension of life expectancy for the hemodialysis patient will increase. Added to this is the role of newer biosensor like FGF 23 and the use of more paricalcitriol and calcicinet to reduce the incidence of CVD which should be beneficial to our patients.

Which Mode of Dialysis will Ensure Adequacy of Dialysis and Also Offers the Best Chances for Longevity?

With the present state of the art, there are several factors one has to consider in order to formulate the best choice for the moment. The mode of dialysis must incorporate high flux membranes in order to remove middle molecules. The peritoneal membrane is also one that can remove middle molecular toxicity. There must be not only adequacy of dialysis in the prescription but nutritional adequacy must also be managed. One of the major problems is phosphate removal. The best way of not having high plasma phosphate is not to consume protein. But to do so will mean malnutrition which will cause the patient to succumb to infections and curtail life. The answer then would lie in extending the hours of dialysis. It would appear then that Nocturnal Dialysis, done 7 to 8 hours every night with the patient asleep would be the answer. Nocturnal HD offers the best KT/V and is ideal for removal of high molecular toxins as well. The patient is in his home environment and does not have to sacrifice his wakeful hours on dialysis. But Nocturnal HD unlike CRRT would still cause myocardial stunning which would contribute to loss of residual renal function as well as cardiovascular morbidity and mortality. Mortality rates have been found to be lower for patients on high efficiency convective modalities (hemofiltration and hemodialfiltration) than in those on conventional HD in the Dialysis Outcomes and Practice Patterns Study (DOPPS) [Canaud B *et al.* Kidney Int 2006, 69:2087–2093].

For now, the consensus would favour Daily Nocturnal Home HD with its benefits of better BP control, regression of left ventricular mass, improved phosphate control despite a liberal phosphate intake and use of low dose or no phosphate binders. There is also improvement in quality of life and cognitive function, decreased sympathetic tone, improved endothelial function and vascular compliance, increased exercise capacity, correction of anemia and sleep apnea and improved nutrition.

REFERENCES

1. Andreas Pierratos. Daily nocturnal hemodialysis — a paradigm shift worthy of disrupting current dialysis practice. *Nature Clinical Practice Nephrology* 2008, 4(11):602–603.

2. Tentori T *et al.* Mortality risk among hemodialysis pateints receiving different vit D analogs. *Kidney Int* 2006, **70**:1858–1865.
3. Patel TV and Singh AK. Role of Vit D in CKD. *Semin Nephrol* 2009, **29**:113–121.
4. Cardus A *et al.* Differential effects of Vit D analogs in on vascular calcification. *J Bone and Mineral Research*, 2007, **22**:860–866.
5. Boudville NC *et al.* C.E.R.A. (Continuous Erythropoeitin Receptor Activator) versus Darbepoeitin Alpfa. *Clin J Amer Soc Nephrol* 2009, **4**:738–750.
6. Levin NW *et al.* C.E.R.A. versus Darbepoeitin Alpfa. *Lancet*, 2007, **370**:1415–1421.
7. O'Hare AM *et al.* When to refer patients with CKD for vascular access: Should age be a consideration? *Kidney Int* 2007, **71**:555–561.
8. Shaldon S. First use of Nocturnal Hemodialysis. *Kidney Int* 2009, **76**:230.
9. Davenport A *et al.* Achieving BP targets during dialysis improves control but increases intradialytic hypotension. *Kidney Int* 2007, **73**:759–764.
10. Szczch L, Anemia trials: Lessons for clinicians, politicians, and 3rd party payers. Editorial, *Kidney Int* 2010, **77**:479–480.
11. Isakova T *et al.* A blueprint for randomised trials targeting phosphorus metabolism in CKD. *Kidney Int* 2009, **76**:705–716.
12. O'Neill WC. The fallacy of the calcium phosphorus product. *Kidney Int* 2007, **72**:792–796.
13. O'Hare AM *et al.* When to refer patients with CKD for vascular access surgery: Should age be a consideration? *Kidney Int* 2007, **71**: 555–561.
14. Andreas Pierratos. Daily nocturnal hemodialysis — a paradigm shift worthy of disrupting current dialysis practice. *Nature Clinical Practice Nephrology*, 2008, **4**(11):602–603.
15. Tentori T *et al.* Mortality risk among hemodialysis pateints receiving different vit D analogs. *Kidney Int* 2006, **70**:1858–1865].
16. Patel TV and Singh AK. Role of Vit D in CKD. *Semin Nephrol* 2009, **29**:113–121.
17. Cardus A *et al.* Differential effects of Vit D analogs in on vascular calcification. *J Bone and Mineral Research*, 2007, **22**:860–866.
18. MacDouggal JC *et al.* Correction of anemia with Darbepoeitin in patients with CKD receiving dialysis. *Nephrol Dial Transpl* 2003, **18**:576–581.
19. Boven K *et al.* The increased incidence of pure red cell aplasia with an Eprex formulation in uncoated rubber syringes. *Kidney Int* 2005, **67**:2346–2353.

20. Cullen P *et al*. Hypochromic red cells and reticulocyte Hb content as markers of iron deficiency in patients undergoing hemodialysis. *Nephrol Dial Transpl* 1999, **14**:659–665.
21. NKF KDOQI guidelines and clinical practice recommendations for anemia in CKD. *Amer J Kidney Disease*, 2006, **47**S:S1–S146.
22. Boudville NC *et al*. C.E.R.A. (Continuous Erythropoeitin Receptor Activator) versus Darbepoeitin Alpfa. *Clin J Amer Soc Nephrol* 2009, **4**:738–750.
23. Levin NW *et al*. C.E.R.A. versus Darbepoeitin Alpfa. *Lancet*, 2007, **370**:1415–1421.
24. McFarlane PA *et al*. International trends in erythropoietin use and Hb levels in hemodialysis patients. *Kidney Int* 2010, **78**:215–223.
25. Lasalle M *et al*. Age and comorbidity may explain the paradoxical association of an early dialysis start with poor survival. *Kidney Int* 2010, **77**:700–707.
26. Komenda P *et al*. British Columbia Provincial Renal Agency, Vancouver, Canada. The cost of starting and maintaining a large home hemodialysis program. *Kidney International Kidney Int* 2010, **77**:1039–1045.

CHAPTER 31

Peritoneal Dialysis

In 1959, Dr ST Boen wrote about peritoneal dialysis (PD) in his PhD thesis in Amsterdam as a means of saving and prolonging lives of patients with AKI and ESRF. Boen's thesis contained details of the techniques of PD. He gave details of PD kinetics and changes in plasma concentrations during dialysis. Dr Gjessing from Uppsala in Sweden in 1967 described new osmotic agents like Amino acids (AA) and Dextran and new indications for PD like severe haemorrhagic pancreatitis, use of PD in acute poisonings and pharmmcokinetics of drugs administered intraperitoneally. Subsequently Popovich and Moncrief presented the first results of continuous ambulatory PD (CAPD) as a new PD option and Oreopoulos presented the first clinical results of CAPD using flexible bags. CAPD was first use in Singapore in 1980 and today about 23% of patients on dialysis at SGH are on CAPD/APD. With the aging population in Singapore and elsewhere, assisted PD as well as automatic PD (APD) offer an equally viable alternative to HD. It is home based and is a popular choice among the frail older patients. PD compared to HD also lessens the financial burden on families [Divino JC *et al*. Back to the future: It does not only happen in Hollywood. Kidney Int 2008, 73S:S1–S4].

PRINCIPLES OF PERITONEAL DIALYSIS

The peritoneum is a membrane lining the stomach and the intestines. It forms an apron that lies freely in the abdominal cavity. Its rich blood supply allows us to use it for exchange of substances in and out of the body. For the purpose of dialysis, the peritoneal membrane acts as the dialysis membrane. Waste products carried in the blood vessels of the peritoneum would diffuse across the membrane into the dialysate which is infused into the abdominal cavity. Again, by means of principles of osmosis and diffusion, waste products like urea, creatinine and excess potassium which are at a higher concentration in the blood of patients with renal failure will diffuse into the dialysate in the abdominal cavity and can be drained out.

A flexible catheter called a Tenckhoff Catheter is used for peritoneal dialysis. It is inserted into the peritoneal cavity by means of a sterile technique with aseptic precautions under anaesthetic. The dialysate fluid is then run into the abdomen via the catheter and out again after exchange of waste products has taken place. Each cycle (run-in and run-out of dialysate plus period allowed for diffusion to take place) takes about 1 hour. Usually after 2 to 3 days the patient feels much better with this treatment.

This form of dialysis can be used for the patient who is awaiting the maturation of his AV fistula prior to haemodialysis. It can also be used for the patient with acute renal failure due to septicaemia or drugs where he only requires a few dialyses before kidney function returns. Acute peritoneal dialysis is seldom practised nowadays, most physicians prefer acute hemodialysis or CRRT.

The Tenckhoff Catheter

For the patient who requires long-term peritoneal dialysis (continuous ambulatory peritoneal dialysis or CAPD), a Tenckhoff catheter is used. It is soft and flexible and is made of non-irritating Silastic. It is inserted under anaesthesia in the operating theatre. The correct insertion is important for long-term catheter survival and for avoidance of infection at the site of catheter insertion.

Dialysate Used for Patients on Peritoneal Dialysis

The dialysate (dialysis fluid) is sterile and it is supplied in 1- or 2-litre polythene bags. It is a buffered solution of salts like the haemodialysis fluid but is different because of its high glucose content. The glucose is necessary for the removal of fluid from the patient.

The presence of glucose in the dialysate will cause water from the bloodstream to be drawn into the peritoneal cavity by means of osmosis. In this way the patient can get rid of excess fluid which causes swelling of his body.

Continuous Ambulatory Peritoneal Dialysis (CAPD)

There are 2 forms of peritoneal dialysis. Acute peritoneal dialysis is used for intermittent or once-only dialysis. Chronic peritoneal dialysis is employed when the patient requires continuous dialysis and is called CAPD (Fig. 31.1).

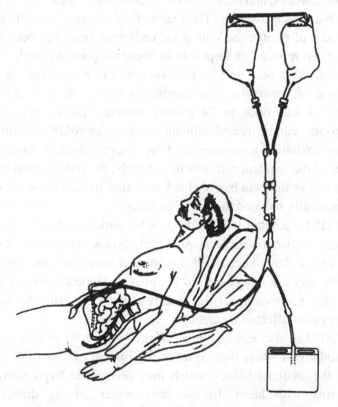

Fig. 31.1   Diagram of patient on peritoneal dialysis

In CAPD, the patient performs a slow but continuous exchange using a Tenckhoff catheter, in contrast to acute peritoneal dialysis where hourly exchange is the rule.

CAPD is a form of treatment alternative to haemodialysis for end stage renal failure. The procedure involves exchanging 2 litres of dialysate 4 times a day. This is done daily and at each exchange the bag is rolled up and worn until the next exchange. The patient walks about and does his work until the next exchange when the bag is disconnected and a new one connected and run in.

It has no capital expenditure as the patient does not require a machine and the only disposables are the bags of dialysate. The monthly recurrent expenditure is about S$1,400.

It is simple to use since a patient usually learns the technique within 2 weeks, and the low intrinsic costs have made CAPD popular with many patients. The major disadvantage is the frequent episodes of peritonitis. With good technique these episodes have now been reduced to 1 episode in about 42 patient months. This is to say that once in about 42 months the patient may get an episode of peritonitis. This compares very well with the past where it was once in 24 patient months. These episodes of peritonitis can be treated with antibiotics. Control of infection by better exchange techniques and by microbiological filters has reduced the incidence of infection. Lately, the introduction of the ultra bag or the twin bag to check infection in CAPD patients has dramatically reduced the infection rates.

CAPD is a better form of dialysis for patients with kidney failure due to diabetes mellitus. A diabetic on haemodialysis runs the risk of blindness because of the heparin used for haemodialysis which may cause bleeding in his eyes, a tendency arising from diabetic retinopathy. This usually occurs in patients whose kidneys are affected by diabetes.

CAPD is also less strenuous to the heart. It is gentler, unlike hemodialysis where there is an initial run-off of 100 ml of blood into the artificial kidney which may precipitate hypotension in patients with heart disease (commoner among diabetics).

Therefore CAPD is recommended for the elderly especially those with ischemic heart disease.

For diabetics on CAPD, there is the additional advantage of administering insulin intra-peritoneally with more physiological absorption compared to subcutaneous route of insulin where there is wider fluctuation of insulin levels.

Automated Peritoneal Dialysis

Apart from CAPD, Chronic Peritoneal Dialysis can also be performed at night when the patient is asleep, using an automated peritoneal dialysis machine. The machine performs the exchanges at night which the patient is asleep. The main advantage is that the patient is free of the burden of dialysing himself in the day time. The expenditure for APD is about $1,600 a month.

Nutrition in PD

1. Prevalance of malnutrition is high and several indices have been used to monitor nutritional status including serum albumin and prealbumin, lean body mass, total body nitrogen and creatinine excretion. The major determinants of serum albumin are protein loss in dialysate and presence of inflammation as indicated by C reactive protein.
2. Measures to help nutritional status include oral nitrogen supplements as well as intraperitoneal amino acids. Some have suggested correction of acidosis since acidosis induces catabolism in ESRF patients.
3. Other measures include anabolic strategies like giving anabolic steroids and even the use of recombinant growth hormones, but these are short term strategies and fraught with side effects.
4. Utimately the best strategy is to eat well, especially protein rich foodstuff to supplement the protein loss in the dialysate which can be considerable. Unfortunately, often it is the poor with comorbidities who cannot afford to eat well and also are

bogged down by a poor appetite, the vicious cycle of the poor dialysis patient dependent on help from VWO for dialysis support and trying hard to make ends meet. How can they afford good quality protein to counter the loss of protein in the dialysate against the background of low serum albumin associated with nutritional edema.

MEDICAL PROBLEMS WHILST ON PERITONEAL DIALYSIS

1. Hyperglycemia

    Glucose absorption due to the glucose used in the peritoneal dialysate can cause hyperglycemia which could exacerbate hyperglycemia in diabetic patients and cause glucose intolererance in non diabetic patients so that they require oral hypoglycemics or insulin. Metformin should be avoided as it causes lactic acidosis in renal failure, but sulphonylureas can be used. For those patients requiring insulin, nowadays we no longer use intraperitoneal insulin even though the absorption of insulin is more physiologic as intraperitoteal insulin requires much larger doses and there is a risk of contamination when the bags are injected.

2. Obesity

    Obesity is a problem, again due to glucose absorption from the dialysate and the average patient could gain weight from about 10% to 20%. The glucose absorption contributes from 500 to 1000 kilocalories per day. This is a lot compared to the recommended daily allowance of 3500 kilocalories per day for the patient. There is a necessity for dietary counselling and exercise and in patients where this is a very significant problem due to excess obesity one may have to resort to the use on non glucose dialysate.

3. Hyperlipidemia

    Most patients on peritioneal dialysis would have elevated LDL Cholesterol and triglycerides. This is related to glucose absorption. Hyperlipedemia contributes to the increased atherogenesis leading to increased cardiovascular morbidity and mortality in these patients. Patients should be prescribed statins for the raised LDL Cholesterol and if the Triglycerides are excessively high despite the use of statins, some may require the use of fibrates. But beware of myositis and rhabdomyolysis when combining the use of statins and fibrates. At this stage there is no conclusive evidence that lowering triglycerides in patients on peritoneal dislysis [PD] will decrease cardiac mortality.

4. Hypoalbuminemia

   Each day during PD, the patient can lose from 5 to 10 gms of protein a day into the dialysate and soon the serum albumin of the patient will decrease [average from 34 to 30 gm/L] associated with edema. Serum albumin of 34 g/l is already very low. They should have serum albumin >38 g/l to 42 g/l. The loss of protein occurs more amongst the high transporters and those with peritonitis or inflammation as evidenced by high C Reactive Protein [CRP]. Patients on PD should be advised by a dietician to increase their dietary protein intake in order to increase the low serum albumin which tends to occur more often among poor patients who cannot afford to eat more meat, especially beef. They should be advised on alternative foods to increase protein intake.

5. Calcium and Phosphate abnormalities

   Patients on PD may have hypercalcemia often due to the calcium acetate and calcium carbonate given as phosphate binders to control high serum phosphate in the patients. Check the serum calcium regularly and decrease dose of these binders if necessary. Generally the phosphate controls are better for PD when compared to HD patients. One of the things to exclude when a PD patient has hypercalcemia is TB peritonitis which can present as hypercalcemia. This is because the macrophages present in the peritoneum in patients with TB peritonitis can produce Vit D causing hypercalcemia.

6. Hypokalaemia

    Hyperkalaemia is not a problem in PD patients as the potassium is constantly removed by the ongoing dialysis. PD patients are in fact more prone to develop hypokalaemia and hence are encouraged to consume more fruit and vegetables unlike their HD counterparts. They can also take more salt and drink more fluids compared to the HD patient. Most patients on PD require potassium supplements in the form of potassium chloride tabs 600 mg a day, some even up to 1200 mg/day. Hypokalemia, especially among the elderly PD patients should be avoided as hypokalaemia is deleterious to the heart in these patients.

7. Hyponatremia

    Patients on PD may have a low serum sodium as they tend to drink more. If they have edema and the serum albumin levels are satisfactory they should take less fluid.

Peritonitis

1. This used to be a serious complication of PD accounting for many failures and much mortality and occasional mortality in the early days when we started the PD programme in Singapore General Hospital but today our rate of peritonitis for both CAPD and APD programme is 1 episode of peritonitis per 48 patient months which is comparable to many of the advanced centres throughout the world. This is especially so after we introduced the twin bag or the integrated double bags. For the APD patient on day dry APD, the effluent dialysate can be collected after a 1 litre dwell collected 1 to 2 hours later. PD cell count for APD is the same as for CAPD.

2. Peritonitis is diagnosed by abdominal pain, cloudy effluent dialysate, effluent dialysate cell count of >100 WBC/ml with or without positive effluent dialysate culture. Sometimes cloudy or turbid dialysate could be due to too much fibrin, protein or chyle [chylous ascites]. Positive cultures are obtained in about 80% of

peritonitis. For those with negative cultures one has to exclude fungal infection or TB peritonitis or sometimes the patients may already have been put on antibiotics before culture.

3. For most patients with PD peritonitis, high fever is unusual and if present one has to do blood cultures to exclude systemic sepsis or septicaemia as the patient may develop septicemic shock with hypotension. In such cases they will require dopamine support as well as antibiotics. Abdominal pain may or may not precede the cloudy PD effluent. Pain is usually mild for Staph epidermidis and dipththeroids but for Staph aureus, Pseudomonas aeroginosa or fungal peritonitis the pain can be very severe.

4. Gram positive organisms account for most of the infections. About one third are mild and often due to coagulase negative Staph related to touch contamination. Staph aureus accounts for another 20% and is often associated with exit site and tunnel infection. Diptheroids and Enterococcus are the causes of gram positive organisms and are mild and easily treated.

5. Non Pseudomonas Gram Negative (NPGN) peritonitis is a frequent, serious complication of PD. Based on the ANZ-DATA registry [Jarvis EM *et al.* Predictors, treatment and outcomes of non-Psudomonas Gram-negative peritonitis, Kidney Int 2010, 78:408–414], over a 39 months period, a total of 837 episodes of NPGN peritonitis (23.3% of all peritonitis) occurred in 256 patients. The most common organism isolated was E coli, but included Klebsiella, Enterobacter, Serratia, Acinebacter, Proteus and Citrobacter with multiple organisms identified in 25% of patients. The principal risk factor was older age with poorer clinical outcome predicted by older age and polymicrobial peritonitis. Overall antibiotic cure rate was 59%. NPGN peritonitis was associated with a significantly higher risk of hospitalisation, catheter removal, permanent transfer to HD and death compared to other organisms contributing to peritonitis. Underlying bowel perforation requiring surgery was uncommon.

6. About 1 in 10 infections are due to Pseudomonas. This often causes severe pain and is difficult to treat and it is our practice to remove the Tenckhoff catheter and treat with antibiotics. Even with treatment the relapse rate is high. It can also be associated with exit site and tunnel infection.

7. Nowadays, in many centres, the prevalence of coagulase negative Staph seems to be on the decline and we are seeing more of the non Pseudomonas gram negative Staph which accounts for about 30% of cases of peritonitis. These are the E coli, Klebsiella, Serratia and Proteus.

8. Fungal infection accounts for about 5% of peritonitis with Candida as the most common. The catheter has to be removed quickly and the patient treated with anti fungal drugs. This is a serious complication which can result in death in about 25% if catheter is not promptly removed and patients treated. Patients should be treated with Amphotericin or Flucytosine and antifungal therapy changed after sensitivity results are known. Fluconazole or other oral antifungal agents may be used to replace Amphotericin depending on culture results. Beware of bone marrow suppression when using Flucytosine. Oral antifungal therapy has to be continued for 2 weeks after removal of catheter.

9. Fungal infections could be the result of repeated infections with frequent usage of antibiotics. The other consequence of antibiotic abuse is the spread of antibiotic resistance, in particular MRSA or Meticillin Resistant Staph Aureus. Treating MRSA infection including MRSA peritonitis is fast becoming a big problem in many hospitals.

10. Tuberculosis causing TB peritonitis, like fungal infection presents as culture negative peritonitis. As mentioned, hypercalcemia can be an associated feature of TB peritonitis because the macrophages in the peritoneal cavity can produce active Vit D. Patients should be treated with rifampicin, isoniazid, pyrazinamide for 3 months and then rifampicin and Isoniazid continued for another 9 months. Pyridoxine supplement is required, 100 mg a day as opposed to the usual 10 mg

we give as a supplement to some patients. Pyridoxine is continued for a few years. Patients can continue on PD while on treatment, but for atypical mycobacteria the catheter should be removed.

11. Removal of catheter is necessary for difficult to treat peritonitis, i.e. those who do not respond within 5 days of treatment, otherwise to continue therapy will cause such severe fibrosis and adhesions that it will be difficult or impossible for the patient to return to PD later on. The other indication for removal of PD catheter is when the patient has frequent PD relapses, i.e. having another infection within 4 weeks of completing antibiotic therapy. Those with exit site or tunnel infection may require removal of catheter. Other indications are fungal or fecal peritonitis. Fecal peritonitis indicates an intraabdominal pathology and exploratory laparotomy would be required. For bacterial peritonitis the catheter can be reinserted after 4 weeks but for fungal peritonitis one may have to wait for 6 weeks. Those with exit site or tunnel infection can have a swing over, i.e. removal and placement of new catheter at a different site. Patients with frequent peritonitis should undergo retraining. For patients with Staph aureus exit site or tunnel site infection the application of mupirocin to the nose or to the exit site can prevent infection.

12. Antibiotic therapy for CAPD peritonitis. Patients are generally given intraperitoneal or I/P antibiotics. With intermittent dosing the antibiotic must dwell for at least 6 hours for cephalosporine, aminoglycosides and vancomycin. For APD patients cephalosporine can be added to each exchange and the others according to dose intervals determined by monitoring of drug levels.

13. For coagulase negative Staph 2 weeks with cephalosporine is enough. Streptococcal and Enterococcal I/P ampicillin can be used together with gentamicin or amikacin. For Staph aureus, cephalosporine is used but if meticillin resistant then use vancomycin. Treat for 3 weeks. Teicoplanin can

be used as alternative to vancomyciin. If vancomycin resistant, use linezolid.

14. For Pseudomonas aeroginosa, use two antibiotics, oral quinolone like ciprofloxacin with I/P cephtazidime or cephapime or tobramycin. Catheter has to be removed.

15. Non Pseudomonas gram negative peritonitis (NPGN). We routinely use cephalosporine plus an aminoglycoside for 2 weeks. If the response is poor after 3 days it is better to remove the catheter if patients's plan is to return to PD. For multiple enteric organisms, suspect a bowel pathology and refer to a surgeon for exploration. Metronidazole will have to be added to cephtazidine plus an aminogylcoside. For those patients with adhesion colic, intestinal obstruction or those suspected to have a collection of loculated pus, a computerised abdominal scan is necessary with a view to exploratory laporatory. Such patients may have to convert to HD thereafter.

ENCAPSULATING PERITONEAL SCLEROSIS

1. This is an uncommon but important and feared complication of PD. In this condition there is widespread sclerosis of the peritoneal membrane which also encapsulates the intestines causing intestinal obstruction leading to anorexia and weight loss. Patients have haemorrhagic ascites with fever, anemia and low serum albumin. Radiologically there is calcification of the peritoneum with encapsulating fibrotic cocoon in the presence of dilated bowel loops with fluid levels indicating obstruction.

2. The etiology is unknown and it occurs after patients have been on PD for some years, about 6% after 10 years and 20% after 15 years [Nomoto Y *et al.* Sclerosing encapsulating peritonitis in patients undergoing CAPD: a report of the Japanese Sclerosing Encapsulating Peritonitis Study Group. Am J Kidney Dis 1996, 28:420–427]. These are usually patients who have

switched from PD to HD and develop progressive ascites with intestinal obstruction. Other conditions which parallel encapsulating peritoneal sclerosis [EPS] are idiopathic EPS which can occur in patients without renal failure like those with autoimmune disease, malignancy and the use of β blockers [Kawanishi H *et al.* Epidemiology of encapsulating peritoneal sclerosis in Japan. Perit Dial Int 2005, **25**(Suppl 4):S14–S16]. Some attribute this condition to the use of non biocompatible dialysates, the glucose or the buffers but so far there is no conclusive evidence. In fact, this has also occurred in PD patients who have never had an episode of peritonitis.

3. Apart from the high occurrence in the Japanese, EPS is uncommon in North America, so there could be a genetic or ethnic basis in its etiology. There have been recent reports among Europeans [Summers AM *et al.* Single centre experience of encapsulating peritoneal sclerosis in patients with end stage renal failure. Kidney Int 2005, 68:2381–2385].

4. Treatment; Steroids and tamoxifen have been shown to be useful. Surgical techniques have improved with Kawanishi reporting better results using enterolysis. Patients have to be fed by total parenteral nutrition.

5. Prevention: Some have advocated switching from PD to HD after 5 or more years. But there is no certainty as others have pointed to the fact that many patients develop this only after switching from PD to HD and in many cases often within 6 months of switching from PD to HD. Unfortunately, EPS is associated with a high mortality rate from 30% to 50% [Nakamoto H *et al.* 2005, Encapsulating peritoneal sclerosis — a clinician's approach to diagnosis and medical treatment. Perit Dialy Int 2005, **25**(Suppl 40):S30–S38].

6. In a recent review [Johnson DW *et al.* Encapsulating peritoneal sclerosis: incidence, predictors and outcomes. *Kidney Int* 2010, 77:904–912] among 7618 patients on the Australian and New Zealand Renal Registry, measures over a period of 13 years, EPS was diagnosed in 33 patients, giving an incidence rate of 1.8/1000 patient years. The respective cumulative

incidences at 3, 5 and 8 years were 0.3, 0.8 and 3.9%. The authors conclude that this is a rare condition affecting 0.4% of PD patients on PD for at least 4.5 years. It is independently predicted by younger age <50 years and longer time on PD >4 years. In their study of patients who were transferred to HD before or immediately after EPS diagnosis, the median survival was 4 years, not different from that of PD controls matched for age, gender, presence or absence of diabetes mellitus and time spent on PD. There is as yet no single rule on optimum time spent on PD to avoid EPS and the decision should be tailored to the individual based on age, prognosis, quality of life and potential risks of HD and suitability for transplantation.

Concerns Regarding the Use of Hypertonic Glucose Exchanges and the Contribution of Combined Crystalloid and Colloid Osmosis to Fluid and Sodium Management in PD

1. Results from earlier studies had suggested the need for elevated clearance targets in PD and these led to the implementation of high dose automatic PD [APD] and CAPD strategies to enhance small solute clearances which required high volumes of glucose based dialysate. This then led to concerns of metabolic consequences for the patient and long term structural damage to the peritoneal membrane [Davis SJ. Kidney Int 2006, 70S:S76–S83].

2. However, the long dwell that can last up to 15 hours at night is not suited to glucose based dialysate since glucose absorption will lead to loss of UF and reduced sodium clearance.

3. It has been demonstrated that 7.5% icodextrin will be beneficial in this respect. **Icodextrin** can induce UF during the long dwell period via colloid osmosis. Using icodextrin will also reduce glucose exposure. There is also increased sodium removal with icodextrin since water movement with icodextrin is through the small pores.

4. But the osmotic effect of 7.5% icodextrin alone is insufficient to achieve fluid balance in many patients on APD without recourse to hypertonic glucose during the overnight exchange.

5. The solution then is to mix or combine colloid and crystalloid osmosis in the same exchange with the possibility that the effects on UF would be additive. The challenge lies in the appropriate concentrations in the combination.

6. The development of combination[bimodal] dialysis solutions for PD based on the Sheffield and the French Experience has enabled PD to achieve a new and enhanced dimension which has revolutionised the whole art of PD [Freida P. Perit Dial Int 2007, 27:267–276].

7. The concept of ultrafiltration efficiency has been defined as the amount of net UF obtained for every gram of glucose absorbed. Applied to the 10 hour dwell of CAPD in 94 patients using alternatively 2.5% dextrose or 7.5% icodextrin for the daytime exchange, this index was shown to be three fold higher with icodextrin than with the glucose based dialysate.

8. In another study of 92 patients on either 4.25% dextrose or 7.5% icodextrin over a 14 hour dwell period in APD, it was again shown that in patients on icodextrin the UF was three fold more than in the hypertonic glucose based dialysate [Freida P].

9. The use of a combination solution in the long dwell will lead to a diminished use of hypertonic glucose based dialysate during the remainder of the 24 hour therapeutic cycle in CADP or APD. This glucose sparing approach will result in better metabolic balance for the patient and better preservation of the peritoneal membrane.

10. The combination PD solution should be formulated according to the individual patients' responses with respect to fluid and sodium removal.

11. Apart from the advantage of equilibrium of sodium and water balance in the patient, the development of efficient UF will mean less salt restriction for the patient and help to improve the food intake in PD patients and thereby optimise their nutrition.

12. The concept of combining colloid and crystalloid osmotic agents shows great promise. It demonstrates efficiency of sodium and water removal and is glucose sparing and addresses one of the biggest concerns in PD.

Newer PD Solutions

1. The clinical use of newer PD solutions containing non glucose osmotic agents (Amino acid, Icodextrin) and more physiological buffer combinations and pH together with the use of cyclers brought PD therapy to a new dimension. These new techniques have resulted in better fluid removal, tighter blood sugar control, attenuation of hyperlipidemia and improved protein synthesis.

2. The leptin/adiponectin ratio is a novel marker for atherosclerosis. Glucose based PD fluids aggravate the adipokine production balance from cultured adipocytes whereas glucose-free PD fluids improve this balance. This balance will reduce the burden of CVS disease in the PD patients [Teta D *et al*. The leptin/adiponectin ratio: peritoneal implications for PD. Kidney Int 2008, 73S:S112–S118].

3. Another new area is PD fluid biocompatibility. Comparing biocompatible PD fluid with conventional fluid, it was found that biocompatible PD fluid could modulate baroreflex sensitivity during glucose containing PD dwell independently of glucose concentration and UF volume. Thus biocompatible PD fluid can influence cardiovascular regulation and function, important in the PD patient prone to CVS disease [John SG *et al*. effects of PD fluid biocompatibility on baroreflex sensitivity. Kidney Int 2008, 73S: S119–S124].

4. The use of icodextrin in diabetic PD patients have resulted in better management and metabolic control.

5. Amino Acid (AA) containing PD solutions compared to glucose based PD solution showed that the AA containing solution

was associated with significant increase in skeletal muscle AA uptake both in the fasting and during insulin stimulation [Asola M *et al.* Amino acid based PD solution improves amino acid transport into skeletal muscle. Kidney Int 2008, 73S:S131–S136].

6. Today, the use of glucose sparing PD solutions offers a totally new dimension for PD, especially with the introduction of biocompatible solutions.

7. In 24 centres in 3 countries (Canada, Greece, Turkey), among 530 PD patients it was shown that PD combined with dietary measures and phosphate binders, was associated with satisfactory serum phosphate control in the majority of patients compared with comparable HD cohorts [Yavuz A *et al.* Phosphorus control in PD patients. Kidney Int 2008, 73S:S152–S158].

8. Finally, to add to the new dimension of PD, APD has been used as a frontline acute therapy option for renal failure patients with severe hyperkalaemia and metabolic acidosis in the Emergency Room [Ilabaca MB. Automatic PD as a life saving therapy in the emergency room: Report of 4 cases. Kidney Int 2008, 73S:S173–S176].

REFERENCES

1. Freida P *et al.* The contribution of combined crystalloid and colloid osmosis to fluid and sodium management in PD. *Kidney Int* 2008, **73S**:S102–S111.

2. Freida P *et al.* Combination of crystalloid (glucose) and colloid (icodextrin) osmotic agents markedly enhances peritoneal fluid and solute transport during the long PD dwell. *Perit Dial Int* 2007, 27:267–276].

3. Davis SJ. Mitigating peritoneal membrane characteristics in modern PD therapy. *Kidney Int* 2006, **70S**: S76–S83

4. Divino JC *et al.* Back to the future: It does not only happen in Hollywood. *Kidney Int* 2008, **73S**:S1–S4.

Adequacy of Dialysis in PD

1. The prescription for PD has to take into consideration PD clearance and volume removal as well as nutritional, cardiovascular and metabolic status. The two indices used are the Kt/V or fractional urea clearance and the creatinine clearance normalized for body surface area [CrCl].
2. Calculation of these indices require 24 hour collections of PD effluent and urine with measurements of urea and creatinine content, a simultaneous blood sample to measure urea and creatinine, and then a simple standard calculation of clearance. For calculation of the residual component of CrCl, a mean of urea and creatinine clearance is used because residual renal clearance is known to substantially over estimate the true GFR.
3. The clearance is then normalized to a measure of body size, which for urea is, by convention, the total body water or "V" to give Kt/V and for creatinine is the body surface area (BSA) to give CrCl. Both BSA and V are estimated from formulae based on height, weight and sex. The resulting daily values are multiplied by 7 and expressed per week.
4. The targets for weekly Kt/V by KDOQI guidelines is 1.7 (previously it was 2) for both CAPD and APD and for all transport types. CrCl has no added value. For CAPD the standard is 4×2L CAPD.
5. CAPD prescription can be modified by raising the dwell volume for 1.5 to 2 to 2.5 to 3 L or from 3 or 4 exchanges to 4 or 5 exchanges if one wishes to increase the clearance. Both are effective, but increasing the dwell volume is usually preferred. For patients who still have Residual Renal Function of 2 to 4 ml/min, the concern for adequate middle molecule clearance is less. For those who are anuric, the addition of a day dwell would be advisable.
6. With regards to volume status, a higher salt and water removal is associated with better cardiovascular outcomes, but daily salt and water removal also reflects salt and water intake and not degree of volume control. Fluid overload is not desirable and we should attempt to normalize BP and remove

edema while avoiding hypotension and dehydration and at same time limit exposure to hypertonic glucose dialysate. The use of loop diuretics for salt removal and use of ACEI and ARBs to preserve RRF may be desirable. Management of hypertension is related to salt and fluid removal.

7. Ultrafiltration failure is defined as fluid overload associated with less than 400 ml of ultrafiltrate after a standardized 4 hour duration dwell with a 4.25% glucose 2-L dwell. Other causes of fluid overload like excess salt and water intake, loss of residual urine output, non compliance with exchanges, incorrect dialysate solution, catheter dysfunction have to be excluded first. True UF failure is rare in the first 2 years of PD. For UF failure, review and restrict salt and water intake and use loop diuretics if a patient still has significant urine output. Avoid long glucose dwells and switch to icodextrin if necessary. If there is no improvement one should convert to HD.

HOW DOES PERITONEAL DIALYSIS [PD] COMPARE WITH HEMODIALYSIS [HD]?

Whilst in the 1980's PD may have been considered a Cinderella as a modality of Renal Replacement Therapy, today most would agree that both HD and PD are equally viable modalities with Kidney Transplantation as the ideal since dialysis only rids the patients with ESRF of the waste products of protein metabolism and to a large extent the uremic toxins which cause all the ravages of ESRF compared to a kidney transplant which would produce hormones, vitamins and many other benefits known and unknown which are the functions of the kidney as the prime regulator of our internal environment.

For the patient therefore, whether he opts for HD or PD he has to consider various factors like cost and convenience since for most patients they are not in a position to realise the medical differences of both modalities in terms of the advantages versus the disadvantages of HD or PD. They have to let their physicians decide if there are any contraindications to either modalities of dialysis peculiar to their personal condition. That apart, for the rest of the 90% of patients it is really up to them to choose the particular modality best suited to their out of pocket expenses which is the balance after the subsidy from Medishield and Voluntary Welfare Organisation (VWO) like the National Kidney Foundation (NKF), the Kidney Dialysis Foundation (KDF) and the Peoples' Dialysis Centre (PDC) as well as the one modality that best suit their personal convenience and lifestyle.

Most would prefer to go to the Dialysis Centre [DC] thrice a week and park themselves there and have the procedure done for them citing the risk of peritonitis and having to do the procedure if they were to opt for PD. For those who choose to have PD, they are the patients who are self reliant, the DIY type, self motivated and like to take charge of their own affairs, depending on themselves and trusting themselves that they would do a good job and not develop peritonitis. They call the shots and are not at the mercy of nurses and DC staff who will control their time and schedule.

For HD, it is usually thrice weekly about 4 hours a session. For PD, the patient can have CAPD where they would do 4 exchanges a day, for example at 8am, 12pm, 6pm and 11pm before bedtime. These times are flexible and for the lunch time session, patients can do it in the office or at home if they come home for lunch. Those who find it a hassle doing CAPD in the day time can have APD or automated PD where the machine does it when the patient is asleep at night. The next morning the patient unplugs the machine and goes to work.

Apart from these factors, in general, an older patient or the one with heart disease should opt for PD which causes less strain on the heart. Diabetic patients who are more prone to heart disease and tend to have vascular access problems would be better off on CAPD as the initial run off of about 100 mls of blood from the patient's circulation into the dialyser circuit may cause the patient to suffer myocardial ischemia with hypotension. Heparin is used in HD and for the Diabetic patient with vitreous haemorrhage, CAPD which does not use heparin may be better for the patient's eyes.

One of the important considerations in support of CAPD is the preservation of Residual Renal Function [RRF]. This is the amount of kidney function still remaining in both the diseased kidneys when the patient goes on dialysis. The RRF may be 5 to 10 mls of eGFR, but it still serves a function of getting rid of toxins which the artificial kidney and the dialysis machine cannot do. It is remaining kidney function every minute of the day within the patient's body, still producing some urine and ridding potassium and other waste products. It is still producing some Erythropoietin to boost up the patient's low Haemoglobin. So overall it is useful to have and to preserve the RRF.

A patient on HD may still have RRF but he soon loses it unlike the patient on CAPD. This is because, during the process of HD, there will be intermittent drop of systolic BP and with each drop the renal perfusion of blood through the 2 remaining diseased kidneys will become less and less and within 6 months to a year, the RRF may drop from 5 to 10 mls to about 1 to 2 mls which is of much less use. For the patient on CAPD, the RRF is usually preserved for a much longer time and this translates into less morbidity and less mortality for the CAPD patient compared to the HD patient. This would explain why the morbidity and mortality for CAPD is better compared to HD, at least for the first 3 years on CAPD [Fenton SS *et al*. Hemodialysis versus peritoneal dialysis: a comparison of adjusted mortality rates. Am J Kidney Dis 1997, 30:334–342]. In contrast, patients on HD have a much higher mortality during the first 2 to 3 years accounting for about 30% deaths of HD patients during the initial years on HD.

At this stage there are no large scale multi centre randomised controlled trials to compare HD and PD simply because patients have refused to be randomised and majority of patients choose to be on HD rather than PD. There are 2 prospective studies so far, the first is the Canadian study on more than 800 patients from 11 centres followed up for 2 years. It showed that patients on PD survived better than those on HD. There were about 50% of patients in each group. But this survival advantage for PD disappeared after correction for baseline comorbidities. [Murphy

SW *et al*. Comparative mortality of hemodialysis and peritoneal dialysis in Canada. Kidney Int, 2000, 57:1720–1726].

The other major study is the Choice Study from the USA where there were more than 1000 patients from 81 centres followed up for a mean duration of 2.4 years. There were less patients on PD. The initial data showed no difference in unadjusted survival, but after adjustment it was found that HD patients had better survival compared to PD [Jaar BG *et al*. Comparing the risk for death with peritoneal dialysis and hemodialysis in a national cohort of patients with chronic kidney disease. Ann Intern Med 2005, 143:174–183].

Even though PD is less expensive compared to HD since it does not incur much capital expenditure and there is less need for manpower support in terms of providing nurses for hemodialysis, in many countries most patients would till opt for HD compared to PD. Many consider HD to be a better modality since HD has been established for a much longer time than PD and patients are more aware of the benefits of HD since fund raisers and VWO would rather canvass for support for HD than PD as they can generate more revenue doing HD and getting insurance reimbursements compared to PD where the financial returns are much less. Institutions and private organisations also would promote HD rather than PD as HD is more attractive financially with a larger profit margin. However in countries where the subsidy has to come from government coffers, we see more patients on PD compared to HD since there needs to be better accountability for usage of funds and patients' placement on either HD or PD may have to be dependent on more objective medical criteria and a little less on patients' choice. With government funding there is more encouragement by administrators of the dialysis programme to have patients opt for the less expensive PD programme. Hence in countries like the United Kingdom, Australia and Canada where there are state supported CAPD programmes, the uptake rates for PD are much higher, about 20% compared to about 10% for many other countries. In Hong Kong it is as high as 80% since PD is the modality of first choice unless there are contraindications to PD, all patients have to opt for PD. In the USA and Japan, the PD rates are very low, about 5% to 8%. This is because the reimbursement is through insurance companies and the dialysis providers consider HD a lucrative source of revenue compared to PD [De Veechi AF *et al*. Healthcare systems and end stage renal failure disease (ESRF) therapies — an international review; Costs and reimbursements/funding of ESRF therapies. Nephrol Dial Transplant 1999, **14**(suppl 6):31–41.

Preservation of Residual Renal Function (RRF) in Patients on Peritoneal Dialysis

1. A residual GFR of 1 ml/min is equivalent to a weekly peritoneal clearance of about 10 litres.
2. Preservation of RRF is associated with better long term survival, a reduction in BP, reduction in LVH, increased sodium removal, improved fluid status, increased serum β 2 microglobulin clearance, higher Hb levels, better nutritional status and decreased circulating inflammatory markers.
3. RRF rather than the delivered dose of PD is an essential marker of patient survival.
4. Incidence of peritonitis was found to be 3 fold higher in patients with GFR <1 ml/min compared to those with GFR >1 ml/min at the start of PD.
5. Factors associated with preservation of RRF included higher calcemia, use of ACEI or calcium channel blockers and PD.
6. Frusemide contributed to the maintenance of residual diuresis, improved natriuresis and volume control, but failed in the objective of protecting RRF, measured as solute clearance.
7. Use of ARBs can slow the progressive decrease in RRF even after 2 years on follow up in PD patients.

REFERENCE

Marron B *et al*. Benefits of preserving residual renal function in PD. *Kidney Int* 2008, **73S**:S42–S51

AWAK or Automated Wearable Artificial Kidney

This is presently a 6 pounds battery operated prototype designed to provide 24 hours daily continuous dialysis. However through development effort, AWAK is targeting towards a weight of 2 pounds. This is a technological breakthrough based on joint research with the University of California, Los Angeles (UCLA) and the Dept of Veterans affairs, USA. Dr Martin Roberts and Dr David BN Lee are the Chief Scientists and Inventors with Dr Gorden Ku as the Chairman of AWAK Technologies. Dr Gorden Ku is also Chairman of the Kidney Dialysis Foundation (KDF) in Singapore. With this invention, Martin feels that patients will be freed from dialytic regimes, freed from stringent dietary and fluid restriction and freed from being bound to a geographical locality. David stated that AWAK is based on the technique of peritoneal dialysis and sorbent- based regeneration of used dialysate in perpetuity. It is seemingly both bloodless and waterless, provides round the clock dialysis and represents the ultimate frequent dialysis which provides a steady state metabolic and fluid regulation. Because both the aqueous and the protein components of the used dialysate are regenerated and recycled, AWAK produces a novel protein containing dialysate that is expected to reduce or eliminate protein loss, with the additional possibility of removing protein-bound toxins. The first prototype is designed to provide a dialysate exchange rate of 4 litres per hour which will translate into a Kt/V of 4, a 100% increase over that used in current practice. This device is in the process of procuring FDA certification and plans are underway for clinical trials in the USA and Singapore in 2010. In the words of Gorden, this device will change the landscape of the dialysis industry.

Other Types of Wearable Artificial Kidneys

The present modalities of dialysis, whether hemodialysis and peritoneal dialysis are still far from ideal. However, apart from renal transplant, many patients with ESRF have to go on dialysis because of the shortage of transplant organs for donation. Between HD and PD, it would appear that HD in the long term may provide better survival. The best data is accrued from patients who are on daily hemodialysis. These patients have better appetite, better serum albumin levels and have better phosphate controls. They have decreased morbidity and mortality from cardiovascular diseases, strokes, improved BP controls, less myocardial stunning and less intradialytic hypotension. CAPD and Automated PD initially offer better preservation of residual renal function for the initial 2 to 3 years but after this period there does not appear to be more advantages compared to daily HD. Patients on PD live in fear of peritonitis and a worst fate awaits them if and when they develop encapsulating peritoneal sclerosis or EPS which occurs in those patients on PD for at least 5 years.

Problems faced by patients on dialysis therefore are high mortality rates almost approaching those with metastatic cancers of lower grade like colon and prostate, but still these are unacceptably high considering that kidney failure is and should no longer be a life threatening disease with the availability of dialysis and renal transplant. Other problems relate to vascular disease and sepsis including septic emboli , worse if they develop MRSA septicaemia.

The bright ray of hope is the recent development of Wearable Artificial Kidneys (WAK). These are the truly WAK, not those of the mammoth days where the WAK were large, heavy, cumbersome, ineffective and inefficient, short battery life and therefore limited hours of dialysis. The present WAK being developed are based on peritoneal dialysis like those mentioned above by Martin Roberts and David Lee or they are based on hemodialysis [Davenport A *et al.* A wearable hemodialysis device for patients with ESRF: a pilot study. Lancet, 2005, 370:2005–2010] and CRRT [Gura V *et al.* Continuous Renal Replacement Therapy for ESRD. A wearable artificial kidney (WAK). Contrib to Nephrol 2005, 149:325–333]. These machines use extracorporeal blood cleansing and charcoal and or sorbents for regeneration of effluent ultrafiltrate. The key is to develop machines using novel sorbent compounds that enable continuous dialysis for 7 days without the need to change cartridges in between. At the same time these machines are light and affordable using minimal amounts of dialysate. Like HD and CRRT, these types of AWAK will still require vascular access [different from those of Martin and David which is PD based].

Vascular access, the way we have it now are still problematic due to high morbidity resulting from sepsis, thrombosis and embolisation. The ideal vascular access for the future would be those with button hole access, biocompatible, non thrombogenic with no need for anticoagulant use and perhaps DNA or RNA compatible with the patient using it. Such technology are already available with the implants or access materials impregnated with compatible DNA/RNA.

PROGNOSIS FOR PATIENTS ON DIALYSIS

Mortality varies from 5% annually for 20- to 40-year-old patients to 10% annually for those over 60 years. Cause of death is usually due to myocardial infarction, stroke or infection. Only 15% of patients are classified as unfit for full or part-time work on medical grounds. Where the typical dialysis patient used to be anaemic and as a consequence cannot sustain hard physical effort today with recombinant DNA erythropoeitin becoming more affordable, anaemia of renal failure is no longer a problem and patients with Hb of about 12 gm or more are able to sustain hard physical effort. One of the main problems remaining is Cardiovascular disease which is related to poor phosphate control and secondary hyperparathyroidism. The use of synthetic Vit D have been associated with a high incidence of vascular calcification resulting in high cardiac morbidity and mortality. With the use of the newer Vitamin D Receptor (VDR) analogs like paricalcitriol, this may be one way we can help our patients. However, the high cost is prohibitory. We should look into ways to incorporate such drugs including the newer calcimimetics like calcicinet into the Medishield Insurance Scheme so that they are within the reach of the poorer patients. This is a sensible and humane way to reduce the number of patients on dialysis dying from cardiovascular diseases every year.

REFERENCES

1. Ronco C, Davenport A, Gura V. A wearable artificial kidney: dream or reality? *Nature Clinical Practice Nephrology*, 2008, **4**:604–605].
2. Nakamoto H *et al* 2005, Encapsulating peritoneal sclerosis — a clinician's approach to diagnosis and medical treatment. *Perit Dialy Int* 2005, **25**(Suppl 40):S30–S38.
3. De Veechi AF *et al*. Healthcare systems and end stage renal failure disease (ESRF) therapies — an international review; Costs and reimbursements/funding of ESRF therapies. *Nephrol Dial Transplant* 1999, **14**(Suppl 6):31–41.
4. Murphy SW *et al*. Comparative mortality of hemodialysis and peritoneal dialysis in Canada. *Kidney Int*, 2000, **57**:1720–1726.
5. Liem YS *et al*. Comparison of hemodialysis and peritoneal dialysis survival in The Netherlands. *Kidney Int* 2006, **71**:153–158.
6. Marron B *et al*. Benefits of preserving residual renal function in PD. *Kidney Int* 2008, **73S**:S42–S51.
7. Szczch L, Anemia trials: Lessons for clinicians, politicians, and 3rd party payers. *Editorial, Kidney Int* 2010, **77**:479–480.
8. Isakova T *et al*. A blueprint for randomised trials targeting phosphorus metabolism in CKD. *Kidney Int* 2009, **76**:705–716.
9. O'Neill WC. The fallacy of the calcium phosphorus product. *Kidney Int* 2007,**72**:792–796.
10. Patel TV and Singh AK. Role of Vit D in CKD. *Semin Nephrol* 2009, **29**:113–121.
11. Cardus A *et al*. Differential effects of Vit D analogs in on vascular calcification. *J Bone and Mineral Research*, 2007, **22**: 860–866.
12. Freida P *et al*. The contribution of combined crystalloid and colloid osmosis to fluid and sodium management in PD. *Kidney Int* 2008, **73S**:S102–S111.
13. Freida P *et al*. Combination of crystalloid (glucose) and colloid (icodextrin) osmotic agents markedly enhances peritoneal fluid and solute transport during the long PD dwell. *Perit Dial Int* 2007, **27**:267–276.

14. Davis SJ. Mitigating peritoneal membrane characteristics in modern PD therapy. *Kidney Int* 2006, **70**S:S76–S83
15. Divino JC *et al.* Back to the future: It does not only happen in Hollywood. *Kidney Int* 2008, **73**S:S1–S4.
16. Johnson DW *et al.* Encapsulating peritoneal sclerosis: Incidence, predictors and outcomes. *Kidney Int* 2010, **77**:904–912.
17. Jarvis EM *et al.* Predictors, treatment and outcomes of non-Psudomonas Gram-negative peritonitis, *Kidney Int* 2010, **78**:408–414.

CHAPTER 32

Renal Transplantation

In Singapore, the first cadaver renal transplant was performed in 1970. The first living related donor transplant was performed in 1976.

For cadaver transplants the graft survival rate is 89% for the first year, 85% for the fifth year, and 77% for the tenth year.

For living related donor transplants the graft survival rate is 98% at one year, 92% at 5 years and 82% at 10 years. Table 32.1 shows the number of kidney transplants performed in Singapore.

Our transplant survivor rates are comparable to those of advanced centres elsewhere.

Parents and siblings sharing 1 or 2 haplotypes are preferred in living donor transplantation as transplants from relatives with zero matched haplotypes have only the success rate similar to those of cadaver kidneys.

Successful live donation is often gratifying to the donor. Apart from the slight inevitable perioperative risk, the donor suffers no shortening of life or adverse effects on the quality of life. We have had living related renal donors from all walks of life and apart from mild hypertension in a few who are over 50 years which could well be unrelated to renal donation, none of our donors have suffered any adverse effects as a result of their donation.

A patient who is to be transplanted should be mentally and physically prepared. All correctable medical and surgical problems should be attended to while the patient is still on dialysis. This may involve treatment for peptic ulceration or dental clearance as such measures will help to minimise morbidity and mortality.

Table 32.1   Number of Kidney Transplants Performed in Singapore (1970–1996)

| | | Cadaveric | | | |
Year	Live Related	Local Transplant	Overseas Transplant	Cadaveric	Total
1970	—	1	—	1	1
1971	—	2	—	2	2
1972	—	3	—	3	3
1973	—	2	—	2	2
1974	—	6	—	6	6
1975	—	3	—	3	3
1976	1	3	—	3	4
1977	2	—	—	—	2
1978	10	2	—	2	12
1979	14	—	—	—	14
1980	18	—	—	—	18
1981	15	—	—	—	15
1982	17	8	—	8	25
1983	18	7	18	25	43
1984	12	16	8	24	36
1985	15	1	—	1	16
1986	14	15	5	20	34
1987	12	16	2	18	30
1988	4	23	2	25	29
1989	1	26	2	28	29
1990	11	45	4	49	60
1991	14	36	4	40	54
1992	18	60	17	77	95
1993	24	32	2	34	58
1994	16	84	45	129	145
1995	11	53	26	79	90
1996	12	44	14	58	70
1997	8	25	—	25	33
1998	15	42	14	56	71
1999	13	42	20	62	75
2000	10	54	14	68	78
2001	18	44	10	54	72
TOTAL	323	695	207	902	1225

LIVING RELATED DONOR

Within a family, HLA typing clearly separates siblings into 2, 1 or 0 haplotype matches. This allows the prediction of 95% or 84%

1-year graft survival for 2 or 1 haplotype matches respectively and hence the selection of the best donor. A transplant from a parent to a child has a 84% 1-year graft survival because a child inherits only one haplotype from each of his parents.

CADAVER DONOR

HLA-A and HLA-B matching confers a small but definite benefit. The B locus is probably more important than the A locus. DR locus matching confers an additional benefit.

A prerequisite for a successful graft is ABO compatibility, and a negative cross-match of donor T lymphocytes and recipient sera using a sensitive direct cytotoxic technique. Kidneys are harvested from brain dead donors. It is important to maintain the blood pressure of the potential donor to ensure adequate urine flow (about 60 ml/hour) as this will increase the likelihood of a viable donor kidney. When a cadaver kidney has been obtained it is cooled by simple perfusion with a hyper-osmolar solution and then left at 4°C prior to transplantation. Over 25% of grafts run a course of acute tubular necrosis for 1 to 2 weeks.

TISSUE TYPING

In our body is a particular series of closely linked genes called the Major Histocompatibility Complex (MHC). In humans, the MHC codes for proteins or antigens called the Human Leukocyte Antigen (HLA) that are important in kidney transplant matching. There are two principal classes of HLA. The class I HLA genes are named HLA-A, HLA-B and HLA-C, and the class II HLA genes are named HLA-DR, -DQ and -DP. Each HLA gene has multiple alternate forms called alleles. Each person inherits one allele of each HLA gene from his father and one allele of each HLA gene from his mother. Thus, each of us will have two sets of HLA gene alleles, i.e. two HLA-A alleles, two HLA-B alleles, two HLA-C alleles, two HLA-DR alleles, etc. Because each gene has many alleles, this leads to an extremely large number of possible combinations, making it difficult to have matching HLA types for unrelated individuals.

PATTERN OF INHERITANCE OF HLA TYPES

Because HLA genes are closely linked, they are inherited as a set of HLA-A, -B, -C, -DR, and -DQ alleles, called a haplotype. Each child will inherit one haplotype from the father and one from the mother. A child will therefore share one haplotype or at least 50% of HLA with each of his parents. Between siblings, they have a one in four chance of identical HLA (inherit the same haplotypes from both parents), a one in two chance of sharing half the HLA (inherit the same haplotype from one parent), and a one in four chance of completely non-identical HLA (inherit different haplotypes from both parents). Apart from parents and siblings, HLA typing matches are less common because of the diversity of HLA gene alleles. In practice, there should be at least a 25% match before living related donor transplant can be done, which would include the parents and some of the siblings (Fig. 32.1).

(Above two sections by courtesy of Diana Teo).

ABO BLOOD GROUPING IN KIDNEY TRANSPLANT

All of us have a certain type of blood group on our red blood cells. For a kidney transplant to be successful the blood group between the donor and the recipient must be compatible, otherwise the transplanted kidney will be rejected very quickly by the recipient's body. Blood grouping rules apply to both cadaver and living related transplants.

The various blood groups are A, B, 0, and AB. 0 is the universal donor and can give to 0, A, B, AB but can only receive from 0.

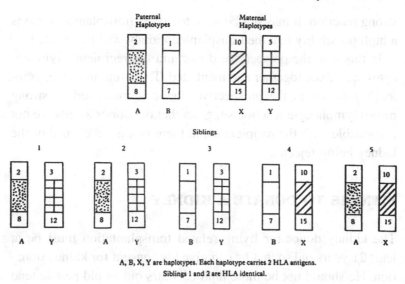

Fig. 32.1　Human Leukocyte Antigen (HLA) segregation within a family

AB is the universal acceptor. It can accept from 0, A, B, AB but can only give to AB.

A can receive from 0 or A and can give to A and AB. B can receive from 0 or B and can give to B and AB.

All this means that if the patient has 0 group he can only receive a kidney from an 0 donor. If he is A, he can receive from 0 and A. If he is B, he can receive from 0 and B. If he is AB he can receive from 0, A, B and AB.

But nowadays, with advances in transplant technology, we now perform living related transplant across blood groups. In other words, ABO blood group incompatible individuals can now be transplanted.

THE MIXED LYMPHOCYTE REACTION

This is a test to determine whether the recipient's lymphocytes will react very strongly to those of the donor's. If there is a very strong reaction, it may not be wise to do the transplant as there is a high possibility that the transplanted kidney will be rejected.

In this test, the prospective donor and the recipient's lymphocytes are mixed together and incubated. The strength of the recipient's reaction to the prospective donor is measured. A strong mixed lymphocyte reaction suggests that the donor's cells are not compatible with the recipient's and there is a good chance of the kidney being rejected.

FITNESS TO DONATE A KIDNEY

The kidney donor for living related transplantation must be at least 21 years old so that he can give his consent for kidney donation. He should not be more than 65 years old as old people tend to have very stiff and thick wall arteries (atherosclerosis). In kidney transplant the blood vessels of the donor's kidney has to be stitched to those of the recipient. If the blood vessels are atherosclerotic it makes the surgeon's job very difficult and dangerous as the vessels are more likely to tear during the operation. In addition, older people tend to have hypertension and kidneys that may be already slightly damaged by the process of ageing.

The donor must be healthy and have no illness or systemic disease like diabetes and hypertension that might already have caused damage to their kidneys. They must of course not have kidney disease themselves.

Is it safe for a parent or sibling to donate a kidney? Will it do any harm? What about people who do heavy work? Can young women marry and have children after giving away one kidney?

These are the questions that are often asked at the same time by several anxious relatives of the patient with kidney failure. A normal person has two kidneys but one kidney is sufficient to enable one to lead a normal life. The other kidney acts like a reserve. It is like a car with 4 spare tyres. If the 4 spare tyres are removed the car can still function normally. Or expressed another way, one can say that the two kidneys represent 200% kidney function. So, after donating a kidney the donor can still lead a normal life with no restriction whatsoever. He can continue to do heavy work. In the case of a woman she can still marry and have babies. However, should the donor meet with an accident and the remaining kidney is damaged he runs the risk of kidney failure, since his other kidney which acts as a reserve has been donated earlier.

Complications of Live Kidney Donation

Apart from the slight unavoidable risk which occurs in any major operation, the donor suffers no shortening of life or adverse effects on the quality of life. We have had living related renal donors from all walks of life and apart from mild hypertension in a few donors who were over 50 years which could well be unrelated to renal donation none of the donors have suffered any adverse effects as a result of their donation.

The donor would experience some pain over the operative wound which can be relieved by injections of pethidine. He has to stay in hospital for about a week and after that would be given medical leave to rest at home. He should be back at work within a month's time. Once a year he has to go for a renal check-up where the blood pressure, urine and blood are checked to make sure that the remaining kidney is well.

Social Pressure on a Relative to Donate Kidney

In Singapore, as we are short of cadaver donors and dialysis is expensive, the patient's relatives (parents, brothers and sisters) have to be approached by the doctors regarding volunteers for living related kidney donation in order to save the life of the patient. A lot of social pressure may be brought to bear upon the potential kidney donor, sometimes conflicting pressures.

A brother or sister may want to donate a kidney to another brother or sister but may face parental objection, especially if the parents tend to be elderly. On the other hand, a brother or sister may be pressurised to donate by the parents. Married people may face objections from in-laws. A sister may want to donate to a brother but her mother-in-law may object. Similarly a wife or husband may object to a spouse donating a kidney to a sibling. Even boy friends, girl friends and fiancees/fiances have been known to object.

In general married people face more social pressure in giving a kidney, particularly when they have dependent children. There is always the fear on the spouse's part that if something should happen to the donor the family may be left without a father (sole bread winner) or mother (home-maker). Family conflicts can result in marriages breaking up. Sometimes between parents and children, loyalties may be divided to provide for a single child who is sick while depriving the other offspring at home of a parent. Also parents would have to face up to the possibility that despite their sacrifice the kidney may not function usefully and all will have been in vain.

Finally, there may be conflict between siblings or even between parents as to who should give a kidney. Some may argue about the effect of donation on a career or the future of child bearing of an unmarried potential donor.

The stand of kidney doctors with regard to living related donor transplantation and what they tell potential donors

Kidney doctors always stress to the family that renal donation is voluntary and there should be no pressure on a particular individual to donate his or her kidney. Any social pressure from relatives on the potential donor is strongly discouraged. Potential donors are informed of the various tests they must pass in order to be considered suitable donors. The doctors cannot guarantee that the transplant will always be successful.

There will be a few transplanted kidneys that will not work. Donors would be told about transplant survival rate. It would also be explained to them that donating a kidney would mean loss of renal reserve.

Successful live donation would of course be gratifying to the donor. He or she would have given a new lease of life to a loved one. Apart from slight perioperative risks the donor should suffer no shortening of life or adverse effects on the quality of life.

Spouse to Spouse Renal Transplant

The Spouse to Spouse Transplant Programme was implemented more than 10 years ago. This allows one spouse to donate a kidney to the other. It is heartening and justifiable as married couples share an emotional bond though they are not blood relatives. With the advent of Cyclosporine A and the improved success rates of cadaver transplant on CyA, as long as there is ABO blood group compatibility, spouse to spouse transplant is justifiable and can be performed.

Assessment of Donor for Living Related Transplantation

The potential donor has to undergo a very thorough and vigorous investigation to make sure that both his kidneys are healthy. If there is the slightest doubt, his kidney will not be taken from him. He must be in good health and have no history of kidney disease, hypertension, diabetes mellitus, cancer or any other disease. He will be assessed psychologically and mentally to ensure that he fully comprehends the nature of the donation, that there are no social pressures on him to donate and that he is donating voluntarily out of love and consideration for the patient. He will undergo a thorough physical examination. The urine and blood tests performed on him must be normal. There must be no protein or blood in the urine. He must have no evidence of renal disease and have normal creatinine clearance.

The ABO blood group between the donor and the recipient must be compatible. The HLA tissue typing should have at least a 25% match. In addition a cross match is performed between the white blood cells (lymphocytes) of the donor and the serum of the recipient. If there are antibodies present in the recipient's serum against the donor's white cells the white cells would be killed by the antibodies. This means that the same antibodies would attack the transplant kidney if it were transplanted in the recipient. Therefore it would not be safe or wise for the donor to donate his kidney which is bound to be rejected by the recipient. All further transplant work-up tests for the particular donor would be discontinued once he is found unsuitable. Another volunteer or the next best volunteer based on the degree of matching of the tissue typing would have to come up for tests.

If the above tests are satisfactory the prospective donor then undergoes an arteriogram to visualise the blood vessels of his kidneys and also to look for any abnormality in the kidneys and to make a decision as to which kidney to remove for the transplant. If all the tests are satisfactory the donor is considered suitable for kidney donation and a date for the transplant operation will be scheduled.

Potential Cadaver Kidney Donors

Donors should not be patients suffering from cancer as cancer may have invaded the kidney and it could be carried over to the recipient with the kidney. The donor should not have infection too as it can be transmitted to the recipient. The cadaver donor should also not be more than 70 years of age. Most donors were patients who had sustained head injuries from road traffic or other accidents. Sometimes bleeding in the brain from various causes can also cause brain death, qualifying the person as a suitable cadaver donor.

The potential donor is therefore someone who has had an accident or damage to the brain with no possibility of recovery and is being maintained on a respirator to ventilate the lungs. It is important that the potential donor be placed on a respirator as it pumps oxygen into the donor's lungs and keeps the heart beating so that blood would flow to the kidneys to keep them functioning, though the donor's brain is already dead (brain dead).

Brain Death

When a person dies it means his brain has ceased to function. The medical term for this is brain death. The beating of the heart and respiration can be taken over by machines but it does not mean that the dead person is still alive. If the machines are turned off the heart and respiration will stop because the dead brain is incapable of supporting these functions.

By testing certain functions of the brain and noting their absence, doctors can pronounce that a person is dead. The criteria for brain death are:

- absence of spontaneous respiration
- fixed and dilated pupils
- no response to pain
- absence of corneal reflex
- absence of gag reflex
- absent doll's eye movement
- no response to the cold calorie test

When all the above criteria are fulfilled the patient can be pronounced brain dead. It means that the brain has been so severely damaged that it is not capable of sustaining life and there is no possibility of its recovery.

Note that the heart can still be beating in a person who is brain dead because the heart muscles can continue to beat for some time after brain death. For the purpose of kidney transplant it is important that the cadaver donor's heart is still beating as it means that blood is still circulating into the kidneys to keep them functioning and producing urine. If the heart has stopped beating for more than an hour, the kidneys which have been deprived of blood during this time would be irreparably damaged and of no use at all in kidney transplantation. This explains why kidneys for transplantation must be removed during the time the person is brain dead rather than wait till the time when the heart stops beating because they will be useless by then.

Kidney Transplant Legislation

In most countries most of the transplanted kidneys are from cadaver donors but in Asian countries most of our transplanted kidneys come from living-related donors. There is sadly a lack of cadaver donors because relatives have not been willing to give consent for kidney donation for various cultural and other reasons. These kidneys which are buried or cremated actually go to waste because they could be used to save many Singaporeans who die needlessly because they are unable to get cadaver kidney transplants. It is a tragedy as the majority are young, aged between 30 and 40. Many are married and are fathers or mothers of very young children. Many are also sole bread winners at the peak of their lives. The majority die due to a lack of cadaver kidneys.

The Medical Therapy, Education & Research Act (MTA) was passed in Parliament in 1972 to enable individuals to will their kidneys for transplantation in the event of death. This is called the Opting-in-law. But even though 28,401 individuals had pledged their kidneys, not a single kidney had become available for transplantation. The average number of kidney transplants averaged only about 5 a year.

The government studied this problem and came out with a solution. In 1986, 128 people died from road traffic accidents. To save 100 patients with kidney failure only 50 brain dead cadavers are required because each cadaver has 2 kidneys and a patient with kidney failure needs only one kidney to survive. A law called the Human Organ Transplant Act (Opting-out-law) or HOTA was passed on 16th July 1987 and implemented in January 1988. The Act allows for the removal of kidneys from Singaporeans and Permanent Residents who die from accidents for the purpose of transplant to kidney failure patients, unless they have specifically objected to this in their lifetime. In some countries like France, Austria, Israel and Belgium where this Act is practised, many patients who suffer from kidney failure have been saved. Since the implementation of HOTA, together with the MTA, the number of cadaveric renal transplants has increased. (see Table 32.1 and Table 32.2)

Key Changes under the Human Organ Transplant (Amendment) Act:

In 2004

1. Inclusion of deaths resulting from non-accidental causes
2. Inclusion of livers, hearts and corneas in cadaveric organ donations
3. Regulation of living donor organ transplants.

In 2008

1. Inclusion of Muslims
2. Provision of enforcement powers to give Ministry of Health [MOH] the authority to investigate offences under HOTA.

In 2009

1. Removal of the 60 year upper age limit on cadaveric organ donors.
2. Allowing donor-recipient paired matching. Put simply, this is a system whereby recipients who have medically incompatible donors exchange their donors so that each recipient receives a

Table 32.2   Number of Kidney Transplants Performed in Singapore

Year	Living Related Transplants	Cadaveric Transplants		Total Cadaveric	Total
		Medical Therapy Act	Human Organ Transplant Act		
1985	21	1	0	1	22
1986	18	20	0	20	38
1987	16	18	0	18	34
1988	8	7	16	23	31
1989	6	11	15	26	32
1990	16	21	24	45	61
1991	20	24	12	36	56
1992	24	37	23	60	84
1993	24	18	14	32	56
1994	18	68	16	84	102
1995	11	38	15	53	64
1996	17	28	16	44	61
1997	15	16	9	25	40
1998	26	32	10	42	68
1999	35	36	18	54	89
2000	30	34	10	44	74
2001	46	28	18	46	92
2002	44	24	6	30	74
2003	26	18	0	18	44
2004	53	14	18	32	85
2005	54	6	37	43	97
2006	61	8	48	56	117
2007	88	2	44	46	134
2008	83	8	38	46	129
2009	87	10	31	41	128

suitable organ. The exchange can be carried out across two or more donor-recipient pairs.

3. Reimbursement of living donors in accordance with international and local ethical practices.

4. Increased penalties for organ trading syndicates and middlemen.

Preparation of the Patient for Renal Transplant

Usually the patient who is to receive a transplant will be on regular dialysis having been registered among a long list of patients awaiting renal transplants. When there is a potential cadaver donor available, the donor's tissue typing will be performed and the two patients with the closest match with compatible ABO blood group will be called up urgently and prepared for the transplant. One cadaver has two kidneys which means that 2 patients can be transplanted at the same time. The patients are checked to ensure that they have been well dialysed and then prepared for the operation. In addition they are given injections of prednisolone and azathioprine. Cyclosporin A is not given preoperatively for cadaver transplants. It is started only after the transplant operation when the graft starts producing urine. In this way the nephrotoxic effects on the ischaemic graft which is still recovering from acute tubular necrosis is minimised.

The Transplant Operation

During the transplant operation, the cadaver kidney which has been earlier harvested and kept on ice is put into the pelvis of the patient with kidney failure (recipient), low down and to one side of the bladder. The blood vessels of the kidney are joined to the internal iliac artery and the common iliac vein of the recipient. The ureter of the donated kidney is then sewn onto the recipient's urinary bladder. The operation itself takes about one and a half to two hours (Fig. 32.2).

What Happens to the Patient (Recipient) After the Operation?

After the operation the patient is under intensive care. All the urine collected is measured and carefully charted to keep a record

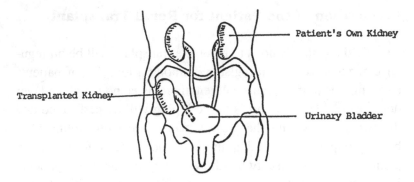

Fig. 32.2   Position of the transplanted kidney

of his progress. Usually cadaver transplants take a few days before they can make urine, sometimes up to two weeks. A few may not work at all. During this period the blood urea, creatinine and serum electrolytes are measured everyday. If there is poor urine production by the transplanted kidney the blood tests will still be abnormal and the patient will still continue to require dialysis 3 times a week until the kidney can put out a good amount of urine.

The patient will also receive daily anti-rejection medicine to prevent his body from rejecting the transplant. These drugs are prednisolone, azathioprine, cyclosporin A or mycophenolate mofetil. If the blood pressure is high he will have to continue taking blood pressure medicine to lower it.

A renal scan is performed the day after the transplant to check that the blood flow through the kidney is adequate and the kidney is well perfused with blood. If there is no blood flow to the kidney the transplant surgeons will have to explore the kidney. Usually the cause is due to a blood clot blocking the blood vessel of the kidney. After removing the clot the kidney will function again.

Even when the kidney is functioning, blood tests have to be performed to watch out for acute rejection which is usually diagnosed by a raised serum creatinine. A renal biopsy of the transplanted kidney may be performed to confirm a diagnosis of acute rejection. If rejection is diagnosed, the patient is given a 3-day course of methylprednisolone. This will usually reverse the rejection process.

Sometimes there may be problems like obstruction of the transplanted kidney or there may be leakage of urine from the ureter of the transplant kidney. An ultrasound examination of the transplanted kidney would have to be performed to determine the cause and site of the obstruction or urinary leakage and if necessary, the transplant surgeon will be called in to explore the kidney with a view to repairing the urine leak or remove the cause of obstruction.

The Donor Nephrectomy on a Live Donor

The kidney is removed from a live donor by means of an operation. The incision is made in the flank to expose the kidney. The blood vessels of the kidney are tied and cut. The kidney is then lifted out of the incision wound, flushed with cold solution and carried to the adjacent operation theatre where the recipient is waiting and then inserted into the recipient's body as for cadaver transplant described before.

The donor's operative wound is sutured and he returns to the ward. The donor should be out of bed after a couple of days and home within 2 weeks.

Immunosuppressive Drugs

During the transplant operation and after, for as long as the transplanted patient is alive, he will have to take his transplant medication faithfully in order to prevent the kidney from being rejected. The medication consists of prednisolone, azathioprine and cyclosporin A. Some patients may be given Tacrolimus [FK 506] instead of cyclosporine A. All these three main immunosuppressive drugs are equally effective. These drugs may predispose the patient to infection. The common sites of infection are in the urine, lungs, skin or bloodstream. The other problem is that there is a definite increase in the tendency to develop cancer in the long term; this risk however is very small.

The other side effects relate to **Prednisolone**, but nowadays, with a tendency to the use of much smaller doses of prednisolone these effects are much decreased. Patients who are on prednisolone develop an increase in the size of their cheeks (moon face). Their appetite increases and they gain weight and become obese. They may also develop high blood pressure, diabetes mellitus, ulcers in the stomach and a condition called avascular necrosis which causes pain in the hip bone, due to necrosis of the femoral head. The pain can be relieved by pain relievers but if it gets worse an operation can be performed to replace the hip with a metal one. In the old days with the use of high dose prednisolone therapy, Femoral Head Necrosis used to be quite common. But today, with the advent of CyA it has become less common, affecting less than 8% of patients in most centres. In fact, patients with SLE are the ones getting more of this form of complication due to steroid therapy.

Cyclosporin A is the most important drug used in preventing transplant rejection and though expensive it is being used in countries all over the world because of the tremendous boost it confers on long-term kidney transplant survival. Among some of its disadvantages, apart from prohibitive cost, are its toxicity to the kidney when too high a dose is given and risk of cancer developing in long-term users. Hence it is important to measure the levels of cyclosporin A in the blood stream so that the dose could be adjusted if the levels are too high in order to try to avoid the toxic effect of the drug. Other side effects of cyclosporin A are increased hair growth (hirsutism), swollen gums, tremors, inflammation of the liver (hepatitis), but the worst as mentioned earlier is nephrotoxicity or toxicity to the kidneys which can cause kidney damage. Hepatitis positive transplant patients should not be put on azathioprine as it is more hepatotoxic than cyclosporin A. They are only on dual therapy with cyclosporine A and prednisolone compared to all the other patients who are on triple therapy consisting cyclosporine A (6 mg/kg BW), azathioprine (1 mg/kg BW) and prednisolone (20–30 mg) daily. For patients who are on dual therapy, the dose of CyA is higher, 8 mg/kg BW.

Azathioprine [Imuran] (50 mg daily) is a purine analog that inhibits DNA and RNA synthesis and inhibits both T and B cell proliferation. Azathioprine is a purine synthesis inhibitor. Its main side effect is bone marrow suppression but given in a dose of 1 to 2 mg/Kg BW/day, it is usually well tolerated. We tend to use a lower dose of 1 mg/Kg Bw/day in Singapore with good results and less side effects. It has served many patients well for more than 3 decades. Remember that Azathioprine is inactivated by xanthine oxidase, the enzyme which is inhibited by allopurinol. Allopurinol is therefore contraindicated in patients with a kidney transplant with gout who are on azathioprine. If these patients are given allopurinol when on azathioprine they will develop severe bone marrow suppression which is life threatening.

Tacrolimus (FK 506) (0.25 mg/kg BW) and Mycophenolate Mofetil (MMF) (1 gm BD) and Sirolimus (Rapamycin) (2 mg OM) are the newer immunosuppressive agents which have been introduced over the past decade. Tacrolimus [FK506] even though its structure is distinct from Cyclosporin A [CyA] its mode of action, drug interaction, side effects including nephrotoxicity is similar to CyA. However its use is associated with lower rates of acute rejection compared to CyA. There are also less cosmetic problems, less hyperlipidemia and hypertension. Refractory acute rejection are also less and easier to treat. However, compared to CyA there are disadvantages in that there are more gastrointestinal side effects and neurotoxicity. There are also more patients developing diabetes mellitus while on it.

Mycophenolate Mofetil [MMF] is a reversible inhibitor of inosine monophosphate dehydrogenase, the rate limiting enzyme in de novo purine synthesis. It is a selective inhibitor of the pathway of de novo purine synthesis. T and B cells are dependent on the de novo pathway for synthesis of guanosine nucleotides, hence the antiproliferative effect on lymphocytes. **Many centres have now switched to MMF instead of using Azathioprine**. The side effects of MMF are nausea and vomiting which are dose related. MMF has been shown to have a 50% reduction in the incidence of acute rejection in the first year after transplantation [Davis C, Amer J Kidney Disease 2004, 43(3):508–530]. **However, It is teratogenic and patients contemplating pregnancy should convert to azathioprine**. Some consider the combination of MMF and Tacrolimus better in preventing acute rejection [Gonwa T *et al.*, Transplantation 2003, 75:2048–2053]. In our Dept, we have also switched over to MMF for all new transplant recipients. The trade off is a lower dose of CyA with less nephrotoxicity and better renoprotection in the way of lower acute rejection rates in the first year post transplant. However, this does not necessarily translate into longer term graft survival because **doctors are still using too high a dose of CyA, hence indirectly inducing CNI nephrotoxicity which constitutes a major cause of graft lost today**. This is **despite the use of so called 'Triple Therapy'** consisting of Prednisolone, CyA and MMF.

Sirolimus (Rapamycin) can also be used to treat refractory acute rejection. It may limit the development and progression of chronic rejection. (Saunders RN *et al.* Kidney Int 2001, 59:3–16). It blocks the proliferative responses of T and B cells, as well as other cell types of cytokines. It binds to the same intracellular protein [FK binding protein] or FKBP as for Tacrolimus, but its mechanism of action is distinct from Tacrolimus. It binds to and inhibits a kinase called the Target of Rapamycin [TOR]. It acts on receptors which control growth factors of the cell cycle. Unlike Cyclosporin [CyA] it is not a calcineurin inhibitor [CNI]. Its side effects are impairment of wound healing, diarrhoea, hyperlipidemia, anemia, thrombocytopenia and interstitial pneumonitis. Sirolimus is associated with a lower rate of acute rejection compared to

Azathioprine [Kahan BD, Lancet, 2000, 356:194–202]. It may have a role as a CNI sparing agent. Sirolimus also has antineoplastic effects.

Everolimus is a derivative of Sirolimus but it has a shorter half life. It is associated with a higher plasma creatinine in patients on steroids and CyA.

Novel Immunosuppressive Agents

We have had more than 40 years experience in the field of Renal Transplantation. Some 10 years ago when I analysed the transplant data of the Prednisolone/Azathioprine Era, I had noted that despite the use of CyA , the long term survival data of patients treated with CyA whether as part of Dual Immunosuppression Therapy using prednisolone and Azathioprine or as part of Triple Therapy, using Prednisolone/CyA/Azathioprine, the results of long term graft survival were no better than what we achieved in the old days using only Prednisolone and Azthioprine. For the small group of patients who cannot tolerate azathioprine on Prednisolone/Azathioprine after about 10 years or so, when they develop thrombocytopenia and necesscitate a change from Azathioprine to CyA , I have observed that these patients begin to lose their graft after a few years, and many after about 5 years or so had to return to life on dialysis again. Also, for those on Prednisolone/Azathioprine, even when they do develop chronic allograft failure after 15 to 20 years post transplant, their grafts can still last another 10 years or so before they reach a serum creatinine of about 400 to 500 micromol which signals the time to re-start dialysis.

I am not alone with this conviction. Whilst some patients may experience a reduction of acute rejection episodes in the first year post transplant, in the longer term this does not translate into longer term graft survival. In the USA, after a mean post transplant period of 7 years, many grafts start to fail. I believe that **many of these graft failures are the result of CNI**

nephrotoxicity induced by CyA and this believe is also held by others [Cooper JE and Wiseman AC. Clinical Nephrol 2010, 73(5):333–343].

We should therefore explore the possibilities of newer immunosuppressive agents with less CNI nephrotoxicity and which offer a promise for long term preservation of renal allograft function. Some of the newer drugs for the future which are now undergoing clinical trials may include:

Voclosporin

This is a semisynthetic structural analog of CyA. It causes immunosuppression by inhibition of the calcineurin signal transduction pathway. It is more robust binding to calcineurin and has faster elimination of metabolites. It has been found to be useful in treating plaque psoriasis. Now undergoing Phase III trials in human renal transplant recipients. [Gaber AO *et al*. Am J Transplant 2008, 8:336].

Sotrastaurin

Activation of T cell receptors plus costimulatory signalling via CD28 leads to protein kinase C activity. Sotrastaurin inhibits protein kinase C activity. Here again in patients with psoriasis, a two week course led to 69% reduction in severity. So far a phase II trial in human renal transplant rejection has not yet shown promise.

Belatacept

Costimulation (Signal 2) is a crucial step in the activation of T cells. T cells undergoing Signalling 1 without a signal 2 response will become unresponsive and undergo apoptosis. Belatacept inhibits signal 2 response, hence its immunosuppressive role. It has been shown to be useful in treating Rheumatoid arthritis. One of its safely concerns is the development of post transplant lymphoproliferative disorder [LPD]. Phase II trials are ongoing for renal transplant.

Everolimus

This is an inhibitor of cell proliferation derived from the naturally occurring immunosuppressant sirolimus. Everolimus blocks mTOR activity as described above, resulting in arrest of cell cycle at the G1 phase, hence inhibiting cell proliferation. Clinical trials are ongoing to explore everolimus based CNI free protocol for renal transplant.

Alefacept

This has been approved by FDA for use of psoriasis plaques. It has been found to reduce T cell infiltration of skin grafts in mice. In humans, apart from psoriasis, it has been shown to be effective in chronic refractory graft versus host disease [Shapira MY *et al.* Bone marrow transplant 2009, 43:339–343]. Phase II trials in renal transplant are ongoing.

Efaluzimab

This is a humanised anti-LFA-1 antibody specific for the CD11a subunit that blocks LFA-I/ICAM interactions and subsequently inhibits T cell activation in vitro. It has been used in cardiac allografts with increased graft survival compared to controls [Poston RS *et al.* Transplantation 2000, 69: 2005–2013]. Phase I/II trials in renal transplantation has been published [Vincente F *et al.* Amer J Transplantation, 2007, 7: 1770–1777].

REFERENCE

Cooper JE and Wiseman AC. Novel immunosuppressive agents in kidney transplantation. *Clin Nephrol* 2010, **73**(5): 333–343.

COMPLICATIONS OF KIDNEY TRANSPLANTATION

Early complications are acute rejection, urinary leaks, infections, stomach ulcers and wound infection. Late complications include chronic rejection, avascular necrosis of bone, transplant renal artery stenosis, cancer, infections and recurrent or de novo glomerulonephritis in the transplanted kidney which in some cases can again lead to kidney failure.

Transplant Rejection

Despite the routine use of cyclosporine A, azathioprine and steroids, the careful selection of donors and recipients and the fulfilment of all the prerequisites for successful grafting, rejection occurs and is the major cause of graft failure. In the first 6 months about 20% of cadaver kidneys are rejected as are 10% of related donor kidneys.

Acute rejection is usually diagnosed by a raised serum creatinine without other obvious cause such as obstruction, sepsis, or uncontrolled hypertension due to renal artery stenosis. Sometimes rejection is accompanied by a swollen graft with tenderness, fever and oliguria. A closed biopsy of the graft readily confirms the diagnosis of rejection.

A renogram is useful in assessing renal perfusion of the graft and is useful in diagnosing renal artery thrombosis as a cause of non-function. Ultrasound of the graft too is useful in excluding obstruction due to hydronephrosis causing renal deterioration.

The usual treatment of acute rejection is to give 0.5 gm I.V. boluses of methylprednisolone for 3 days. Antithymocyte or anti-lymphocyte globulin or OKT3 (monoclonal antibody) is used for severe acute rejection. These are expensive but nonetheless useful in severe acute rejection. Plasmapheresis, graft irradiation, and thoracic duct drainage have been used by other centres but none of these have gained an established place.

Chronic rejection occurs from about 3 to 6 months after transplant. It causes a slow deterioration of graft function and progresses often relentlessly to end stage graft failure over months to years. It is usually associated with proteinuria and hypertension. On biopsy the lesions are usually vascular as opposed to the cellular lesions in acute rejection. There is no treatment for chronic rejection.

Nowadays most centres are using a low dose steroid regimen, i.e. 30 mg/day prednisolone initially and reducing to 10 mg/day by the end of 3 months. This is in contrast to the old regimen that starts at 60 mg/day of prednisolone, reducing to 30 mg at 3 months post-graft, and to 10 mg/day at 6 months. Patients on low dose steroids have less morbidity and less avascular necrosis and the long-term graft survival is just as good.

Monoclonal anti-T cell antibody: The use of monoclonal antibody to T cell subsets has been reported to assist the early diagnosis and prediction of rejection. They have also been used to treat acute rejection. But their usefulness may be limited by antibody formation to the monoclonal antibody apart from cost and availability. It should be reserved for patients with severe acute rejection which has not responded to pulse therapy with methylprednisolone.

Anti-Thymocyte Globulin (ATG) is another useful agent for treatment of severe acute rejection.

Urinary Tract Infection

UTI is the commonest infection occurring in the transplant patient. This is because of urinary catheters introduced into the urinary bladder in the initial 1 to 2 weeks following the transplant to prevent over distension of the bladder and leakage of urine at the site where the donor ureter is tunnelled into the bladder. The insertion of stents in some patients may also contribute to infection. This includes aggressive immunosuppression which make the patient more prone to infection. The incidence of UTI is nowadays less as many patients are put on prophylactic bactrium or septrin [half tab nightly] against pneumocystis carrinni which causes a life threatening pneumonia in the transplant patient. The use of septrin or bactrium also serves as prophylaxis for UTI. Fever, pain and tenderness over the transplant kidney [graft] with leukocytosis and pyuria usually indicate pyelonephritis. Sometimes acute graft rejection can also cause pain and tenderness with a low grade fever but the pain and tenderness in rejection is milder with rejection. The diagnosis is based on urine culture and empiric antibiotic therapy should be commenced. The renal function [serum creatinine] may rise with UTI but decreases with response to antibiotic therapy. Recurrent UTI may indicate an underlying abnormality and an intravenous pyelogram plus a micturiting cystogram may be required to exclude transplant vesico-ureteric reflux. An ultrasound of the kidneys may also show urinary obstruction due to ureteric stenosis which can cause UTI. A urinoma or lymphocele can also cause urinary obstruction with UTI.

Urine Leaks

Urine leaks usually occur during the first few weeks of the transplant and could be anywhere from the renal calyx, the ureter and the urinary bladder. Often it is due to infarction of the ureter due to disruption of its blood supply. Another source of leakage is at the vesicoureteric junction between the bladder and the ureteric implantation. Other causes include obstruction from any source causing leakage of urine. Patients would present with pain with abdominal swelling associated with raised serum creatinine. Ultrasound examination may reveal a urinoma or collection of urine. Renal scintigraphy may show extravasation of the tracer from the urinary system and help localise the site of the leakage. An antegrade pyelogram will also render a precise diagnosis and localisation of the leak. Surgical exploration is warranted as soon as possible to solve the problem and repair the leakage.

Obstruction of the Urinary Tract

Urinary obstruction would cause pain over the transplanted kidney with little or no urine output associated with raised serum creatinine. An ultrasound examination demonstrate hydronephrosis and reveal the source of the obstruction, often due to a collection of lymph or lymphocele or urinoma.

A lymphocele should be drained and marsupialised. Other causes of obstruction include a sloughed ureter due to ischemia and fibrosis or rejection. Occasionally an intraluminal clot may cause ureteric obstruction. In an elderly male patient, an enlarged prostate gland due to prostatomegaly should be excluded as a cause of obstruction. Obstruction can cause leakage of urine and as hydronephrosis progresses, renal function will worsen. An antegrade pyelogram will demonstrate the source and site of obstruction and in the same setting the radiologist can also perform balloon angioplasty for a fibrosed ureter or a stent inserted to bypass the blockage. Complicated cases will need surgical intervention. An enlarged prostate can be managed with bladder catheterisation and the use of medication like α adrenergic blockers.

Transplant Renal Artery Stenosis

This may present as difficult to control hypertension which may be severe and often associated with raised serum creatinine. An

MR angiography or duplex sonography can diagnose transplant renal artery stenosis quite readily though the standard technique is the use of a renal ateriogram which will show the site of the stenosis. The commonest site of a transplant renal artery stenosis is at the site of anastomosis of the donor renal artery with the recipient artery [internal iliac or other artery]. Mild cases can be treated by controlling hypertension and giving aspirin. A blockage of the arterial lumen by 70% or more constitutes functionally significant stenosis and mandates intervention. A percutaneous transluminal renal angioplasty [PTRA] can be performed sometimes at the sitting following the renal arteriogram if the patient has been prepared for the procedure. Difficult cases may not be amenable to PTRA and surgery may be required to fashion a new anastomosis after resecting the stenotic portion. Other site of stenosis are pre or post anastomotic. Cases where there are stenoses which are intrarenal may be related to transplant rejection and not amenable to angioplasty or surgery. Anti rejection therapy may help in some cases.

Infections

UTI is the commonest form of infection due to catheterisation of the bladder. This has been discussed above. Respiratory tract infection is the next commonest, both upper and lower respiratory tract infections are common like influenzae, including H1 N1 influenza. A renal transplant patient should therefore be immunised against influenza including H1N1 infuenza. They are also more susceptible to Pseudomonas Pneumonia and Erythromycin should be avoided in these patients as Eyrthromycin interferes with the liver enzyme Cytochrome P450 which metabolises CyA causing CyA levels to increase resulting in CyA toxicity to the kidney. Legionaires disease is also more common in the transplant patient causing pneumonia. Patients are prone to viral, bacterial and fungal infections because of immunosuppression. Infections can be grouped into the post transplant period from 0 to 1 month, 1 to 6 months and more than 6 months.

In the first month, patients may have surgical wound infection, UTI and respiratory tract infection. From 1 to 6 months, Cytomegaloviral infection, Pneumocystitis carinni pneumonia [PCP] and fungal infections are common. After 6 months they are still prone to the above infections including the usual viral and other bacterial infection common in the general population, except that these occur more often in the renal transplant patient as he or she is on immunosuppression which affects his ability to mount the usual immune response against viral, bacterial, fungal and other infection, unlike a healthy person who succumbs less readily. Fungal infection common in the transplant patient includes candida infection presenting as oral thrush or moniliasis appearing as white patches in the throat with severe pain on swallowing indicating oesophagitis. In the female patient it may cause vaginitis with itch and vaginal discharge sometimes with urethritis requiring fungal vaginal pessaries.

If a transplant patient complaints of headache, one should always be alert to the possibility of Cryptococcal or Torula Meningitis. The patient should be admitted and have a CT scan of the brain followed by a lumbar puncture. An early diagnosis would result in a cure. Otherwise the disease will prove deadly. In a patient who has diarrhoea, always send off fecal cultures for Salmonella typhi which is common in the immunosuppressed patient.

The transplant patient may also have herpes zoster infection or shingles which causes very painful vesicular eruptions along the dermatome representing the particular nerve root infected. The patient will require therapy with acyclovir and depending on the severity some patients may require intravenous gancyclovir. Remember to reduce the dose of gancyclovir given, otherwise the standard dose may cause ganciclovir neurotoxicity causing confusion and even coma in some patients.

Cytomegalovirus [CMV] Infection

Exposure to CMV varies with age and in practice one may find that about two thirds of adult renal transplant adult donors and recipients are already infected with CMV even before the renal transplant operation. Infection is evidenced by the presence of CMV antibodies [CMV IgG]. A renal transplant patient is deemed to have CMV infection post transplant if there is a rise in CMV IgG titres after transplant or if CMV is demonstrated in body fluids or tissue.

This infection may arise from 3 possibilities [1] reactivation of latent recipient virus, [2] primary infection passed by the donor allograft or blood products, or [3] reactivation of latent donor derived virus. A patient is said to have CMV disease when he has symptoms of CMV infection or there is presence of CMV tissue invasion or both. Risk of CMV infection is highest in CMV positive donor/CMV negative recipient pairings, followed by CMV positive donor/CMV positive recipient pairings and lower with CMV negative donor/CMV positive recipient pairings. Risk is lowest with CMV negative donor/CMV negative recipient pairing. Patients treated with OKT3 polyclonal antibody for rejection are more likely to develop CMV infection subsequently.

CMV infection occurs within the first 6 months of renal transplant. Patients present with fever and general malaise with myalgia and leukopenia. There may be respiratory, gastrointestinal and hepatic features as evidenced by pneumonia, oesopahgitis, gastritis and colitis. Retinal involvement would cause blurring of vision and flashes and floaters. Detection of CMV should be pursued in blood and body fluids, including procedures like bronchoscopy and endoscopy. One should look for CMV antigenemia and tissue diagnosis with immunohistochemistry. Treatment consists of reduction of immunosuppression together with antiviral therapy with intravenous ganciclovir and the newer valganciclovir. CMV can be prevented by giving CMV prophylaxis to all patients who are at risk, like when both donor or recipient are positive. Alternatively one can monitor the recipient and treat only when there is evidence of active viral replication. Valganciclovir is often preferable for prophylaxis.

Pneumocystitis Carinni Infection

Patients with Pneumocystitis carinni pneumonia [PCP] presents with fever, cough and severe breathlessness. The chest Xray will show bilateral widespread interstitial alveolar infiltrates, often to the extent where both lungs appear wiped out with these changes. Referal to a chest physician is urgent as the patient will require a bronchoscopy with bronchial alveolar lavage so that the diagnosis can be confirmed and the patient started on SMX-TMP [bactrium or septrin]. SMX-TMP is the treatment of choice. Nowadays, renal transplant patients are routinely offered prophylaxis against PCP using half a tablet [480 mg] of SMX-TMP and this practice has helped prevent many patients form PCP infection.

Human Polyomavirus Infection

The polyomaviruses are DNA viruses, of which the BK virus, JC virus and SV40 virus are the better known ones. Many healthy adults have serologic evidence of past subclinical exposure. Over the past decade or so, BK virus has been recognised as one of the important causes of renal allograft infection and loss. This may be related to the use of more potent immunosuppressants like MMF and tacrolimus. Replication of the BK virus with shedding of infected uroepithelial cells (decoy cells) into the urine occurs in about one third of renal transplant recipients. The clinical features associated with such replication are acute and chronic allograft dysfunction with haemorrhagic cystitis. The renal dysfunction is due to interstitial nephritis. A kidney biopsy is necessary in order to make a diagnosis. The presence of intranuclear tubule cell inclusion by light microscopy is suspicious and is confirmed by immunohistochemistry. Treatment consists of major reduction of immunosuppressants. Other therapies include low dose cidofovir, IgG and the use of fluroquinolones. Most transplant centres now screen for subclinical infection so that dose reduction of immuno-suppressants may prevent severe nephritis. Patients who are positive should have dose reduction of immunosuppressants and a renal biopsy.

Cancer

Patients with renal allografts have decreased tumour surveillance mechanisms and are therefore more prone to developing cancers compared to the general population. Hence transplant patients should not have excessive immunosuppressant drugs. The more the drugs and the bigger the doses, the higher the chances of cancer developing. Patients who are on CNI like cyclosporine A are more prone to developing cancer of the skin, though often not fatal. Once a patient with a kidney transplant develops cancer, the dose of immunosuppressant should be reduced to the minimal dose. For the transplant patient there should be heightened alertness to the possibility of cancer occurring. Patients should have routine and regular breast examination, mammogram, cervical smear and colonoscopy.

They should eat less meat and not smoke.

1. Skin cancers are among the commonest cancers. Fortunately for our patients in Singapore, the incidence of skin cancer is low compared to other countries where it is much higher. It may be due to the generally smaller dose of immunosuppressants used by local doctors and also, unlike Australians, perhaps Singaporeans do not go for sunbathing as often as the Australians. After 30 years of transplant, about 70% of Australian transplant patients will have developed skin cancer. The forms of skin cancers are squamous cell carcinoma, basal cell carcinoma and melanomas. Patients are counselled about too much exposure to the sun and they should wear protective clothing and apply sunblocking creams. Retinoid creams may be useful and any suspicious skin lesion should be removed.

2. Anogenital cancers are also common in the transplant patients, including cancer of the cervix, vulva, uterus, scrotum, penis, anus and the perianal region. Such cancers tend to be multifocal and those with certain human papillomavirus are more prone. Patients and physicians should check regularly for suspicious looking lesions and have them removed.

3. Kaposi's sarcoma may also occur more commonly in transplant patients, apart from those patients who have HIV disease. It is more common amongst Arabs, Jews and those of Mediterranean origins. Patients who have human herpes virus B infection are also more prone. Visceral forms occur in the lungs, GI tract and lymph nodes and the non visceral forms occur in the skin, conjunctiva and the oropharyngx. Treatment consists of surgical excision, radiotherapy and chemotherapy.

4. Post Transplant Lymphoproliferative Disorder [PTLD]. The incidence is 1% to 2% in the transplant population. Hodgekin's lymphoma occur in 90% and most are of recipient B cell origin. Risk factors for development of lymphomas are 1. Epstein-Barr virus [EBV]–positive donor and EBV- negative recipient 2. CMV-positive donor and CMV-negative recipient and 3. Aggressive immunosuppression. Gastrointestinal and Central Nervous System as well as extranodal involvement is more common in the transplant population compared to the general non transplant lymphomas. Rituximab is being increasingly used as it has been reported to yield good results.

Recurrence of Glomerulonephritis

1. Sometimes, the original kidney disease may recur. We do not have the actual incidence as many patients do not have renal biopsies performed and present to us as Chronic GN. In about 7% of patients presenting with ESRF the cause of renal failure is also unknown.

2. Since IgA nephritis is a very common GN occurring in Singapore, many recurrences would be expected from IgA nephritis. The histologic recurrence of this disease is about 35%, very common compared to other GN. But fortunately, the recurrent disease is mild and patients generally do not lose the graft.

3. Lupus nephritis as a recurrent disease is uncommon, either systemically or as a GN because the disease as well as the GN is often burnt out by the time of transplantation and nephrologists generally wait for about 1 year after the disease is quiescent before embarking on a kidney transplant to reduce the risk of recurrence.

4. Membranous Glomerulonephritis does recur in about 30% or it can arise as a de novo GN. These patients present as proteinuria or as nephrotic syndrome. Other causes of membranous GN like Hepatitis B and C infection have to be excluded. If the patient has active hepatitis they should be treated with lamivudine for Hepatitis B and interferon for hepatitis C. If hepatitis is not related to the recurrence of Membranous GN, one is faced with the choice of increasing immunosuppression. In cases with biochemical or asymptomatic nephrotic syndrome they should not be treated and for those with full blown symptoms one has to consider various factors and in most cases one should opt for non immunosuppressive therapy like ARB and Aliskiren with diuretics and statins.

5. Focal Segmental Glomerulosclerosis (FSGS) has a high recurrence rate in first renal allograft, at least around 30%, even higher in subsequent allografts. The frequent recurrence of this disease is caused by a circulating factor secreted by an abnormal clone of T cells causing podocyte injury. This is thought to be a circulating factor bound to protein A with molecular weight of 50 kDalton. The permeability factor induces redistribution and loss of nephrin as well as reduced expression of podocin giving rise to massive proteinuria. The risk of recurrence is similar for both the classic FSGS as well

as the collapsing variant, but the collapsing variant is associated with more severe vascular abnormalities, higher serum creatinine and higher degree of graft failure. Treatment consists of high dose CyA therapy together with ACEI or ARB. Use of anti tumour necrosis factor alpha agents (infliximab and etanercept) has been reported with success. Intensive plasmapheresis for 14 days with high dose CyA and high dose steroids with continuing P/P for up to 9 months have resulted in complete remission in 9 out of 10 patients with recurrent FSGS (mean proteinuria 0.19 g/day at 12 months). Another patient who lost 2 previous grafts became P/P dependent remained in partial remission at 12 months [Canaud G *et al.*, Intensive and prolonged treatment of FSGS recurrence in adult kidney transplant recipients; a pilot study. Amer J Transplant 2009, 9:1081–1086].

Preemptive P/P or immunoadsorption may help in preventing recurrence. Post transplant increase in proteinuria heralds recurrence. If proteinuria >2 g/day, P/P is indicated. Additional support with ACEI/ARB and statins. Rituximab may be worth attempting.

Reference: Ponticelli C. Recurrence of focal segmental Glomerular sclerosis (FSGS) after renal transplantation. Nephrol Dial Transplant 2010, 25:25–31.

6. Wegener's Granulomatosis, an ANCA associated small vessel vasculitis has about 10% recurrence rate. This is despite CyA immunosuppression for kidney transplant. Like lupus nephritis, patients should wait at least a year after disease is quiescent before transplantation. Recurrent WG responds well to cyclophosphamide just like the original disease.

ADVANTAGES OF TRANSPLANTATION

The quality of life is much better for the patient who has been transplanted as opposed to one on regular haemodialysis. There is greater mobility as he is no longer tied to a kidney machine three times a week. The spouse or partner assisting him on dialysis is also freed of the burden of dialysis. Dialysis only rids the patients of waste products of protein metabolism but it does nothing in terms of the hormonal role of the kidney like producing 1,25-dihydroxycholecalciferol, erythropoietin, and prostaglandins which the transplanted kidney would be capable of doing. The family and working life of the patient is also less disrupted with a transplant compared to the long hours spent on haemodialysis. The patient is also freed from paying for the machine as well as the monthly maintenance.

The only medication required by the patient are prednisolone, azathioprine and cyclosporin A or mycophenolate mofetil or FK 506 in the case of some patients. It is imperative that he remembers to take his medication faithfully, as the omission can cause a prompt rejection of the grafted kidney. Some patients after transplantation may also have to continue taking medication for the control of hypertension. Surely these are minor inconveniences for someone who has been given a new lease of life. An additional bonus is that most men will regain their potency after successful transplantation and women will become fertile and can bear children.

Living Kidney Donor Transplant

The number of living donor transplants has grown vastly over the past decade with 62% of countries worldwide reporting an increase of 50%. The greatest numbers on a yearly basis was highest in the USA [6435], Brazil [1768], Iran [1615], Mexico [1459] and Japan [939]. Saudi Arabia has the highest reported living kidney donor transplant rate at 32 procedures per million population (pmp), followed by Jordan (29), Iceland (26), Iran (23) and the USA (21). Rates of living donor transplant have increased all over the world. There is a need to put in place safety and ethical considerations [Lucy Diane Horvat *et al.*, Global trends in the rates of living related donation. Kidney Int 2009, 75(100):1088–1098]. In addition, larger transplant centres with long waiting times are increasingly likely to see patients returning with newly transplanted kidneys from overseas. These patients need urgent attention especially with regards to infectious complications [Cohen DJ. Transplant Tourism; A growing phenomenon. Kidney Int 2009, 5:128–129].

The Unsolved Cyclosporine Induced Kidney Injury: Is Paricalcitriol a Feasible New Renoprotective Option?

Flavio NF Reis. Kidney Int 2010, 77:1055–1057.

One of the main concerns in kidney transplantation today is nephrotoxicity of the immunosuppressive agents resulting in loss of graft function. Chronic allograft nephropathy is an independent risk factor for graft loss and mortality. Sirolimus (SRL) an inhibitor of mTOR is a new option but the cardiorenal side effects of SRL plus other SE like lipid abnormalities and thrombocytopenia as well as nephrotoxicity and proteinuria and lack of long term validation in large cohorts doses not inspire or instill confidence [Rangan GK. SRL associated proteinuria and renal dysfunction. Drug Safety 2006, 29:1153–1161]. CyA has been long and well tested and has been used as an anchor immunosuppressant in renal transplant for decades. However, its intrinsic nephrotoxicity (CNI toxicity) proves a great disadvantage. CyA directly upregulates TGF $\beta1$ expression in tubular epithelial cells Recently, Park [Park JW *et al.*, Paricalcitriol attenuates CyA induced kidney injury in rats. Kidney Int 2010, 77:1076–1085] *et al.* has proposed that the renoprotective activity of paricalcitriol was due to inhibition of nuclear factor kappa B and nitric oxide signalling and that this anti inflammatory action causes a reduction of TGF $\beta1$ expression and the restoration of renal tubular cell damage. The efficacy of paricalcitriol in the prevention and attenuation of CyA induced nephrotoxicity needs to be confirmed by more research and then tested in randomised prospective clinical trials.

REFERENCES

1. Cooper JE, Wiseman AC. Novel immunosuppressive agents in kidney transplantation. *Clin Nephrol.* 2010, **73**(5):333–343.
2. Lucy Diane Horvat *et al.* Global trends in the rates of living related donation. *Kidney Int.* 2009, **75**(100):1088–1098.
3. Hirsh HH *et al.* BK Virus in solid organ transplant recipients. *Amer J of Transplantation.* 2009, S41:S136–S146.
4. Kotton CN *et al.* International consensus guidelines on the management of cytomegalovirus in solid organ transplantation. *Transplanation.* 2010, **89**:779–795.
5. Ponticelli C. Recurrence of focal segmental Glomerular sclerosis (FSGS) after renal transplantation. *Nephrol Dial Transplant.* 2010, **25**:25–31.
6. Sayegh M. Looking into the crystal ball: Kidney transplantation in 2025. *Nature Clinical Practice Nephrology.* 2009, **5**:117
7. Cohen DJ. Transplant Tourism; A growing phenomenon. *Kidney Int.* 2009, **5**:128–129.
8. No authors listed. The declaration of Istanbul on organ trafficking and transplant tourism. *Nephrol Dial Transplant.* 2008, **23**:3375–3380.
9. Rudge CJ. Organ Donation in the United Kingdom. Editorial. *Kidney Int.* 2006, **70**:2945–2046.
10. Flavio NF Reis. The unsolved cyclosporine induced kidney injury: Is paricalcitriol a feasible new renoprotective option? *Kidney Int.* 2010, **77**:1055–1057.

CHAPTER 33

The Aging Kidneys

The aging kidneys like all other organs in the human body, whether it is the heart, brain or the bones and joints would with time deteriorate as the whole human body undergoes the process of wear and tear and senescence or what is referred to as old age. There is a proportionate decrease in the structure, form and function of the kidneys consistent with the rest of the other organs. By age 70 there could be a loss of 30% to 50%. About one third of the adult population over the age of 60 years would have eGFR less than 60 ml/min or they would be classified as Chronic Kidney Disease or CKD Stage 3.

The kidneys themselves would have decreased in weight, size and volume from the fifth decade onwards, for example, from 250 gm to 200 gm or less from a young adult to a 70 year old man. Up to 10% of glomeruli would become globally sclerotic in normal subjects younger than 40 years. The aging kidney also has mesangial matrix expansion and thickening of the GBM. With some glomeruli already sclerosed as part of the aging process, the surviving nephrons would be subject to Glomerular Hyperperfusion or Hyperfiltration giving rise to proteinuria, further glomerulosclerosis and tubulointerstitial atrophy.

As the larger blood vessels throughout the body age and harden due to arteriolosclerosis with rise in systolic BP causing systolic hypertension, this adds to further compromising whatever renal structure and function remains contributing to a steady decrease in GFR. The generalised arteriosclerosis also affects the renal blood vessels including the smaller intrarenal vasculature which leads to ischemic wrinkling and narrowing of the afferent and efferent arterioles of the glomeruli. All these lead to progressive glomerular sclerosis and tubulointerstitial fibrosis with concommittant loss of renal function.

Parri pasu with the antecedent injury and loss of glomeruli and tubular structure and function related to the ongoing aging process, as a result of ischemia and inflammation, various other inflammatory mediators including cytokines and growth factors contribute to further injury. There is activation of the Renin Angiotensin System with release of vasoconstrictive peptides. Noxious cytokines like transforming growth factor and platelet derived growth factors, nitric oxide depletion and advanced glycosylation end products [AGE] would cause further ongoing injury. Nitric Oxide [NO] helps to decrease fibrosis but in the aging kidneys, oxidative stress induces NADPH oxidase –mediated NO scavenging and NO depletion which in turn leads to further ischemia of the renal tubulointerstitium. AGE and RAGE [AGE–receptor] deposition in the kidneys also lead to increased mesangial matrix production and basement membrane thickening together with increased vascular permeability and induction of TGFβ and PDGF injury.

In the aging kidneys there is also presence of excess or increased levels of reactive oxygen species [ROS] which is associated with lipid oxidative injury. Also excess cholesterol deposition in the aging kidneys may further contribute to increasing glomerulosclerosis and tubulointerstitial injury with proteinuria. Hence tissue injury in aging can be attributed to free radical production and antioxidant enzyme deficiency with subsequent lipid peroxidation and oxidative stress. It has been shown that the ARB losartan can prevent renal injuries in aged spontaneously hypertensive rats by enhancing NO bioavailability and ameleriorating oxidative stress [Zhou XJ *et al.*, Kidney Int 2002, 17:1096–1098].

ACUTE GLOMERULONEPHRITIS

Acute Glomerulonephritis in the elderly commonly present as Rapidly Progressive Glomerulonephritis [RPGN] with more than

50% crescents on renal biopsy. The immune histology can be: Type 1 due to anti GBM antibodies, Type 2 due to granular immune deposits and Type 3 with no immune deposits seen but circulating anti-neutrophilic cytoplasmic antibodies (ANCA) may be present. Type 2 and 3 are more common among the elderly. Some studies have suggested that pauci immune crescentic GN is more common presenting as RPGN with acute renal failure among patients over 60 years old. The use of pulse methylprednisolone, plasmapheresis and cyclophosphamide must be carefully considered because of the side effects which could be lethal among the elderly [Bergesio F *et al.*, Contrib Nephrol 1993, 105: 75–80]. Post Infectious or Post Streptococcal GN occur in about 22.6% among those age over 55 years. The prognosis is good without resorting to immunosuppressants.

CHRONIC GLOMERULONEPHRITIS

Among the elderly who present with nephrotic syndrome, the commonest form of GN is Idiopathic Membranous GN followed by Minimal Change GN. Cyclosporine A therapy is safer than prednisolone in this age group. One must always exclude the possibility of an underlying malignancy which occurs in about 20% of these cases [Moorthy AV *et al.*, Clin Nephrol 1980, 14:223–229]. Other causes of nephrotic syndrome are amyloidosis and multiple myeloma and for this group, a bone marrow stem cell transplant is usually curative.

RENAL FUNCTION AND THE PATHOPHYSIOLOGY OF THE AGING KIDNEYS

Although the mean decline in Creatinine Clearance [CrCl] was taken as 0.75 ml/min/year from age 30 years, 36% of the subjects did not have a decrease in CrCl and a few subjects actually showed an increase. Clearly this is multifactorial. The true GFR measured by inulin clearance in healthy elderly subjects, although lower than the young, remains within the normal range and is underestimated by the CrCl and even more so by the Cockroft Gault [CG] equation [Levy AS *et al.*, Ann Intern Med, 1999, 130:461–470]. The MDRD formula for calculating GFR yielded higher estimates for GFR than the CG equation among the elderly. This is important when calculating drug dosage as overdosage could result using the MDRD equation. Hence we should use the CG equation for estimating GFR for drug dosage for the elderly [Zhou ZJ *et al.*, Kidney Int 2008, 74(6):710–720].

Aging causes a reduction in urinary sodium excretion in response to dietary sodium chloride deprivation. Hence the elderly are more susceptible to volume depletion. The elderly have impaired lithium clearance which is an indicator of proximal tubular function. They cannot handle a potassium load and are prone to hyperkalaemia. This is due to impaired potassium secretion due to tubular atrophy.

Hyponatremia is a common geriatric problem. Enhanced osmotic AVP release and impaired diluting capacity predisposes the elderly to a higher incidence of hyponatremia. The idiopathic form of syndrome of ADH secretion can be readily found in many clinics where there are elderly patients. Thiazide used in the elderly further impairs an already present dilution defect and is implicated in about 30% of these cases of hyponatremia. Decreased prostaglandin synthesis in the elderly also impairs water diuresis and causes hyponatremia. Drugs like NSAIDS, tolbutamide, chlorpropamide also potentiate AVP action and decrease water excretion. Drugs causing a nonosmotic release of AVP like nicotine, histamine, morphine, epinephrine, angiotensin, bradykinin, cyclophosphamide can worsen or exacerbate hyponatremia. Prompt action is required with identification and removal of the offending drugs.

Hypernatremia is also common in the elderly due to impaired renal concentration and sodium conserving ability. Usually thirst followed by water intake would be adequate to protect against hypernatremia and free water loss. However, the thirst mechanism may be blunted in the elderly due to clouded sensorium, sedatives, immobility or disability. Use of high protein or high glucose feeds or laxatives must be monitored to ensure the elderly patient is not dehydrated and has access to water. Medications that cloud the sensorium like sedatives and tranquilisers can inhibit thirst and those that inhibit AVP action on the renal tubules like lithium and demeclocycline should be avoided.

With decreasing renal function there is **decreased erythropoietin production** and they are prone to anemia. Similarly they lack Vit D due to a diminished conversion of 25hydroxyvitamin D to 1,25 dihydroxyvitamin D by the aging kidney. A CrCl of less than 65 ml/min is associated with falls and fractures in the elderly. Calcitriol therapy can reduce the number of falls by 50% due to increase in 1,25 dihydroxyvitamin D. It induces an upregulation of vitamin D receptors in the muscle and contributes to an improvement of muscle strength [Gallagher JC *et al.*, J Ster Biochem Mol Biol 2007, 103:610–613].

Insulin secretion is also impaired in the elderly due to decreased β cell secretory reserve. So even though the total body insulin clearance is lower in the elderly than in younger patients, the geriatric population is still at a higher risk of glucose intolerance.

Arterial stiffening of blood vessels in the elderly predisposes to systolic hypertension which also contributes to declining renal function.

Caloric restriction has been shown to achieve a longer life span in rats [McCay CM *et al.*, Nutrition 1989, 5:155–171]. Long term caloric restriction slows the aging related decline in physiological processes and slows the development of age related diseases. Caloric restriction over a few years have produced reduction in body weight, BP, blood sugar, blood cholesterol as well as reduce the development of atherosclerosis and ameliorated the decline in diastolic function [Fontana L *et al.*, Proc Natl Acad Science USA, 2004, 101:6659–6662].

AGING AND END STAGE RENAL FAILURE
AND KIDNEY TRANSPLANTATION

About 6.6 million elderly people have Stage 3 CKD with eGFR < 60 ml/min [[K/DOQI clinical practice guidelines for chronic kidney disease. Am J Kidney Dis 2002, 39:S1–S266]. This is due to diabetes mellitus, hypertension, chronic GN, renovascular disease and obstructive uropathy. Both modalities of dialysis, hemodialysis and peritoneal dialysis are equally viable in the elderly. One advantage of PD is the preservation of residual renal function which is soon lost during HD due to intermittent drop in BP during HD. Residual GFR contributes to less morbidity and mortality for the PD patient compared to HD. PD also allows a more liberal diet in terms of fluid, vegetable and fruit [Potassium] intake.

Among the 300,000 and more patients on dialysis in the USA, the prevalence rates are highest for those in the 7th and 8th decade of life. The question asked is whether an elderly patient with comorbidities and an average life expectancy of 10 to 15 years should be given a kidney over a younger patient. The fact is, the relative risk of renal allograft failure, adjusted for comorbidities, is statistically similar for renal transplant recipients older than 65 years and their younger counterparts. Many of them die with the grafts intact and functioning and the death is related to the comorbidities. So if we could screen these elderly patients carefully for comorbidities like cancer, cardiovascular diseases, diabetes mellitus, chronic obstructive airway disease we should be able to minimise early post transplant morbidity and mortality. The "**expanded criteria donor**" kidneys allow for the use of **donors over the age of 60 years** or donors over the age of 50 years with two comorbidities including hypertension, death from cerebrovascular accidents or terminal serum creatinine levels greater than 1.5 mg/dl or 135 micro mol/l.

In the USA there are two renal transplant lists. One for standard criteria and the other for expanded criteria donors with the latter list recommended for older patients, patients with diabetes as the primary cause for renal failure and patients with difficult vascular access. In Europe, a comparable Eurotransplant Senior Program allows for local allocation of kidneys from donors over 65 years of age to recipients over the age of 65 ["old for old" kidney allocation] [Ruggenenti P *et al.*, Am J Transplant 2006, 6: 2543–2547].

PATHOGENESIS OF AGING

Women tend to outlive men simply because they age better and this is related to the female hormone. Much of the age related renal damage in males is related to androgen. **Castration can limit age related changes** and therapy with estrogen related products can protect the males against age related changes [Maric C *et al.*, J Amer Soc Nephrol 2004, 15:1546–1556]. The problem of aging is receiving immense attention and is considered one of the priority areas for research in many well known centres.

There has been much interest in the **anti–aging gene Klotho** [Zhou XJ *et al.*, The aging kidney. Kidney Int 2008, 74(6): 710–720]. In rats, a reduced expression of the Klotho gene leads to the developing of an aging- like syndrome, whereas an overexpression of the gene suppresses aging-related organ degeneration. This Klotho protein is a hormone that mediates its cellular effect by binding to a cell surface receptor and repressing the intracellular signals of insulin and insulin growth factor I [Kuro-o M *et al.*, Nature 1997, 390:45–51]. The Klotho protein can facilitate the neutralisation of ROS and confer protection against oxidative stress [Kuro-o M *et al.* Biol Chem 2008, 389:233–241]. A hydrogen peroxide induced stress led to reduced expression of Klotho. Angiotensin II can downregulate renal expression of Klotho in a rat model [Saito K *et al.* FEBS Lett 2003, 551:58–62]. **Klotho is also involved in vitamin D, calcium and phosphate metabolism**. It is also an **essential cofactor for stimulation of fibroblast growth factor receptor** [Razzaque MS *et al.* J Endocrin 2007, 194:1–10]. Klotho is highly expressed in the human kidney in the distal renal tubular cell and its gene polymorphism has been associated with bone mineral density in women [Kawano k *et al.* J Bone Mineral Research, 2002, 17:1744–1751] and with decreased longevity [Arking DE *et al.* Proc natl Acad Sci USA 2002, 99:856–861].

Global gene expression using cDNA microarray analyses have yielded more than 500 genes form young and old and among the old kidneys it has been shown that there are declining expressions involving respiratory electron transport, glucose and lipid metabolism, protein and amino acid turnover as well as altered expression of cytoskeletal genes. Genes which encode for immune response and inflammatory mediation have also shown age related changes including those involved in collagen catabolism. Note however that most of these data on senescence are derived from animal studies and there is as yet no parallel human studies.

In the Health ABC study which is a prospective cohort study designed to evaluate the relationships between body composition and weight related health conditions with incidental functional limitations among well functioning black and white adults aged 70–79 in the USA, it was found that Cystatin C has a linear association with inflammatory biomarkers in an ambulatory elderly cohort with eGFR > 60 ml/min, associations particularly strong for TNF-α and the STNF-R. [Kerrel Cr *et al.* Kidney Int 2007, 71:239–244].

SYNDROME OF NOCTURNAL POLYURIA IN THE ELDERLY

1. By age 60 to 70 years, about 11% to 50% of individuals would have nocturia. By 80 years about 80% to 90% would have it. About 30% of these people have two or more episodes nightly.
2. Nocturia is associated with 1.8 fold increase in hip fractures among the elderly. Those with more than three times nocturia nightly have two fold increase mortality compared to those with less than thrice a night.

3. Aging affects both the urinary system and the kidney function. Post void urine increases with age, from zero in young adults to more than 100 mls in those over 80 years. Voiding frequency is due to diminished bladder compliance and detrusor overactivity with ageing. Uterine fibroids, enlarged prostate and fecal impaction are some of the causes. Age related diabetes mellitus and spinal stenosis can also lead to detrusor dysfunction.

4. The proportion of sclerosed glomeruli increases to 35% to 50% by 70 years. The GFR declines from 120 ml/min at age 40 to 60 to 70 mls/min by age 85 years. These elderly people have decreased urine concentration and diluting ability of the kidneys.

5. The elderly also experience a shift in circadian rhythm. They retire and rise earlier than the young. Old people have more frequent sleep arousals than the young. It is important to distinguish between actual nocturia and night time frequency when taking the history in the elderly. Did they arise because they have to pass urine at night or was it because they were waiting to return to sleep? Elderly also have less time in REM sleep. REM sleep is associated with decreased urinary flow rate and increased urinary osmolality. This altered pattern would affect the production of urine at night.

6. In nocturnal polyuria 33% of the 24 hours urine output occurs at night. In some the urine output at night exceeds that in the day. Normal urine output about 1 to 1.5 litres a day.

7. Saito *et al.* [Saito M *et al.*, Br J Urol 1993, 72:38–41], after excluding those with enlarged prostate, neurogenic bladder, cystitis, diabetes mellitus or CKD found that nocturnal polyuria was the commonest cause accounting for 37% and detrusor overactivity, 34% was the next common cause. It is postulated that ADH levels which are typically high during sleep are very low in these people with nocturnal polyuria.

8 The typical functional bladder capacity is about 350 to 400 ml but decreases with age.

9. Non Pharmacological Treatment Options include reducing fluid intake 6 hours before sleep, avoid alcohol, caffeine and diuretics before bedtime. Treat underlying medical conditions like

correcting hyperglycemia in diabetics, treat fluid overload in congestive heart failure and offer continuous pressure therapy for those with obstructive sleep apnea.

10. Pharmacological options in men include the use of α Adrenergic blockers for those with prostatic enlargement as this will benefit the urinary symptoms when combined with 5-α-reductase inhibitors such as finasteride. For women with detrusor overactivity, bladder relaxant therapies like oxybutynin, propantheline and solifenacin have been shown to be helpful in the nocturia. In women, combination hormone replacement therapy can reduce nocturnal voids. Topical estrogen creams can improve atrophic vaginitis and alleviate associated symptoms of urgency and nocturnal frequency.

11. Oral desmopressin have been shown to reduce nocturnal voiding and is generally well tolerated. The side effects include headache, nausea, dizziness and peripheral edema were seen in less than 5 to 10% of cases. Hyponatremia occurred in 14% of patients but was asymptomatic (serum sodium >130 mmol/l). Intranasal desmopressin is less successful because of unpredictable absorption. However, hyponatremia introduces a new set of problems like the FDA report of seizures in 61 patients, of which 2 were fatal. Most of these patients had intranasal formulations of desmopressin. Many were also using tricyclic antidepressants that affect water excretion. Patients should be initiated on a small dose, half of a 0.1 mg tablet in the evening with a check of serum sodium after 3 days. Majority of patients respond at a dose of 0.2 mg and less. Above 0.2 mg the additional benefit is minimal and the risk of complications higher.

12. Nocturia in the elderly is a common complaint in the elderly which is associated with increased morbidity and mortality and is due to interacting effects of aging and sleep on renal and urinary function. Careful management to relieve these symptoms are necessary using various therapeutic options including pharmaceutical and even electrical neuromodulation

[Kujubu DA and Aboseif SR. An overview of nocturia and the syndrome of nocturnal polyuria in the elderly. Nature Clinical Practice Nephrology 2008, 4:426–435].

ASYMPTOMATIC HYPONATREMIA IN THE ELDERLY

1. Hyponatremia is characterised by the equilibrium of water across cell membrane into cells which leads to their swelling.
2. If chronic hyponatremia is corrected rapidly (with increases of sodium more than 10–12 mmol/l over 24 hrs), brain damage and even death can occur.
3. The term:Asymptomatic hyponatremia refers to symptoms of mild or moderate hyponatremia (<125–135 mmol/l) like lethargy, restlessness, disorientation, headache, nausea and vomiting, cramps and depressed reflexes. When hyponatremia is <125 mmol/l the condition becomes more severe and patients manifest with seizures, coma and cardiopulmonary arrest.
4. In a study of patients with hip fractures [Renneboog B *et al.*, Amer J Med, 2006, 119:71.e1–71.e8], it was found that those patients had a 6 to 7 fold higher risk of being hyponatremic than being normonatremic and these patients had associated gait disturbances, decreased reaction time like people with alcohol excess.
5. In another study, mild hyponatremia defined as serum sodium about 131 mmol/l was associated with risk of bone fracture (odds ratio 4.16) in elderly patients [Gankam K *et al.* QJ Med, 2008, 101:583–588].
6. Another placebo controlled study of 448 patients with hyponatremia had significant rise of serum sodium after 30 days of vasopressin V2 receptor with improvement in mental ability [Schrier RW *et al.*, N Engl Med 2006, 355:2099–2112].

7   Schrier contends that with the growing elderly population, including those with subclinical and clinical dementia about 30% have been reported to have asymptomatic hyponatremia. Some are on thiazide diuretics. Yet others are on anti-depressants, all these making them prone to hyponatremia. He is of the opinion that in individuals with a range of serum sodium 130–135 mmol/l, we should offer treatment for hyponatremia the same way we treat patients with hypokalaemia. We should consider hyponatremia as a serious clinical issue like hypokalaemia. The following options in therapy should be considered: Fluid restriction, frusemide, hypertonic saline, demeclocycline or V2 receptor antagonists. [Shrier RW. Does "asymptomatic hyponatremia" exist? Editorial, Kidney Int 2010, 6:185].

REFERENCES

1.   Zhou XJ *et al*. The aging kidney. *Kidney Int* 2008, **74**(6):710–720.
2.   Keller CR *et al*. Kidney function and markers of inflammation in elderly persons without chronic kidney disease: The health, aging and body composition study. *Kidney Int* 2007, **71**:239–244.
3.   Kujubu DA and Aboseif SR. An overview of nocturia and the syndrome of nocturnal polyuria in the elderly. *Nature Clinical Practice Nephrology* 2008, **4**:426–435.
4.   Shrier RW. Does "asymptomatic hyponatremia" exist? Editorial, *Kidney Int* 2010, **6**:185.

CHAPTER 34

Research in Kidney Diseases

IgA NEPHRITIS: A CLINICAL RESEARCH JOURNEY FROM PLATELETS TO GENOMICS (1976–2006)

I Clinical Research

Translational Research (TR) can be defined as research where a discovery made in the laboratory (bench) can be applied in the diagnosis, treatment or prevention of a disease. In a broader definition, TR can refer to any form of research which embraces new technological or biomedical advances including clinical trials (both drug and non drug) which contribute to an improvement in patient care in the clinical setting.

There is an elite group of medical researchers known as clinician scientists who are best positioned to do work involving TR or Translational Medicine (TM). Basically these group of researchers are trained clinicians who are also trained researchers. But because of their medical training they would be best poised to ask the critical research question to formulate the research hypothesis needed to address a particular problem which they encounter in clinical practice. The research question therefore could be a basic research question pertinent to a particular disease or it could be a clinical question raised at the patient's bedside which seeks a research solution from the lab (bench). Hence the terminology in TR, from bench to bedside and bedside to bench.

What about basic research or clinical research done by the scientist or the clinician? Both the scientist and clinician can do basic research so long as they have received the necessary training in bench work. Whilst the current medical research focus is on TR, one must remember that current TR is built on the foundations of fundamental basic research. The difference is that much of basic medical research is often undirected and have no immediate clinical impact. However supporting basic research is important since we cannot predict which of today's extraordinary ideas in basic science will lead to clinical applications in the future.[1]

Apart from TR and basic research, most of the bulk of the research work undertaken by doctors today would be considered Clinical Research which can be further classified into purely clinical (non-lab) based research and lab based research. Clinical (non-lab) based research could involve incidence studies of diseases, epidemiology, clinicial trials (drug and non-drug), natural history of diseases and documentation of interesting case reports or successful therapy.

Lab based clinical research refers to research conducted in the lab using patient material (blood, body fluids, tissue samples) to find answers or solutions to clinical questions raised at the patient's bedside. Hence the terminology "from bedside to bench" would seem more appropriate as opposed to "bench to bedside" in the case of TR.

II A Journey in Clinical Research

In this chapter, most of the work would focus on IgA nephritis (IgANx) which is the commonest form of glomerulonephritis occurring world wide and in Singapore as well. This work spans almost 30 years or 3 decades involving lab based research, clinical trials and in the later part, genomics of IgANx.

Professor Chan Soh Har, Director of the WHO Immunology Lab then based in MacAlister Road was my first Research

Teacher (1976). One of the early projects we did was to address the question of whether the uremic factor was in the serum or the cell (lymphocyte). In the paper "The Mixed Lymphocyte Reaction (MLR) and the response to Phyto-hemagglutinin in patients with renal failure" we reported that cell mediated immunity was impaired in patients which chronic renal failure and that the MLR in renal allograft recipients could serve as a sensitive monitor of the dose of immunosuppressant.[2]

After a 6 months attachment at the WHO lab with hands on lab exposure (protected time for research from my kind boss Dr Lim Cheng Hong), I spent a year at the Royal Melbourne Hospital with Professor Priscilla Kincaid Smith on a Colombo Plan Fellowship for a Clinical and Research attachment. At that time Professor Kincaid-Smith's focus was on the role of platelets in Glomerulonephritis. She had devised a Combination Therapy of Cyclophosphamide, Persantin and Warfarin (CPW) known as the Melbourne Cocktail which she utilised in the treatment of many patients with various forms of glomerulonephritis (GN) with good results. My task was to look for platelet involvement in glomerulonephritis to support the role of persantin in the Melbourne Cocktail. Together with Professor Judith Whitworth (my Research Mentor), we found supporting evidence for platelet involvement through the Circulating Platelet Aggregate Ratio (CPAR) and elevation of Plasma Beta Thromboglobulin, as in-vivo index of platelet aggregation in patients with Membranoproliferative GN and Focal Sclerosing GN.[3]

Back in Singapore in 1979 we were faced with the task of treating patients with IgANx. We asked the following questions : Are platelets and thrombogenecity involved in IgANx? What is the Natural History of IgANx? How do we treat this disease which was the commonest cause of kidney failure in Singapore then? We started several projects at almost the same time. We studied the Natural History of IgANx. We embarked on a controlled Clinical Trial using a modified CPW regimen. And we looked for lab evidence of platelet involvement (Beta thromboglobutin or BTG) and Thrombogenecity (Anti-Thrombin-III or AT III) in IgA nephritis. Our studies showed that plasma BTG was elevated in IgA nephritis and was correlated with the degree of glomerular sclerosis and could form a basis for anti-platelet therapy.[4] We also found that Anti-Thrombin III was also elevated in IgANx due to a constant thrombogenic tendency as well as increased platelet aggregation and degranulation with release of AT III from platelets. The increased levels were correlated with proteinuria, glomerular sclerosis and crescents on biopsy, suggesting that low dose warfarin therapy could be useful.[5]

Meanwhile our study of the Natural History of IgANx involving 151 patients followed up for 50 ± 34 months had shown that the patients had 2 clinical courses, one was a slowly progressive course with ESRF at 7.7 years, while the other a more rapid course with ESRF within 3.3 years. The poor prognostic indices were proteinuria >2 gm a day, hypertension and presence of crescents on renal biopsy.[6]

Our paper on the effects of a 3 year Triple Therapy (modified CPW) in IgANx was published in 1987[7] which reported a control trial of 104 patients. The entry criteria depended on renal function, degree of glomerular sclerosis and proteinuria. Those in the treatment group had delayed progression to ESRF by about 8 years. This trial subsequently using only persantin and low dose warfarin was repeated successfully by Grace Lee *et al.*[8] in 1989. Today this therapy is classified as level 1 evidence supporting a grade A recommendation for treatment of IgANX.[9] The evidence base for the therapy was provided from further work by Grace Lee[10] and Lina Choong[11] from their work on mesangial cells and umbilical cord endothetial cells. Both showed the effects of persantin and warfarin on the suppression of cell proliferation through cytokine (PDGF) inhibition.

Further work in the WHO Immunology Lab with Prof Chan Soh Har showed that patients with IgANx have abnormal Suppressor T cell function.[12] This paper was accepted for oral presentation at the International Society of Nephrology Meeting in Greece (1980). It was at this historic meeting that I met my 3 IgA Friends, Hideto Sakai, Yasuhiko Tomino and Endoh. We were to share information on our work on IgANx over the next 2 decades. Our immunological studies provided the basis for the use of steroids and cyclophosphamide.

In 1987 our work in IgANx was formally recognised and we were invited to the International IgANX club where we presented our work in Bari, Italy in 1987.[13] Our papers were published, students and visitors came to visit our centre and we were invited to present our work at various scientific meetings. In 1996 Singapore hosted the 7th International Symposium on IgANx.

The study of Proteinuria formed another significant aspect of our work in IgANx. We had reported the pattern and behaviour of proteinuria in IgANx through our papers on Protein Selectivity,[14] SDS-PAGE[15] and Iso-Electric Focussing.[16] We had documented 4 patterns of proteinuria in IgANx and produced data to confirm that it is not the quantity but also the quality of proteinuria in IgANx which determined progression and prognosis in IgANx. We also documented Low Molecular Weight (LMW) proteinuria as a bad prognostic marker.[15] This is now widely accepted.

At the turn of the century (2000) we published one paper "ACEI/ATRA therapy decrease proteinuria by improving glomerular permselectivity in IgANX.[17] This was a controlled therapeutic trial in IgANX which showed that the therapy decreases proteinuria, improves renal function and converts non-selective to selective proteinuria. We showed that 8/21 (38%) patients had improved renal function with 3 of them who had mild renal failure normalising renal function. Hitherto the use of ACEI/ATRA was only aimed at protein reduction with a view to retard progression of renal function. But here we had reported that therapy can not only improve renal function but also restore normal renal function among those patients with mild renal failure. Subsequently from our further work we showed that it was the ATRA and not the ACEI which contributed to improved renal function.[18] Present evidence now supports that ATRA causes amelioration of renal lesions and remodelling of renal architecture by reducing TGF Beta production in the glomerulus, thus decreasing mesangial cell proliferation and sclerosis.[19] This form of therapy offers a new outlook compared to our earlier therapy with CPW which only aimed at retarding the progression of renal failure. With ATRA therapy we are geared towards restoration of normal renal function in patients with mild renal impairment.[20]

One of the questions we sought answers to was why some patients with IgANX respond to therapy with ACEI/ATRA and others do not? Our hypothesis was that individual antiproteinuric response to ACEI/ATRA therapy varies depending on ACE gene polymorphism. Vleming[21] and Yoshida[22] had postulated that those with the D-allele of ACE gene polymorphism respond better to the antiproteinuria effect of ACEI therapy.

We therefore decided that we had to embrace the new science of genomics to look for our solutions to our patients' problems. In 2002, we published "IgA Nephropathy: Effects of Clinical Indices, ACEI/ATRA therapy and ACE Polymorphism on disease progression.[23] In a study of 118 Chinese patients with IgANX and 94 healthy Chinese subjects we found that (I) ACE DD genotype was associated with IgANX and (ii) DD genotype was associated with progression to ESRF.[23,24]

III Disease Progression and the Influence of Genomics in IgA Nephritis

(i) *Role of ID Polymorphism of the ACE Gene*

Human genetic studies revealed that all genes comprising the renin-angiotensin system (RAS) have several forms of polymorphism, raising the possibility that activity of Renin-angiotensin system (RAS) may vary among individuals according to their genetic make-up. One such polymorphism is the deletion/insertion (I/D) polymorphism of the ACE gene. Individual anti proteinuric response to ACEI/ATRA therapy varies depending on ACE gene polymorphism.[21,25] In this controlled trial, patients were followed up for 5 years to determine their long term renal outcome to ACEI/ATRA therapy and to ascertain if their ACE gene profile (ID Polymorphism) could play a role in determining their response to therapy.

Seventy five patients with biopsy proven primary IgANX entered a 5 years controlled trial, with 37 in the treatment and 38 in the control group during the period from Oct 1999 to Dec 2000. Their ACE gene ID genotypes were studied in order to compare the effects of ID polymorphism on the response to ACEI/ATRA therapy. In the control group, hypertension was treated with atenolol, propranolol, hydrallazine or methyldopa. The patients in the treatment group were treated with ACEI/ATRA therapy or both and reviewed at 3 monthly intervals. Patients were initially prescribed 5 mg Enalapril (ACEI) or 50 mg Losartan (ATRA) which was increased to 10 mg or 100 mg respectively if proteinuria had not decreased to less than 1 gm a day.

Genomic DNA was extracted from peripheral leukocytes and PCR amplification of the DNA sequence containing the polymorphism was performed using sense and anti sense primers. DNA fragments were then separated and viewed on 2% agarose ethidium bromide gel. Genotypes were identified by the absence or presence of DNA fragment obtained. There are 3 ACE genotypes: DD, II and ID.

The post trial, serum creatinine in the control group was significantly worse than the treatment group (5.0 ± 2.8 mg/dl versus 2.4 ± 2.0 mg/dl, $p < 0.001$). The post-trial proteinuria in the control group was also worse than in the treatment group (1.9 ± 1.0 gm/day versus 1.1 ± 0.9 gm/day, $p < 0.002$). With regards to renal outcome, there were 21 patients with ESRF in the control group compared to only 7 in the treatment group ($x^2 = 5.4$, $p < 0.005$). Treatment does seem to reduce the number of patients progressing to ESRF. For those with II genotype, there was significantly less patients with ESRF in the treatment group when compared to the control group ($p < 0.02$). For those with the ID and the DD genotype, there was no significance in the renal outcome between the treatment and control group.

Contrary to what earlier workers have postulated, that patients with the ACE gene respond best to ACEI therapy,[21] our data have shown that indeed those with the D allele do poorly, have a higher incidence of ESRF and progress to ESRF much faster compared to those with the II genotype. We conclude that ACEI/ATRA therapy was effective in retarding disease progression in IgANX. However, treatment significantly reduced the incidence of ESRF only in patients with the II genotype but not in those with ID or DD genotype.

(ii) *ACE Gene Sequencing, Nucleotide Variants and Haplotypes*

Association studies with single nucleotide polymorphism (SNP) have been contradictory. Haplotype (block of more than 1 SNP on the same chromosome) studies may be more useful. Employing gene sequencing, one can detect relevant SNPs for haplotype construction. In this study we investigated the complete genomic sequence of the ACE gene in Chinese subjects with IgANX to determine the role of the ACE gene haplotypes and their influence on response to ACEI/ATRA therapy.

For ACE gene sequencing, EDTA blood samples were collected for extraction of genomic DNA using QIA amp DNA blood extraction kit. Overlapping primer sets were used. These spanned the whole genomic sequence of ACE, about 24 kb in length. Genomic data was subject to PCR amplification in an automated thermocycler. PCR amplicons were sequenced using Big Dye Terminator cycle. All variants inspected were reconfirmed by additional PCR and sequenced Haplotypes were identified by Clark's subtraction algorithm.[26]

A cohort of 40 patients with IgA Nx, 20 on treatment with ACEI/ATRA and 20 not on treatment (control group) were followed up for 5 years and long term outcome to continuing ACEI/ATRA therapy correlated with genotype (ACE gene pattern, SNPs, Haplotype), to ascertain if the genetic profile plays a role in determining the response to ACEI/ATRA therapy and long term renal outcome at end of 5 years. These 40 patients were the first 20 patients from the Treatment and Control group of the previous study.

At the end of the trial (60 ± 5 months), the mean post trial serum creatinine in the control group was significantly worse than in the treatment group (5.08 ± 3.15 mg/dl versus 2.72 ± 2.07 mg/dl, $p < 0.01$). The post trial proteinuria in the control group was also worse than in the treatment group (2.1 ± 1.1 gm versus 1.0 ± 0.9 gm, $p < 0.002$). There were 11 patients with ESRF in the control group compared to only 5 in the treatment group ($X^2 = 3.8$, $p < 0.05$). ACE gene was sequenced (24,000 base-pairs) in IgA Nx patients and normal subjects. 55 nucleotide variants were found; 19 were unique, 17 in IgA Nx patients and 2 in normal controls ($X^2 = 8.1$, $p < 0.001$). There were 5 nucleotide variants which were significantly different between patients with IgA Nx with renal impairment and those with ESRF in both genotype and allele frequencies. Using Clark's subtraction algorithm,[26] 5-loci haplotypes were constructed from these 5 nucleotide variants. Comparing patients with renal impairment versus those with ESRF, only 2 haplotypes were distinct, haplotypes 3 and 5. Haplotype 3 associated with a high odds ratio (14.0, $p < 0.02$) was indicative of high risk of ESRF. In contrast, haplotype 5 with a low odds ratio (0.07, $p < 0.02$) was protective against ESRF.

In the treatment group there were significantly more patients with Renal Impairment who have haplotype 5, ($p < 0.05$). Those with ESRF tend to have more haplotype 3 ($p < 0.01$). In the control group irrespective of ACE gene haplotype, whether it was haplotype 3 or haplotype 5, there was no relationship to clinical outcome regarding final renal status: normal renal function, renal impairment or ESRF.

Those with renal impairment with haplotype 3 are at risk of ESRF ($p < 0.01$). Those with renal impairment with haplotype 5 are protected ($p < 0.05$) from ESRF. However for patients in the control group haplotype 3 and 5 did not influence progression of renal failure. This supports our earlier hypothesis[17] that individual response to ACEI/ATRA therapy is influenced by ACE haplotypes. Present data suggest that in IgA Nx, regarding ACE gene haplotypes, the 2 linked haplotypes 3 and 5, do influence response

Table 34.1 Comparing Clinical Data Between Treatment and Control Groups

	Treatment (N = 20)	Control (N = 20)	p values
Sex M/F	9/11	9/11	ns
Age years	40 ± 8	36 ± 10	ns
Trial duration months	60 ± 5	56 ± 8	ns
Hypertension Yes/No	13/7	13/7	ns
Serum creatinine mg/dL			
Before	1.52 ± 0.42[a]	1.45 ± 0.47[c]	ns
After	2.72 ± 2.07[a]	5.08 ± 3.15[c]	<0.01
Urinary protein g/day			
Before	2.0 ± 0.9[b]	2.8 ± 2.1	ns
After	1.0 ± 0.9[b]	2.1 ± 1.1	< 0.002
Blood pressure			
Systolic before	139 ± 13	136 ± 9	ns
Diastolic before	85 ± 6	84 ± 6	ns
Systolic after	138 ± 9	136 ± 8	ns
Diastolic after	83 ± 5	80 ± 6	ns
ACE Alu I/D genotype			
II	8	8	ns
ID	7	7	
DD	5	5	
Outcome			
ESRF	5	11	<0.05
non-ESRF	15	9	$(X^2 = 3.8)$

Intra-group paired t test: a..a $p < 0.02$, b..b $p < 0.002$, c..c $p < 0.001$

of patients to ACEI/ATRA therapy, in terms of decreasing proteinuria and retarding progression of renal failure.

These 2 haplotypes are in absolute linkage with the Alu I/D variant where we had earlier shown that the II genotype was associated with a better renal outcome compared to the ID and the DD genotypes which were associated with a higher incidence of ESRF.

The present data suggest that patients with the II genotype and haplotype 5 of the ACE gene have a lower risk of developing ESRF compared to those with the ID/DD genotype and haplotype 3 who have a higher risk of ESRF.

ACKNOWLEDGEMENT

This Chapter was presented as the 3rd College of Physicians Lecture on 22nd July 2006 and was entitled: Translational Research — From Bench to Bedside and From Bedside to Bench. Section III of the paper was presented at the 3rd World Congress of Nephrology in June 2005 entitled: Disease Progression and Genomics in IgA Nephritis.

The research projects were supported by grants from the Medical Clinical Research Committee, Dept of Clinical Research, SingHealth Cluster Research Funds, National Medical Research Council.

Reference

See references at end of this chapter.

UROTENSIN 2 AND RETINOIC ACID RECEPTOR ALPHA (RARA) GENE EXPRESSION IN IGA NEPHROPATHY

Abstract

IgA nephropathy is a disease where the pathogenesis is still poorly understood. DNA microarray technique allows tens of thousands of gene expressions to be examined at the same time. Commercial availability of microarray genechips has made this powerful tool accessible for wider utilization in the study of diseases. Seven patients with IgA nephropathy, 6 with Minimal Change Nephrotic Syndrome as patient controls and 7 normal healthy subjects were screened for the differential expression of genes, genome-wide. The Human Genome U133 Plus 2.0 Arrays (Affymetrix, USA) were used to quantitate the differential expression of 38,500 well-characterized human genes. A total of

7761 gene expressions were identified that have an IgAN/Normal gene expression ratio of 0.06-fold to 5.58-fold. About 35% of the altered gene expressions have no gene title or just a hypothetical protein label such as FLJ30679. Most of the remaining 65% are identified proteins where their importance to IgAN are not immediately apparent at this time. Among the 30 most up-regulated and 30 most down-regulated genes are Urotensin 2 (up-regulated 3.09-fold, $p < 0.05$) and Fatty-acid binding protein 6 (down-regulated to 0.12-fold, $p < 0.05$). Retinoic acid receptor alpha (vitamin A receptor) was also found down-regulated to 0.41-fold ($p < 0.005$).

Taqman real-time PCR for urotensin 2 and RARA were performed on 20 patients with IgA nephropathy and 11 with Minimal Change Disease and the data correlated with various clinical indices. The findings suggest that there may be a therapeutic role for RARA in IgA nephropathy and a clinical monitoring role for urotensin 2 in Minimal Change Disease.

Introduction

IgA nephropathy (IgAN) is the most common primary glomerulonephritis in Singapore [1] and in many parts of the world [2], contributing significantly to the pool of end-stage renal failure patients annually. Despite more than 3 decades of research, the pathogenesis of the disease is still poorly understood. DNA microarray technique allows tens of thousands of gene expressions genome-wide to be examined together simultaneously. This advance in gene expression profiling has given rise to immense potential for the characterization and prognostication of disease, and for analyzing the complex biological processes involved which would allow a better understanding of the molecular basis of diseases [3,4]. With the aid of bioinformatic tools, sophisticated questions in research can also be answered. Now the commercial availability of microarray genechips has made this powerful tool more accessible for wider utilization in the study of diseases. In this study we analyse the genome-wide gene expressions in 7 IgAN patients, 6 with Minimal Change Disease as patient controls and 7 normal subjects by using the GeneChip Human Genome U133 Plus 2.0 Arrays from Affymetrix. Individual specific gene expression of interest was confirmed using Taqman real-time PCR method.

Discussion

The data show that patients with IgAN have up regulation of Urotensin 2 [URT2] gene expression and down regulation of Fatty Acid Protein 6 [FABP6] as well as Retinoic Acid Receptor Alpha [RARA] gene expression. Urotensin 2 (URT2) was up-regulated 3.09-fold in IgAN patients compared to patient and normal controls

URT2 is the most potent mammalian vasoconstrictor identified. Its receptor UT, exhibits increased expression in cardiac tissue and in plasma of patients with congestive heart failure. It is believed that URT2 plays a hypertrophic role in cardiac hypertrophic remodelling but does not affect cell proliferation or apoptosis [8]. Apart from its potent vasoconstrictor actions, URT2 has also been found to have trophic and profibrotic effects. Recently, some investigators [6] have examined the expression and localisation of URT2 and UT in renal biopsy tissue samples from patients with diabetic nephropathy using quantitative RT-PCR [Reverse Transcriptase-Polymerase Chain Reaction] and determined the intrarenal distribution of their peptides by means of immunohistochemistry. In human diabetic tissue, gene expression of URT2 and UT were increased 45 and almost 2000 fold in comparison to nephrectomised tissue [$p < 0.0001$]. The authors [6] concluded that in the context of its known biological actions, the dramatic over expression of URT2 and UT implicate the vasoactive peptide as having a role as a possible novel factor in the pathogenesis of diabetic nephropathy. Balat *et al.* [9] reported that plasma URT2 levels were decreased in children with Minimal Change Nephrotic Syndrome, compared to those during remission [$p < 0.05$] whereas the urinary URT2 levels were increased during relapse compared to those during remission [$p < 0.05$]. It was concluded that the higher urinary URT2 levels during relapse could be the result of heavy proteinuria.

In our study URT2 was up-regulated 3.09-fold in IgAN patients compared to patient and normal controls. Taqman RT-PCR data showed that URT2 values was positively correlated with the level of both systolic and diastolic BP in patients with IgAN. These findings suggest that URT2 is involved in the pathogenesis of hypertension in IgAN. IgAN is the commonest form of glomerulonephritis in Singapore and hypertension is a well documented poor prognostic index. [1,2]. The patients in this study had their BP as well as blood samples for genomic studies collected at the same time, hence a temporal relationship between the raised BP and the elevated URT2 levels, implying a role for URT2 as a marker of vascular activity. However, based on absence of correlation between URT2 and serum creatinine and proteinuria in patients with IgAN our data do not support URT2 as a predictive or prognostic index in IgAN. For Minimal Change Disease [Patient Control Group] there was a positive correlation between URT2 and diastolic BP suggesting a role for vascular activity for URT2 as in IgAN. We also found that URT2 was correlated with the serum creatinine and proteinuria of patients with Minimal Change Disease despite the fact that these patients were studied when they were in remission in the absence of renal failure or nephrotic syndrome and while on small doses of maintenance prednisolone. This data is in agreement with the findings of Balat *et al.* [9] who also found low levels of URT2 for children with Minimal Change Disease while in remission. In our cases with Minimal Change Nephrotic Syndrome, they had low levels of protein as they were in remission and these levels correlated with the low URT2 levels.

Retinoids (vitamin A derivatives) are signalling molecules important in regulating cell proliferation, differentiation and apoptosis. Retinoids act through receptors such as retinoic acid receptor alpha (RARA) which are ligand-dependent transcription factors in the nuclear. There is an over-expression of RARA in intrinsic ageing of human skin [10] and reduced levels of RARA per gram of brown adipose tissue in mice chronically fed a vitamin A-deficient diet [11].

Our finding of down regulating of mRNA expression for RARA in IgAN may suggest a new therapeutic approach for IgAN, a disease where hitherto there is no known therapy. Shaier's model of Thy-GN mice [12] is akin to the human disease of IgAN since the Thy-GN mice have Mesangial Proliferative Glomerulonephritis [GN] like human IgAN where there is also Mesangial Proliferative GN. In Shaier's report [12] Thy-GN mice treated with RARA agonist had reduced proteinuria and normalisation of blood pressure. We postulate that RARA specific retinoids may provide a therapeutic approach to the therapy of IgAN. RARA belongs to the steroid hormone superfamily of nuclear receptor proteins which exert their effects by binding specific DNA response elements, thus regulating gene expression I target cells [10, 11]. Regulating or normalising RARA mRNA expression in patients with IgAN may thus offer a novel therapeutic approach in terms of gene therapy. This is especially relevant to IgAN which has hitherto no known specific therapy. However, apart from finding low levels of RARA in patients with IgAN, we subsequently found no correlation between RARA and any of the clinical indices studied using Taqman RT-PCR.

Microarray technology together with the aid of bioinformatics softwares is now widely employed for rapid investigation into the complex biology in health and in disease [13–16]. In IgA nephropathy, Preston *et al.* [17] had shown that gene expression profiles of circulating leukocytes correlate with renal disease activity in IgA nephropathy by combining microarray technology with clustering statistics. Genome-wide scan technique had also been applied in a mouse model of IgAN with rapid results in the identification of a susceptibility locus in chromosome 10 [18]. In this study, we found that a literature search on genes with altered expression can also be very useful in providing interesting information on novel biological processes and pathways which may shed new light on the pathophysiology of IgAN.

To summarise, our data suggest that URT2 is a marker of vascular disease in IgAN as patients with raised BP (systolic BP and diastolic BP) tend to have higher levels of URT2. URT2 levels were low in patients with Minimal Change Nephrotic Syndrome in remission. This is consistent with the findings of Balat *et al.* [9]. The diastolic BP and proteinuria were also correlated with URT2 in Minimal Change Disease. Our data showed that patients with IgAN had downregulation of RARA expression. Accordingly, based on the studies by Shaier *et al.* [12] where Thy-GN rats with Mesangial Proliferative GN were reported to respond to RARA agonist with reduction of proteinuria and normalisation of BP, there may be a role for clinical trials with RARA specific retinoids in patients with IgAN since IgAN is also a Mesangial Proliferative GN like Thy-GN.

Conclusion

Thousands of genes remain to be explored. Furthermore, with the gradual identification of the many untitled and hypothetical proteins, the list of identified genes may be repeatedly visited for more information. Assayed simultaneously on the same microarrays, these genes are linked in expression, be it up- or down-regulation. Such linkage information on gene-gene interactions genome-wide may be integrated into a panoramic view of disease pathways to explain the origin and development of IgAN. The present preliminary analysis of genome-wide gene expressions has implicated urotensin 2 up-regulation and retinoic acid receptor alpha down-regulation in the pathogenesis of IgA nephropathy. These may be relevant targets for further research and perhaps development of new drug therapy.

Acknowledgement

This study is supported by a grant from the Dept of Clinical Research P34/2006 with IRB approval from the IRB of the Singapore General Hospital.

Reference

Woo KT and Lau YK *et al.* Urotensin2 and Retinoic Acid Receptor Alpha (RARA) Gene Expression in IgA Nephropathy. *Ann Acad Med, Singapore*, 2010, **39**(9):705–713.

PARALLEL GENOTYPING OF 10,204 SNPS TO SCREEN FOR SUSCEPTIBLE GENES FOR IgA NEPHROPATHY

Abstract

Aim: IgA nephritis (IgAN) is the commonest glomerulonephritis worldwide. We aim to genotype SNPs (single nucleotide polymorphisms) genomewide in patients with IgAN to search for genetic clues to its aetiology. **Methods**: Genotyping for 10,204 SNPs genomewide was done with the Gene Chip Human Mapping 10K Microarray (Affymetrix). Twenty-eight patients with IgAN and 30 normal subjects were screened and analysed for differences in genotype frequency, allele frequency and heterozygosity reduction. **Results**: Among the most significantly associated SNPs, 48 SNPs were found mapping directly to the intron of 42 genes that localised in 13 somatic chromosomes and chromosome X. Genotype distribution of these SNPs did not deviate from the Hardy-Weinberg equilibrium in normal subjects. The most significantly associated gene, glial cells missing homolog 1 (GCM, $\chi^2 = 13.05$, $P = 0.000$) is a transcription factor mapped to 6p12.2. GCM1 reported decreased in placenta of patients with pre-eclampsia. The second gene, Tenascin-R (TNR, $\chi^2 = 9.85$, $P = 0.002$) is a glycoprotein and extra-cellular matrix component mapped to 1q25.1. Tenascin-R was associated with motor coordination impairment and enhanced anxiety profile in deficient mice. Interestingly, Triadin (TRDN, $\chi^2 = 9.16$, $P = 0.01$) is an integral membrane protein mapped to 6q22.31 within the IgAN1 locus. Triadin was shown to participate in cardiac myocyte arrhythemia. However there is no published study of these genes in IgAN. **Conclusion:** Forty-two associated genes (particularly GCM1, TNR and TRDN) are identified as possible susceptibility or marker genes for IgAN. Knowledge of their mesangial expression and binding capacity for IgA-containing complexes may help elucidate the pathogenesis of IgAN.

Introduction

Worldwide, IgA nephropathy (IgAN) is now recognised as the commonest form of primary glomerulonephritis.[1,2] It is an important cause of chronic kidney disease and up to 30% to 40% of patients progress to end-stage renal failure within 20 years after diagnosis.[3] Its causes remain unknown and treatment is symptomatic.[4] The lesion is characterised by the predominant deposition of IgA in the mesangium and para-mesangial regions. These deposits may be immune-complexes with a wide range of antigens. They may be aggregates of abnormal IgA1 with aberrant galactosylation in the hinged-region.[5] Such depositions conceivably activated the renal cells to express various cytokines and growth factors.[6] The results are mesangial cell proliferation and expansion of the mesangial matrix, both characteristic histological features of the disease. Damage to the glomerular structure can lead to leakage of serum proteins and red blood cells giving rise to proteinuria and haematuria which are frequently observed in the urine of patients with IgAN. The proteinuria, if heavy and left unchecked will lead to further damage in the tubules and progression to end-stage renal failure.[7,8]

A locus for familial IgAN called "IgAN1" on chromosome 6q22–23 had been described in man[9] and in mice.[10] The European IgAN Consortium in a genome-wide scanning of 22 multiplex families identified 2 regions with the strongest evidence of linkage, 4q26–31 and 17q12–22.[11] However, no identification of any responsible gene was made. Nevertheless, there is great potential in genetic studies that might reveal new insights in the aetiology and mechanism of pathogenesis. New data in this area may suggest more specific approaches in seeking preventive measures and better treatment for IgAN. The GeneChip Human Mapping 10K Xba 142 Array genotypes 10,204 SNPs on a single array. It allows rapid, accurate, cost-effective and whole-genome scan for susceptibility genes in the genetic study of diseases. Using this chip, we had screened 30 patients with biopsy proven IgAN and 30 normal subjects for differences in their genetic composition.

Discussion

In both patients and normal subjects, absolute linkage between members in all 6 SNP-pairs that mapped to the same gene confirmed reproducibility of genotyping with the GeneChip Mapping 10K Arrays. The low overall error rate of 0.1% had been reported for this GeneChip.[16] The normal population showed Hardy-Weinberg equilibrium in genotype distribution in all the 48 identified SNPs. Normals also showed allele and heterozygote frequencies that were similar with the Affymetrix frequency data for Asians in all the associated SNPs. These observations showed that the Affymetrix microarray procedure was robust and our study population was homogenous.

There are few genetic studies that search for susceptibility genes in IgAN using high-throughput SNP technologies. A locus for familial IgAN had been described with strong evidence of linkage to "IgAN1" on chromosome 6q22–23.[9] Two other loci were reported at 4q26–31 and 17q12–22.[11] However, none of these reports identified the gene responsible. In a large Lebanese family with 38 members,[17] found no evidence of linkage to the loci, 2q36, 4q22–31 and 6q22–23. In our study, 6 SNPs were mapped to chromosome 6. The SNP-pair (Affymetrix Prob Set-ID: SNP_A -1510472/SNP_A-1519262) mapped to Triadin (TRDN) at 6q22.31 which is within the IgAN1 region of 6q22–23. There were 3 SNPs mapping to chromosome 2 but none to the region of 2q36. No associated SNP mapped to chromosomes 4 and 17. Thus besides the IgAN1 locus, association with other reported loci had not been detected here. However, we had only screened 10,204 SNPs or about 0.3% of the estimated 3 million SNPs in the whole human genome of 3 billion base pairs. Therefore it is highly likely that the chromosome regions of these known loci may not be covered by the SNPs included in the GeneChip Human Mapping 10K Array.

Detected by all 3 analyses, the most significantly associated gene identified is glial cells missing homolog 1 (GCM1, a neural transcription factor in Drosophila) which is expected to regulate gliogenesis. However in mice, GCM1 is placenta-specific and is necessary for placental development. Its absence causes abnormal placental labyrinth formation that resulted in embryo death.[18] In human being, decreased placental GCM1 expression was found in pre-eclampsia and may contribute to the aetiology.[19] A complication of pregnancy, pre-eclampsia shared common features with the IgAN lesion. Both are believed to be multisystem disorders with presence of proteinuria and elevated blood pressure. GCM1 has not been investigated in IgAN. Tenascin is a large glycoprotein component of the extracellular matrix. It increases rapidly after inflammation or injury. For this reason, Masaki T *et al.*[20] investigated and reported that Tenascin protein expression may be an indicator of chronicity and Tenascin mRNA expression may be an indicator of disease activity in IgAN. However in this early study, it was not specified which member of the protein family was involved. Also detected by all analyses, the second most significantly associated gene is Tenascin-R, a family member known to express exclusively in the central nervous system. Its deficiency in mice caused motor coordination impairment and consequently an enhanced anxiety profile in elevated plus maze test.[21] Specifically, family member Tenascin-R has not been investigated in IgAN. Triadin (TRDN) is detected by genotype analysis only, ($\chi^2 = 9.16$, $P = 0.02$) and is 31st on the list of associated genes. It is an integral membrane protein with a role in cardiac myocyte arrhythmia.[22] Though mapped to the IgAN1 locus, whether it is the gene responsible or just a marker of gene close-by remains to be investigated.

Examination of the combined effects of GCM1 and TNR gene polymorphisms showed no great synergistic effects on the strength of association. This may be because the 2 polymorphisms are on separate chromosomes and are randomly linked in inheritance. This observation seems to support the hypothesis that IgAN is a complex disease probably with pathology involving the interactions of many genes[23] and environmental factors such as infections and dietary antigens.[24,25] With significant association demonstrated (at significant level $P < 0.05$), all 42 identified genes are legitimate targets for further study in IgAN. A unique feature of IgAN is the mesangial binding and deposition of IgA immune-complexes or abberant IgA molecules with defect in O-glycosylation. In this respect, it is noted that many associated genes code for proteins that are integral of membranes, cytoskeleton or extra-cellular matrix, many with protein-binding properties. These genes have not been studied in IgAN. It would be of interest to study their expression in the mesangium and to test their binding capacity for IgA-containing complexes. Nevertheless, priority should go to GCM1 and TNR, the top 2 genes with the highest significant values from all 3 analyses. GCM1 and TNR may have better chance of success in being established as genetic marker of disease or having a role in the aetiology. At the rate of 2 per 10,204 SNPs, approximately 600 more target genes may be identified from the estimated 3 million SNPs in the human genome for further study. Affymetrix already have a 500K GeneChip in the market for genotyping 500,000 SNPs in one microarray. Computerised analysis technique is available for examining hundreds of proteins and their network of interactions.[26,27] All the tools needed are now at hand to search for genetic clues to the causes of IgAN. In conclusion, 42 associated genes (particularly GCM1, TNR and TRDN) are identified as possible susceptibility genes or as marker genes. Knowledge of their mesangial expression and binding capacity for IgA-containing complexes may help to elucidate the pathology of IgAN.

Conclusion

At the end of our search we found among the patients with IgA nephritis 48 SNPs which mapped directly to the intron of 42 genes which were significantly different from normal healthy controls. This offers an avenue for further investigation of the 42 genes which may be associated with IgA nephritis. Future studies may show that some of these associated genes may play a role in the pathogenesis of IgA nephritis, the commonest form of glomerulonephritis of unknown etiology with an elusive cure. This is a pilot study on a small group of patients. What is needed is a larger cohort of patients with much funding to study a wider array of genes. A large consortium may have to be engaged for this.

Acknowledgement

This study is supported by a grant from the Department of Clinical Research, Singapore General Hospital, Grant No: P34/2006.

Reference

Woo KT and Lau YK *et al.* Parallel Genotyping of 10,204 SNPs to screen for Susceptible genes for IgA Nephropathy. *Ann Acad Medicine, Singapore*, 2009, **38**(10):894–899.

ACE GENE SEQUENCE AND NUCLEOTIDE VARIANTS IN IgA NEPHROPATHY

Abstract

Introduction: Association studies with single nucleotide polymorphisms (SNPs) have been contradictory. Haplotypes (blocks of more than 1 SNP on the same chromosome) may be more helpful. With gene sequencing all SNPs can be found for construction of haplotypes. **Methods**: The ACE gene was sequenced in 4 healthy Chinese subjects and 20 patients with IgA nephritis (IgAN) to observe if differences exist among single nucleotide polymorphisms (SNPs) and haplotypes. **Results**: IgAN patients had 53 variants of which 17 were unique; whereas normals had 38 variants of which 2 were unique ($p < 0.005$). No unique variant was significant as a risk factor for IgAN. Among thirty-six shared variants, 11 were in absolute linkage disequilibrium with the Alu variant. Significant genotype and allele frequency differences in 5 variants (11447 G > A, 13230 A > G, 14094 I > D, 14521 A > G and 15214 G > A) were observed between IgAN patients with renal impairment and those with end stage renal failure (ESRF) ($p < 0.02$). **Conclusion**: It is possible that multiple interacting genes are involved in the pathogenesis of IgAN and further studies may be more fruitful by haplotying SNPs across many genes, genome-wide.

Introduction

IgA nephropathy (IgAN) is a complex human disease characterized by mesangial cell proliferation, mesangial deposition of IgA immune-complexes, proteinuria and haematuria. It is also the most common form of primary glomerulonephritis in Singapore and in many parts of the world,[1-3] contributing significantly to the population of patients with end-stage failure requiring expensive and life-long dialysis. First described by Berger and by Hinglais,[4] the aetiology and pathogenetic mechanism of IgAN is still poorly understood to-day after more than 3 decades of studies.

In 1986, Anderson *et al.*[5] demonstrated that an angiotensin 1-converting enzyme inhibitor (ACEI) can reduce proteinuria and limit glomerular damage in rats with experimental reduction of renal mass. Since then, there have been numerous reports of ACEI therapy for retarding progression of renal failure in patients with various renal diseases[6,7] including IgAN.[8] Another important discovery in ACE was the insertion/deletion (ID) polymorphism which seems to account for half the variance of serum enzyme level in rats.[9] This deletion polymorphism was subsequently shown to be a potent risk factor for myocardial infarction and left ventricular hypertrophy.[10] The DD genotype has also been shown to be associated with the progression of diabetic and nondiabetic nephropathies.[11-12] In IgAN, the ACE ID polymorphism and other single nucleotide polymorphisms (SNPs) in angiotensinogen (M235T) and angiotensin type 1 receptor (A1166C) have also been studied[3,8,11,13] but results have been conflicting.

Recently Narita,[13] reported that certain haplotypes (blocks of more than 1 SNP inherited together on the same chromosome) of the angio-tensinogen gene can influence therapeutic efficacy of renin-angiotensin system blockade in IgAN. It seems possible that more than 1 SNPs of a haplotype acting in synergy may be a better predictor than the individual SNP.[14] Nucleotide sequencing of a gene may reveal all available SNPs for the construction of haplotypes. In this study, we determined the entire genomic sequence of the ACE gene (about 24,000 base pairs) in 24 Chinese subjects (20 patients with IgAN and 4 healthy controls). All identified nucleotide variants and haplotype constructs were tested for predicting disposition to IgA nephropathy and for prognosticating disease progression to ESRF. IgAN.[3,25] The patients were genotyped to see if their genetic profile could play a role in determining their outcome to therapy with ACEI/ATRA therapy.

In the later part of the study, The 20 patients in the Treatment group on ACEI/ATRA therapy were compared with another 20 patients who were not treated with ACEI/ATRA (Control group).

The two cohorts of patients were followed up for 5 years to determine their renal outcome (normal renal function, renal impairment and end stage renal failure) in response to ACEI/ATRA therapy as various studies have shown that genomics like ACE gene polymorphism may play a role in the response of patients to therapy and progression to end stage renal failure (ESRF).

Discussion

Rieder *et al.*[19] reported sequence variations in the human angiotensin converting enzyme from a study of 5 African-American (AA) and 6 European-American (EA). The EA sample had 44 varying sites of which 4 were singleton (variant with a single occurrence only in the entire study). The AA sample had 70 varying sites of which 22 were singletons. The difference in the proportion of singleton variants was significant (χ^2 = 7.7, p < 0.006) but not in their overall nucleotide diversity values of 9.7 ± 4.9 versus 7.3 ± 3.8 respectively (Means ± SD × 10^{-4}). These were similar to our values calculated for the 4 normals (6.1 ± 3.1), 40 patients (5.2 ± 1.7) or 44 combined (5.1 ± 1.6).

Among the 55 variants, 11 were in absolute linkage disequilibrium with the Alu I/D variant. This block of variants are concentrated in a region of about 4,000 base-pair between 10314 C > T in exon 13 and 14094 I/D, Alu variant in intron 16. Recombinant rate must be very low in a small region and hence they stayed in absolute linkage. Each of these SNPs can replace the Alu variant as the genetic marker in disease association study. With the advantage of high through-put and lower cost, SNPs may be genotyped within minutes of PCR completion by measuring the increase in fluorescence of the dye-labeled DNA probes with no downstream processing by using TaqMan real-time PCR for allele discrimination technique; whereas genotyping the Alu I/D polymorphism (distinguished by the presence or absence of a 287 base pair sequence) involved PCR amplification followed by incubation with an enzyme and electrophoretic gel separation of cleavage products and final staining for identification. Furthermore DD cases needed confirmation with an insert specific forward primer in a second PCR.[20] Presently there is much redundancy in association studies with genotyping of polymorphisms that are highly linked or in absolute linkage. Therefore prior to genotyping multiple polymorphisms in a particular gene, it is useful to sequence it to identify all variants and to determine the condition of linkage among them to avoid redundancy.

The frequency of SNPs is high in the human genome and it is not cost effective to genotype all SNPs.[21] From a block of common (absolute or closely linked) SNPs, a single haplotype-tagging SNP (htSNP) maybe selected for genotyping without loss of power.[22] Our findings with the ACE gene were similar. Two of the 6 haplotype constructs from 5 significant-variants had predictive value for risk or low-risk of ESRF (haplotype 3 and 5 in our study). However the predictive power of the individual component SNPs were quite similar. Thus a single SNP may be selected for genotyping without lost of power for prediction. Again the obvious reason for such redundancy was that these variants were highly linked. Between each of the 4 variants and the Alu variant, the correlation of genotype was highly significant, all r values >0.9 and $p < 0.001$. Keavney et al.[22] reported similar findings.

Hence a reasonable proposition for future development is finding a haplotype of non-redundant SNPs from many genes genomewide.[23] In this respect Bantis et al.[24] reported synergistic effect in the combined analysis of AGT-M235T and ACE I/D polymorphism. Yoon et al.[25] also reported interdependent effects of ACE and PAT-AH polymorphisms on the progression of IgAN. It is possible that multiple interacting genes may be involved in the pathogenesis of IgAN.

Conclusion

The ACE gene was sequenced in 20 IgAN patients and 4 normal subjects. Fifty-five variants were found, 19 were unique but none were significant risk factors for the development of the disease. Each of the 11 variants in absolute linkage may replace the Alu I/D variant as a genetic marker and be more rapidly and cost effectively genotyped by real-time PCR. Despite the limitation of the small numbers of patients studied, our data suggest that at least in the ACE gene, haplotyping SNPs within a single gene seems to have no added advantage over genotyping the individual component SNPs. It is possible that multiple interacting genes are involved in the pathogenesis of IgAN and further genetic studies involving haplotyping SNPs across many genes, genome-wide may be more fruitful.

This is a preliminary study and further studies of randomised clinical trials involving larger cohort of patients with control groups will be required to confirm the clinical significance of our study. We could in future proceed to determine specific SNPs of interest in larger numbers using the rapid technique of TagMan real-time PCR for allele discrimination. In previous studies of IgAN[26-28] in relation to ACE gene I/D polymorphism, sample size of a hundred patients or more are readily achievable as the polymorphism studies are less labour intensive and quite readily performed in contrast to gene sequencing work like the ACE gene which has 24,070 bp (base pairs), which is labour intensive. We believe that this modest study involving ACE gene sequencing in Chinese patients with IgAN is worthwhile documenting in our local journal.

Acknowledgement

This study was supported in part by grants from Singapore General Hospital Research Fund SRF#33/00 and Singhealth Cluster Research Fund CC009/2001, IRB Ref No:131/2001.

Reference

Woo KT and Lau YK *et al*. ACE Gene Sequence and Nucleotide Variants in IgA Nephropathy.

REFERENCES

1. Pizzo P. Tanslational Research. http://mednews.stanford.edu/stanmed/2002fall/letter.html.
2. Woo KT, Heng SH, Chew TS, Chan SH, Lim CH. The mixed lymphocyte reaction and the response to phytohemagglutinin n patients with renal failure. *Ann Acad Med, Singapore*, 1978, **7**(1):32–37.
3. Woo KT, Junor BJR, Salem H, d'Apice AJF, Whitworth JA, Priscilla, Kincaid-Smith. Beta-Thromboglobulin and Platelet Aggregates in Glomerulonephritis. *Clinical Nephrology*, 1980, **14**:92–95.
4. Woo KT, Tan YO, Yap HK, Lau YK, Lim CH. Beta-Thromboglobulin in IgA Nephritis. *Thrombosis Research*, 1982, **24**(3):295–262.
5. Woo KT, Lee EJC, Lau YK, Lim CH. Antithrombin III in IgA Nephritis. *Thrombosis Research*, 1985, **40**:483–487.
6. Woo KT, Edmondson RPS, Wu AYT, Chiang GSC, Pwee HS, Lim CH The Natural History of IgA Nephritis in Singapore. *Clin Nephrol* 1986, **25**:15–21.
7. Woo KT, Yap HK, Edmondson RPS, Wu AYT, Chiang GSC, Lee EJC, Pwee HS, Lim CH. Effects on Triple Therapy on the progression of Mesangial Proliferative Glomerulonephritis. *Clin Nephrol* 1987, **27**:56–64.
8. Lee GS, Woo KT, Lim CH. Controlled Trial of Dipyridamole and Low Dose Warfarin in Patients with IgA Nephritis with Renal Impairment. *Clin Nephrol* 1989, **31**:276.
9. Woo KT, Lee GSL, Pall AA. Dipyridamole and low dose Warfarin without Cyclophosphamide in the management of IgA Nephropathy. *Kidney International* 2000, **57**:348–349.
10. Lee GSL, Choong HL, Chiang GSC, Woo KT. Three-year randomized controlled trial of Dipyridamole and low dose Warfarin in patients with IgA Nephropathy and renal impairment. *Nephrology* 1997, **3**:117–121.
11. Liem LK, Choong HL, Woo KT. Action of dipyridamole and warfarin on growth of human endothelial cells cultured in serum-free media. *Clin Biochem* 2001 Mar; **34**(2):141–147.
12. Woo KT, Tan YO, Lau YK, Ng SL, Chew TS, Chan SH, Lim CH. Suppressor Cell Function in Mesangial IgA Nephritis. *Australia New Zealand Journal Medical* 1982, **12**:208–210.
13. Woo KT, Chiang GSC, Lau YK, Lim CH. IgA Nephritis in Singapore: Clinical Prognostic Indices and Treatment. *Seminars in Nephrology* 1987, **7**:379–381.

14. Woo KT, Wu AYT, Lau YK, Lee EJC, Edmondson RPS, Pwee HS, Lim CH. Protein Selectivity in IgA Nephropathy. *Nephron*, 1986, **42**:236–239.

15. Woo KT, Lau YK, Lee GSL, Wei SS, Lim CH. Pattern of Proteinuria in IgA Nephritis by SDS-PAGE: Clinical Significance. *Clin Nephrol* 1991, **36**:6–11.

16. Woo KT, Lau YK, Wong KS, Chin YM, Chiang GSC, Lim CH. Isoelectric focussing and protein selectivity index as predictors of response to therapy in IgA Nephrotic Syndrome. *Nephron* 1994, **67**:408–413.

17. Woo KT, Lau YK, Wong KS, Chiang GSC. ACEI/ATRA Therapy Decreases Proteinuria by Improving Glomerular Permselectivity in IgA Nephritis. *Kidney International*, 2000, **58**:2485–2491.

18. Woo KT, Chan CM, Tan HK, Choong HL, Foo M, Vathsala A, Lee EJC, Tan CC, Lee GSL, Tan SH, Lim CH, Chiang GSC, Fook-Chong S, Wong KS Beneficial effects of high dose Losartan in IgA nephritis. *Clinical Nephrol* 2009, **71**:617–624.

19. Nakajima M, Hutchinson HG, Fujinaga M, Hayashida W, Morrishita R, Zhang L, Horiuchi M, Pratt RE, Dzau VJ. The angiotensin II type 2 (AT2) receptor antagonizes the growth effects of the ATI receptor: Gain-of-function study using gene transfer. *Proc Natl Acad Sci USA* 1995, **92**:10663–10667.

20. Woo KT, Lau YK, Chan CM, Wong KS. ATRA therapy restores normal renal function and renal reserve and prevents Renal Failure. *Ann Acad Med, Singapore*, 2005, **34**:52–59.

21. Vleming LJ, van Kooten C, van Dijk M, Amj Hollander D, Paape ME, Westendorp RGJ, van Es LA. The D-allele of the ACE gene polymorphism predicts a stronger antiproteinuric response to ACE inhibitors. *Nephrology* 1998, **4**:143–149.

22. Yoshida H, Mitarai T, Kawamura T, Kitajima T, Miyazaki Y, Nagasawa R, Kawaguchi Y, Kubo H, Ichikawa I, Sakai O. Role of the deletion polymorphism of the angiotensin converting enzyme gene in the progression and therapeutic responsiveness of IgA nephropathy. *J Clin Invest* 1995, **96**:2162–2169.

23. Woo KT, Lau YK, Choong HL, Zhao Y, Tan HB, Cheung WW, Yap HK, Chiang GSC. IgA nephropathy: Effect of clinical indices, ACEI/ATRA therapy and ACE gene polymorphism on disease progression. *Nephrology*, 2002, **7**:S166–172.

24. Lau YK, Woo KT, Choong HL, Wong KS *et al.* Renin-Angiotensin System Gene Polymorphisms: Its impact on IgA nephritis and its progression to ESRF among Chinese in Singapore. *Nephron Physiol* 2004, **97**:1–8.

25. Hunley TE, Julian BA, Phillips JA, Summar ML, Yoshida H, Horn RG, Brown NJ, Fogo A, Ichikawa I, Kon V. Angiotensin converting enzyme gene polymorphism: Potential silencer motif and impact on progression in IgA nephropathy. *Kidney Int* 1996, **49**:571–577.
26. Clark AG: Inference of haplotypes from PCR-amplified samples of diploid populations. *Mol Biol Evol* 1990, **7**:111–122.
27. Yorioka T, Suehiro T, Yasuka N, Hashimoto K, Kawada M. Polymorphism of the angiotensin converting enzyme gene and clinical aspects of IgA nephropathy. *Clin Nephrol* 1995, **44**:80–85.
28. Harden PN, Geddes C, Rowe PA, McIlroy JH, Boulton-Jones M, Rodger RS, Junor BJ, Briggs JD, Connell JM, Jardine AG. Polymorphisms in angiotensin-converting enzyme gene and progression of IgA nephropathy. *Lancet,* 1995, **345**:1540–1542.

CHAPTER 35
Poisoning

1. In the early 1970s, nephrologists at the Singapore General Hospital also have to take care of patients admitted for acute poisoning, often suicidal with the occasional accidental poisoning. Most of the cases were due to salicylate poisoning especially ingestion of oil of wintergreen or Kwan Loong Medicated Oil which contains salicylate. The other common form of poisoning is the ingestion of barbiturate used as a sleeping tablet for insomnia. Other forms of poisons were due to ingestion of weed killers like organophosphates such as malathion. The most lethal was paraquat, a weed killer which appears like Coca Cola.

2. Nowadays the common classes of drugs involved are analgesics, antidepressants, sedatives, hypnotics, stimulants, anti psychotics and cardiovascular drugs.

3. The intoxicated patient would require prompt resuscitation and stabilization of the respiratory and cardiovascular system with supportive therapy including intubation and inotropics if necessary. Gastrointestinal decontamination in the form of gastric lavage may be performed if appropriate. After collection of clinical specimens for lab and toxicology, if available, the appropriate antidote could be administered. Various decontamination techniques are then employed depending on the type of drugs consumed.

4. For salicylate poisoning in the 1970s forced alkaline diuresis would be employed. This consisted of intravenous infusion of: 500 mls of 5% dextrose plus 50mls of 8.4% sodium bicarbonate, 500 mls of 5% dextrose plus 20 mls of 10% potassium chloride and 500 mls of normal saline. These fluids were infused at a rate of 500 mls an hour. The 3×500 mls infusion

constitute one cycle. The number of cycles needed depended on the general condition of the patient and the amount of "poison" still in the body. If the urine output lags behind the infusion, 40 mg of intravenous frusemide would be given at the end of each cycle and the infusion rate adjusted until the urine output had increased. Forced diuresis is no longer practiced today because of the many complications like fluid retention and pulmonary edema as well as electrolyte imbalance like hyponatremia and hypokalaemia and metabolic alkalosis. Acute Peritoneal Dialysis was also used for salicylate poisoning but again is no longer practiced today though recently, some reports have surfaced regarding the usefulness of using Automated PD as a life saving therapy in the Emergency Room [Ilabaca MB *et al.* Kidney Int 2008, 73S:S173–S176].

5. Today, if necessary, hemodialysis would be the modality employed for removal of poisons. The elimination of a drug by extracorporeal therapy depends on its molecular weight, degree of protein binding, volume of distribution and degree of redistribution. The methods employed are hemodialysis, hemofiltraion and hemoperfusion.

6. Intermittent hemodialysis [IHD] is useful for removal of alcohols, salicylates, lithium and theophylline.

7. Hemoperfusion refers to the circulation of anticoagulated blood through an extracorporeal circuit equipped with an adsorbent cartridge usually containing activated charcoal, sometimes a resin is used as adsorbent. A drug like theophylline has an affinity for the adsorbent and is bound and removed. This method is not useful for alcohol and lithium overdose.

8. Hemodialysis–Hemoperfusion removes toxin by both diffusion and adsorption and is useful for theophylline, barbiturates, mushroom poisoning [Amanita phalloides], organophosphates and antidepressants.

9. Continuous Renal Replacement Therapy [CRRT] using CAVVH or CAVHD. This is useful for slow continuous

removal of poisons which possess avid tissue binding in large volumes of distribution and where rebound phenomenon exists. Drugs like lithium, methotrexate and procainamide would fall into this category.

10. SLED or Slow Low Efficiency Dialysis is useful for the patient who has become hypotensive or has underlying cardiovascular instability and still requires sustained fluid and toxin removal. SLED actually combines the features of IHD and CRRT in that it uses conventional HD at slower blood flow rate [Q_b 200 ml/min] and reduced dialysate rate of 300 mls to 350 mls/min. It is useful for salicylate toxicity [Lund B *et al.* Efficacy of sustained low efficiency dialysis in the treatment of salicylate toxicity. Nephrol Dial Transpl 2005, 20:1483–1484].

TYPES OF POISONS AND TREATMENT

1. Alcohols
   (a) The toxic alcohols include ethylene glycol, methanol and isopropanol. Ethylene glycol causes tissue destruction from calcium oxalate deposition and severe acidosis due to its metabolites. Systemic calcium oxalate deposition occurs in the kidneys causing AKI due to acute tubular necrosis. Patients are inebriated with no odour of alcohol in the breath. They have GI symptoms like nausea, vomiting and haematemesis. Seizures and coma come on later. AKI occurs within 24 to 72 hours presenting with loin pain, hypocalcemia, haematuria and AKI. Ethanol is the traditional antidote. Fomepizole is a recent introduction as an antidote. It is a competitive inhibitor of alcohol dehydrogenase and blocks formation of toxic metabolites. Hemodialysis is effective in removal of ethylene glycol.
   (b) Methanol or wood alcohol is a clear colorless liquid with an alcohol scent used as a solvent for varnishes, paints and thinners in the furniture industry. The patient has

CNS depression, initially inebriated, then drowsy. As a result of the effects on the putamen, patients have ocular symptoms and complain of headache and vertigo. Always consider methanol poisoning whenever the patient has visual changes and abdominal pain with a high anion gap metabolic acidosis. Treatment consists of stabilization of the airway with cardio–respiratory support. Aggressive therapy with sodium bicarbonate is required. Folic acid supplementation plays a key role as the rate limiting step of methanol intoxication is mediated by 10-formyl tetrahydrofolate synthetase which is folic acid dependent. Hemodialysis effectively removes methanol and formic acid and corrects the metabolic acidosis. Continue hemodialysis until serum methanol is undetectable and anion gap metabolic acidosis is corrected.

(c) Isopropanol or Isopropyl alcohol is a clear colorless bitter liquid found in rubbing alcohol, skin lotion, hair tonic, after shave lotion, solvents, cleaning products and products incorporating acetone and glycerine. Intoxication occurs through ingestion or inhalation of vapours especially in infants. Clinically patients present with CNS, cardiovascular and GI symptoms. Patients are confused, have poor coordination, are lethargic, dizzy, have ataxia, stupor, eventually become comatosed and succumb with respiratory arrest. There is myocardial depression with myocyte toxicity; hypotension is present with severe cardiac depression. AKI results from hypotension and or myoglobinuria. Treatment consists of gastric lavage with supportive respiratory and cardiac therapy including the use of IV fluids and dopamine support. Hemodialysis is effective in removal of isopropanol and acetone.

2. Salicylate Poisoning
Salicylate is found in analgesics and is used widely for cardiovascular disease as aspirin. It is also used as a liniment in Oil of Wintergreen for muscular aches and pains. It is a component of Kwan Loong Medicated Oil used for pain and headaches

and various ailments. Poisoning present in the patient as a mixed respiratory alkalosis and high anion gap metabolic acidosis. Clinically patients have nausea and vomiting due to induced gastritis and later develop seizures, hypoglycemia, hyperthermia, AKI. Fatalities are due to severe metabolic acidosis with AKI and non cardiogenic pulmonary edema. If ingestion has occurred within the hour a gastric lavage is useful. Forced alkaline diuresis is no longer practiced because of the risk of pulmonary edema due to fluid overload. Nowadays hemodialysis is the modality of choice for removal of salicylates. CRRT and SLED have also been used for those with cardiovascular instability.

3. Lithium Toxicity

   Lithium has been used to treat Depression since the 1950s to the 1960s and is still in use today. Lithium overdose may occur as accidental ingestion or with suicidal intent or as chronic or gradual lithium intoxication especially among the elderly. Mild or early symptoms of lithium toxicity include lethargy, drowsiness, tremors, weakness, nausea, vomiting and diarrhoea. Those with moderate toxicity present with neurological features like confusion, nystagmus, ataxia, myoclonic jerks and dysarthria. Severe cases will have seizures going into coma and eventually death. Gastric lavage or nasogastric suction may be appropriate depending on the circumstances. Alternatively one may consider bowel irrigation with polyethylene glycol solution. Hemodialysis is an effective method of lithium removal. SLED is an alternative among the hemodynamically less stable.

4. Barbiturate Poisoning

   It is important to know the type of barbiturate ingested. Long Acting barbiturates like barbitone [veronal] act for 12 to 24 hours, medium acting like amylobarbitone [amytal] acts for 8 to 10 hours and the short acting ones like quinabarbitone [seconal] acts for 4 to 6 hours. The medium acting barbiturates are most dangerous [Amytal or Amylobarbitone] and act for a relatively long period at an unsafe blood level. They often cause coma, hypotension and respiratory failure. Absence of Doll's eye sign is an indication of severe poisoning as the brain stem is affected. Barbiturates also affect the myocardium and musculature of the blood vessels leading to peripheral venous pooling and hypovolaemia. Treatment consists of gastric lavage, maintainance of vital functions and hemodialysis. SLED may be required for those with cardiovascular instability. Forced diuresis is no longer practiced though in the old days it was useful for those with long acting barbiturate poisoning as it shortened the period of coma.

5. Organophosphate Poisoning

This is an insecticide sold as parathion and malathion. It causes restlessness, fibrillary twitches, fits, abdominal colic, salivation, hypotension, coma and death. All further exposure should be curtailed, hence the removal of contaminated clothing. The skin should be cleaned, including the mucosa. Gastric lavage where appropriate should be done. Cardiorespiratory support is given when necessary. The symptom complex of the patient will give a clue as to the severity of the poisoning. Serum cholinesterase levels also measure the severity and progress of treatment. Therapy consists of the administration of P.A.M. or 2 Pyridine-Aldoxamine Methiodide. Give I.V. P.A.M. 1 gm over 3 mins. Repeat dose of 0.5 gm after ½ hour. If the response is still poor, repeat the dose of 0.5 gm after another hour. Limit total dose to 20 mg/Kg BW.

Atropine: When cyanosis is absent, give 1st dose immediately 3.6 mg or 6 mls. If cyanosis is present give 1st dose after treating cyanosis with oxygen, otherwise there is danger of ventricular fibrillation. The second dose of 3.6 mg is given 5 to 10 mins later. Repeat dose at 5 to 10 mins intervals until adequate atropinization is achieved.

6. Paraquat as Gramoxone [20%] or Weedol [2.5%] is an insecticide which is rarely used nowadays and in the old days used to be available across the causeway in Malaysia where it was commonly used in the rubber estates as an insecticide and a

weedkiller. It is no longer available in Singapore. Most of the patients who came in were workers from the rubber estates. The minimal lethal dose is 10 mls of Gramoxone or one sachet [1.5 gm of paraquat] of weedol. Ulcers appear in the oral cavity and pharynx in the first 24 to 48 hours followed by renal and hepatic decompensation. Death occurs in the early period from pulmonary edema or pulmonary haemorrhage. Even if patient survives the 1st week he may still eventually succumb to progressive respiratory failure due to pulmonary fibrosis. Mortality is 80% for Gramozone and 10% for Weedol. Treatment consists of gastric lavage and leaving a mixture of 500 ml of bentonite and 25 gm of magnesium sulphate at the end of the washout. Give 250 mls of this mixture every 2 to 4 hours for the first 24 to 48 hours. Check arterial blood gases but do not give oxygen unless paO$_2$ is less than 40 mm Hg as oxygen enriched atmosphere may make pulmonary injury worse. Hemodialysis is not effective. Hemoperfusion may be of some use. Prognosis is poor in most cases.

7. Paracetamol Poisoning

Paracetamol poisoning causes GI symptoms like nausea and vomiting. In addition to liver failure it also causes renal failure. Death from paracetamol poisoning has occurred in 10 to 20% of patients with paracetamol overdose. 10 gms [20 tabs] is a dangerous dose and liver damage can be expected if the blood paracetamol level is > 250 μ g/ml 2 hours after ingestion or > 100 μ g/ml 8 hours after ingestion. Paracetamol by itself does not cause coma. If the patient has coma, it means he has taken another drug or he is in liver failure. Liver failure is the result of the metabolite paracetamol epoxide. Liver failure is evident from the 2nd and 3rd day of ingestion. Besides the liver function tests, the Prothrombin Time is of value in detecting early liver impairment. Other biochemical abnormalities are raised blood urea and creatinine, hypoglycemia and hemolysis. Treatment consists of gastric lavage and administration of IV Cysteamine 2 gm over 5 mins followed by 400 mg [by infusion] over 4 hours, 8 hours and 12 hours to a total dose of 2 to 3 gms. This should only be given if patient is seen within 10 hours of ingestion. Oral methionine 2.5 gm 4 hourly up to 10 gm is given if patient is seen within 10 hours of ingestion. Hemodialysis — Hemoperfusion is of benefit. If the patient does not recover and goes into liver failure, a liver transplant would be required. The patient can then be sustained using liver dialysis until he or she can be transplanted.

8. Opium Alkaloids and Morphine Derivatives

This group includes morphine, heroin, pethidine and codeine. In the old days where opium dens used to thrive underground there were some who could obtain opium which they would swallow as little black balls of opium. Patients present with impaired consciousness, pin point pupils, convulsions and muscle flaccidity. Codeine causes muscle twitching. There is respiratory depression and hypotension as well as hypothermia. Methaemoglobinemia is a sign of codeine poisoning. Death is due to respiratory failure. Treatment consists of gastric lavage, and I.V. Lethidrone 15 mg or Nikethimide [25% w/v] To give 2 mls every 15 mins until consciousness and respiration normal. Supportive therapy as required.

9. Mushroom poisoning

The effects may be due to rapid or delayed poisoning. In rapid poisoning, prompt supportive treatment is required. If muscarinic effects [of acetylcholine] predominate, sweating, lachrimation, salivation and bradycardia occur. Treat with atropine.

In delayed poisoning, this occurs 6 to 12 hours after ingestion. Symptoms include diarrhoea, vomiting and abdominal pain. The following day, liver and kidney failure will become manifest. Mortality can be up to 75%. Treatment consists of gastric lavage, intensive supportive therapy and Hemodialysis-Hemoperfusion.

10. Theophylline Poisoning

Theophylline is an oral methylxanthine bronchodilator used in asthma and chronic obstructive airway disease. Theophylline is extensively metabolized by the liver by several hepatic cytochrome P450 isoenzymes. As a result of extensive metabolism by the liver, the kidney only gets to excrete about 10%. Intoxication results from acute ingestion or chronic usage. Patient presents with anxiety, tremors, tachycardia, abdominal pain, vomiting and diarrhoea. In moderate poisoning they may have supraventricular tachycardia and premature ventricular contractions. Severe cases have focal lip smacking with ocular deviation with hyperthermia, hypotension, ventricular tachycardia, rhabdomylysis and AKI. Serum theophylline concentration should be measured. Treatment consists of cardiac and hemodynamic stabilization. Activated charcoal in multiple doses should be administered to decrease serum elimination half life to 1 to 3 hours. Hypotension and arrhythmias are due to catecholamine excess in the blood stream and low dose β adrenergic antagonists like propranolol or metoprolol should be used to slow heart rate and control arrhythmias.

Diazepam could be used for seizures. Hemodialysis — Hemoperfusion is effective. CRRT using CVVH as well as hemodialfiltration have also been reported to be effective [Hendeles L *et al*. Revised FDA labeling guideline for theophylline oral dosage forms. Pharmacotherapy 1995, 15:409–427].

REFERENCES

1. Fock KM. Acute poisoning. Handbook of Acute Medicine, Third Edition. Feng PH (ed.). Medical Society, University of Singapore 1980, Pgs 143–165.
2. Hendeles L *et al*. Revised FDA labeling guideline for theophylline oral dosage forms. *Pharmacotherapy* 1995, **15**:409–427.
3. Chao TC. Paraquat poisoning. *Annals Academy Medicine Singapore* 1972, **1**:68–73.

Index